IN OUR CONTROL

IN OUR CONTROL

THE COMPLETE GUIDE TO CONTRACEPTIVE

CHOICES FOR WOMEN

Laura Eldridge

Foreword by Jennifer Baumgardner

SEVEN STORIES PRESS
New York

Copyright © 2010 by Laura Eldridge

A Seven Stories Press First Edition

This book is not intended to replace the services of a physician. Any application of the recommendations set forth in the following pages is at the reader's discretion. The reader should consult with her own physician concerning the recommendations in this book.

All rights reserved. No part of this book may be reproduced, stored in a retrieval system, or transmitted in any form or by any means, including mechanical, electric, photocopying, recording, or otherwise, without the prior written permission of the publisher.

Seven Stories Press
140 Watts Street
New York, NY 10013
www.sevenstories.com

In Canada: Publishers Group Canada, 559 College Street, Suite 402, Toronto, ON M6G 1A9

In the UK: Turnaround Publisher Services Ltd., Unit 3, Olympia Trading Estate, Coburg Road, Wood Green, London N22 6TZ

In Australia: Palgrave Macmillan, 15–19 Claremont Street, South Yarra, VIC 3141

College professors may order examination copies of Seven Stories Press titles for a free six-month trial period. To order, visit http://www.sevenstories.com/textbook or send a fax on school letterhead to (212) 226-1411.

Book design by Jon Gilbert

Library of Congress Cataloging-in-Publication Data

Eldridge, Laura.
In our control : the complete guide to contraceptive choices for women / Laura Eldridge.—Seven stories press 1st ed.
     p. cm.
ISBN 978-1-58322-907-1 (pbk.)
1. Contraceptives—Popular works. I. Title.
[DNLM: 1. Contraception. 2. Contraceptive Agents, Female. 3. Contraceptive Devices, Female. 4. Women's Health. WP 630 E37i 2010]
RG137.E43 2010
613.9'43—dc22

                                          2009037886

Printed in the United States of America

9 8 7 6 5 4 3 2 1

To Barbara Seaman (1935–2008)
A true heroine, a great activist, a fearless writer, a generous guide,
a wonderful teacher, and an even better friend.

Contents

Foreword
by Jennifer Baumgardner

When it comes to birth control, I fear I'm like an ostrich—I long ago stuck my head in the sand. You'd think I would have faced up to it by now. I'm a feminist who was raised on *Our Bodies, Ourselves*. I'm thirty-nine, I have two kids, and I don't think I want more. I live with my second son's father and have sex a few times a week. All that is good.

The problem is I have always been intimidated by my birth control options. Thus, I have often avoided using anything to prevent pregnancy. In the two decades in which I've had sex, I spent six years with two girl-friends. During the other fourteen years with men, I was often frustrated with erection-deflating condoms, scary IUDs, and the nausea-inducing birth control pill. Sometimes I look at the array of birth control devices available and think, "Hand me my rabbit pearl." I'm not alone in wondering if masturbation beats sex, all things considered. All of my straight female friends fantasize about better birth control. My friend Christine used to fetishize "the shot" (Depo-Provera)—"Three times a year! You get it and forget it!"—but then she learned that the side effects were atrocious and, further bummer, Depo often didn't work. Many have dreamed a nasty feminist dream about a male pill, but few of those women would trust a guy to take it. My sister uses condoms, but she claims it's because she rarely has intercourse. "Why take a pill all month for that one time you're going to have sex?" she asks. "I wish I were kidding."

To be honest, I never found a contraceptive method that satisfied my contraceptive and sexual needs, and I never found a feminist guide that inspired me to make that search a priority. Until now.

Laura Eldridge is young, savvy, and smart. She worked intimately for most of the past decade with Barbara Seaman, the pioneering women's health activist. Seaman (who married into her last name but knew it was perfect for a health journalist writing about birth control) was a thirty-something mother of three in 1968 when she discovered, via her column at *Ladies' Home Journal*, that women were suffering terrible, often fatal, side effects to the original high-dose Pill. Several pathbreaking books (including *The Doctor's Case Against the Pill*) and campaigns against drug companies later, Barbara succeeded in getting birth control pills to carry warning labels and making the Federal Drug Administration accept input from patients as part of the drug's regulation. She came into my life when she swept into the offices of *Ms.* magazine. Within months of meeting her, I was off the Pill. *In Our Control* makes me see that my ceasing to take the Pill isn't where I should stop—it's just the beginning of figuring out how to find birth control that works for me.

The trouble with most advice out there for women and girls about preventing pregnancy and STIs is that the "experts" never give the full picture, and they don't take into consideration the unique situation every unique woman is in. Contraception is not a one-size-fits-all scenario. It is about options. There are many, and they all have their triumphs and caveats, and each woman needs to figure out what works best for her in her current sexual life. The message of *In Our Control* is an important one: there *is* an option out there for you, and your best option might change throughout your life. This book sets out to keep women in control of their sexual health by equipping them with all the information they need and trusting them to make their own decisions.

Yet, *In Our Control* does more than just offer a survey of contraceptive choices. It brings us into the fascinating history behind this hot topic. Laura Eldridge traces the historical and political roots and ramifications of birth control development, noting how times of social power for women are often met by hostility to birth control, and how middle class and rich women were always able to buy secrecy around their reproductive mishaps. Besides providing a cogent overview of everything from fertility awareness to female condoms, she analyzes why birth control is such a sticky wicket. Is the Pill liberating for women—or dangerous? Are condoms the least effective form of birth control—or the best, given that they also prevent the spread of STIs? Eldridge stays away from either/or prescriptions, concluding, "If you aren't happy with your birth control, there is no reason not to try another method." And with this book, you can figure out how to best do that, armed with health information and political context.

I realized after reading *In Our Control* that there was a lot I didn't know. We have more alternatives than I was aware of, for instance, and birth control options that may be annoying in some ways are powerful in others. Most of all, I learned that contraception does not have to be a damper on your sex life. With Eldridge's astute work in hand, I might just get my head out of the sand and face the facts of life.

Introduction

Three years ago, at twenty-seven, I ended my long-term relationship with the Pill. I had used it off and on for about nine years. Things hadn't been good for a long time, and I had desperately been looking for a way to leave, but felt trapped. It turned out the answer I'd been looking for was there all along.

I first went on the Pill when I was eighteen. I had been in a relationship for almost a year and was thinking about having sex. Of course I planned to use condoms as well, but I was heading off to college in New York City in the fall and didn't want to jeopardize my future in any way. A good child of the 1990s, I had sat through tons of sexual education classes. They all conveyed the same message: birth control pills were the way to go. I also knew what my friends were saying, what the girls who had become sexually active before me whispered over French fries in the cafeteria of my small Utah Catholic high school. The only way to be really safe, pregnancy-wise, was to take matters into your own hands.

Being eighteen, I didn't march up to the family doctor and ask for the Pill, although thanks to good marketing on the part of pill makers, I probably could have. I could have feigned bad periods or claimed that I wanted to erase the blemishes that had danced farther and farther down my forehead toward my eyebrows as puberty progressed. But I didn't. Instead, I did what savvy young people in the Salt Lake Valley did when they were in my situation: I went to the small Planned Parenthood located about two blocks from my high school.

Kids went there because it was cheap, and more importantly, because of its precious "don't ask, don't tell" policy. I knew girls too afraid to ask for pelvic exams who went there out of concern for basic health, and of course I knew those who went for pregnancy tests and abortions. I was pretty nervous on that desert-hot July day when I parked my beat-up red car next to the clinic and walked furtively into the small lobby, praying that none of my friends' parents would see me. I read over a brochure that listed the dif-

1

ferent contraceptive methods next to their respective efficacy rates as I sat and waited for my consultation, but in truth I had decided what I wanted long before I darkened the clinic doors. A kind, soft-spoken staff doctor gave me my first pelvic exam and wrote me a prescription for a popular tricyclic pill.

The first few weeks I was on the Pill, not much happened. My breasts swelled up and became painful, and I found that though I hadn't really had PMS before, I was suddenly inconsolable for two or three days before a bleed. Otherwise, I was pretty happy.

I went off to school in the fall and dropped the Pill. I rarely saw my boyfriend and remembering to take it was too much of a pain. I would go back on periodically over the next six or seven years, always struggling to take it regularly but never considering that otherwise unexplained changes in my health—for example, migraine headaches I had never experienced before—were due to Pill use. And I can honestly say I didn't think much more about it.

In 1999, the way I thought about contraception changed. I had the tremendous honor of meeting and working with the great author and activist Barbara Seaman. Barbara died recently after a short battle with lung cancer and nearly fifty years of battling with drug companies, doctors, and scientists over dangerous drugs, including hormonal contraception and hormone replacement therapy.

I met Barbara as part of an internship for a women's studies class. I fancied myself a serious feminist and jumped at the chance to work with an author who, a friend explained to me, had been an active member of the second-wave women's movement. Imagine my surprise when on my first day of work she told me that her first book, *The Doctors' Case Against the Pill*, critiqued a drug that I had come to see as synonymous with the gains feminism had made. I was about to learn that while the Pill has indeed revolutionized and improved women's lives, the story is much longer and more complicated.

Even as I continued working and eventually writing with Barbara, I stayed on the Pill. When I found myself in a new and increasingly serious relationship with the man who is now my husband, it seemed like the natural choice. But this time, the minor inconveniences that had whispered their presence in years past began to shout at me. My moods became erratic and overwhelming. My breasts swelled unrecognizably, and I shuddered to put on a bra, let alone have them touched by my partner. Most upsetting was that I began to spot each month, right around the middle of my cycle. When I spoke to my gynecologist, she suggested I switch from a low-dose to a regular-dose Pill. (I have since spoken to friends and other women in my life and have learned that an extremely high number of women spot on low-dose hormones, despite what company material suggests.)

Things weren't much better for me on the regular dose. I began putting on weight and my moods were worse than ever, to the point where it was affecting my relationships. I felt like I was standing outside of myself, watching a body that used to be mine and that was now occupied by an emotionally charged, easily angered monster. Every time I spoke to my doctor, her answer was the same: try another Pill. And so I gradually went through five different varieties, each of which brought new problems.

Why didn't I go off? Mostly, if I am honest, because I was scared. Not scared that I would get pregnant using another method, but scared that going off the Pill would change my sex life in a negative way. I liked the freedom the Pill gave me. And I had heard horror stories from friends about other methods.

The truth was (with the notable exception of Barbara) I was surrounded by amazing ignorance on all sides. None of my friends used anything but the Pill and condoms and none had even considered that there were other possibilities. When I began to ask about diaphragms, I couldn't find a single girl among my friends who had used or tried one. Nor had they tried female condoms or IUDs (intrauterine device); they hadn't even tried other hormonal alternatives, like Depo-Provera. This wasn't because my friends were all happy with the Pill—on the contrary, most had complaints that ranged from minor to more severe—but none considered that they had other acceptable options. When people encountered problems, their response (prompted by their doctors) was, like mine, to try another brand. It wasn't just that doctors had only one answer to the birth control problem; it was that they didn't even like the question.

The last straw came when, on my third Pill variety in a year, I stopped bleeding altogether. I know some women might like this "side effect," but for me it was scary. Each month, I wondered if I was pregnant. I felt terrible, like my body desperately wanted to bleed and just couldn't—yet I still had side-splitting cramps. It was at this point that I marched into my gynecologist's office and said, "I want to get off the Pill!"

My gynecologist, a lovely, bright young woman, wasn't thrilled about my new conviction. She told me again that I probably just needed to try another brand. But I had finally realized that when doctors switch brands, they are enlisting you in an experiment. Prescribing the Pill is not like prescribing an antibiotic. With antibiotics, it is known which variety effectively treats specific bacterial strains. With the Pill, it is simply guesswork: if you do poorly on one progestin, try another. If you spot on one dose, try a higher one. You can try a dozen brands, but at what point do you say enough is enough?

When I asked for a diaphragm, my doctor looked at me as though I had requested a chastity belt. "Well I *guess* we can fit you for one," she said reluctantly. "But it's not as reliable." She pulled a dusty brochure out of a bottom drawer in her office and handed it to me. Almost embarrassed, she said, "This is a little old . . . but I don't think anything has changed." When I went to pick up the diaphragm—your doctor writes you a prescription, just like for any drug, which you fill at a pharmacy—the man behind the counter rolled his eyes and told me in an exasperated tone that they would have to order it for me, and it would take a couple of days. But when it came, I was glad to have it.

I don't share this experience to talk women out of using the Pill. I believe that oral contraception is the right choice for many women, and I would never tell a friend who is happy on the Pill to get off it. Our birth control choices are private, and we as individuals dictate which factors—safety, efficacy, expense, ease of use, degree of sexual interference, and so on—are most important to us when we make our decisions. But it is important to realize that these decisions are not independent from the social forces that have directed the contraceptive conversation since it began. When it comes to contraception and sexual health, there is no magic bullet that works equally well for everyone—but that is not the message we receive. We are told that doctors, scientists, and experts know what's best for our bodies, and we are discouraged from seeing our own experience as a source of legitimate knowledge. We are often closed to the idea of trying different methods, a problem that seems to have more to do with the success of pharmaceutical marketing and the alliance of doctors with drug companies than with the safety and efficacy of alternatives. To be informed consumers, to truly exercise our freedom of choice, we must trust ourselves. And to build that trust, we must understand how our birth control works in and on our bodies; research the available contraceptive options independently of advertisements and doctor's visits; and take into account the complicated, sometimes disturbing, history of how birth control came to exist as it does today.

How can we talk about contraception in a way that ensures women have as many options as possible? First, we need to make the conversation intergenerational. As we move through our lives, what we want and need in a contraceptive changes. Our priorities, relationships, economic and vocational situation and biological realities are very different at age eighteen than they are at twenty-five, and different still at forty. For example, at eighteen, the single most important thing in contraceptive decision-making may be pregnancy prevention. By the time you are thirty, even if you aren't planning children, you may not weigh this benefit as strongly against other risks. At forty, the health risks of the Pill are different than they were at eighteen, making this option less appealing. Too often, we act is if birth control is a subject for young women just initiating sexual intercourse. It needs to be an evolving, dynamic, multi-decade discussion.

Your particular health profile impacts pregnancy prevention options. Whether you are under- or overweight, whether you have a history of blood clotting or migraine headaches, even the size of your vagina and whether you have had a baby can change the safety and efficacy of different methods. And class factors into the equation, too: whether or not you have health insurance will have a significant impact on your contraceptive choices. You may not be able to pay out of pocket for expensive methods and may have other barriers to getting the birth control you want on your terms.

When women fought for the right to legally use birth control in the twentieth century, they saw contraceptive access as the answer to women's social problems. Second-wave feminists made the right to abortion and birth control central goals of their activism. Many feminists in the 1970s didn't want to hear that the birth control pill was unsafe, because it meant facing the hard truth that the drug wasn't simply something that enhanced women's power. But decades of experience have taught us that gaining reproductive rights is not a simple answer to the bigger problem of ensuring reproductive justice for all women. The authors of *Undivided Rights*, a comprehensive and instructive study of reproductive justice groups organized by and for women of color, note that all too often "mainstream movements for contraception and abortion . . . have been unable to see how what may be reproductive freedom for them is reproductive tyranny for others."[1] In American history, reproduction has always been a place where racial inequality has been institutionalized, where the control of women by men has been constantly reaffirmed, and where middle-class and wealthy women have been valued over the poor.

Putting women in control of reproduction means addressing these social issues. Building reproductive freedom, including the ability to make contraceptive decisions, means working to give *women*—not the many cultural forces and people in positions of power around them—the ultimate right to make individual choices about pregnancy.

Letting people make up their own minds often means accepting other women's values even when we don't share them. If we are open to understanding others' choices, we can benefit from the unique wisdom that various communities bring to our collective knowledge. Katie Singer, a writer and teacher of the Fertility Awareness Method (FAM) of birth control, learned the technique from leaders of Catholic family groups near her home in the American Southwest with whom she had serious ideological differences on many fronts. But Singer was open to what they could teach her, and with their help she has worked to bring technical knowledge of how fertility works to a wider secular community of women. If Singer had dismissed the information that Catholic leaders had to offer because she disagreed with their position on, for example, extramarital sex, she would never have found her ideal contraceptive method, and she would never have been able to share it with other women.

Limiting access to contraceptive knowledge is as dangerous a form of coercion as preventing physical access to methods. Young women today sit at the epicenter of many cultural battles, and their access to knowledge about all their birth control options is often foreclosed by those arguing that abstinence—not having sex—is the only acceptable form of pregnancy prevention for young adults. Programs insisting on abstinence-only education have been gaining huge amounts of political and financial support for close to three decades in the United States and abroad. Besides seeking to prevent young people from becoming educated about contraceptive health, these programs promote religious values in public schools, decline to address the needs of students with diverse sexual identities, and insist on dangerous essentialist ideas about women and gender. Simply put, they instruct young people that "gender is your destiny."[2] In addition, laws and policies that insist on parental consent to obtain certain types of health care and threaten to limit confidentiality for young women seeking reproductive services violate the civil rights of young women and reinforce a dangerous double standard. Women—even young women—should be given the respect and knowledge needed to make their own decisions.

Women in the twenty-first century have the best birth control in history. They can use methods that promise to work more than 99 percent of the time. And yet, since the hormonal innovations of the 1950s and 1960s, little has changed on the contraceptive landscape. In many ways, female consumers can't win when it comes to birth control innovation. If we insist on safety, it discourages pharmaceutical firms from advancing new and potentially dangerous methods because they are afraid of lawsuits. If we embrace innovation, it often means taking big safety risks. It means accepting that we won't always get comprehensive information from companies with an economic stake in concealing the dangers of undertested and profitable methods. Understanding the ways that protecting consumer safety has prevented birth control innovation can help us to open up the important question of why, after half a century and countless scientific advances, there are no truly new methods of pregnancy prevention.

The obvious gender inequities in birth control are also important to explore. Why is it that—other than condoms, withdrawal, and vasectomies—all methods of contraception involve women's bodies? In what ways has scientific innovation and sexism in medicine prevented the development of male options, and to what extent do women fail to involve male partners in the choices and responsibilities of pregnancy prevention?

Looking at birth control through these many lenses isn't easy. It means asking questions that often breed more questions than answers. It means challenging ourselves to reconsider our choices and to think outside our comfort zones. It means dealing with painful cultural histories and sometimes standing up to doctors we respect, partners we love, and a culture that can make us feel like we aren't in charge. Let's move forward in this difficult but valuable journey together, and work to place contraceptive health firmly in our control.

Chapter One

Past Tense: Contraceptive History Before the Twenty-first Century

Some things that happened for the first time,
Seem to be happening again.
—Lorenz Hart, "Where or When"

Slowly the girl shuffles into the drugstore. It is cold, even for February, and she unwinds a plaid scarf slowly from around her neck as she waits at the pharmacy counter. She is twenty-two years old, and she carries a prescription for low-dose birth control pills in the pocket of her jeans. As she waits, she notices rows of products aimed at consumers for promoting sexual health. There are condoms, female condoms, contraceptive sponges, film, and spermicidal jelly. Some products openly exist to promote pleasure, not just pregnancy prevention: lubricants in alluring purple wrappers and flavored condoms sit alongside more practical products on the store's shelves. When the girl finally gets to the front of the line and hands her script to the pharmacist, she watches as he checks for her particular brand of pill alongside a plethora of other hormonal options, including patches, rings, and even chewable tablets.

It wasn't always like this. Flash back one hundred years to 1910 and the scene would have looked very different for our young woman. While we have dealt with some serious gaps in birth control innovation in the second half of the twentieth and early part of the twenty-first century, we now live in a world that, contraceptively speaking, would have seemed almost unthinkable to our great-great-grandmothers. How it got that way is a story worthy of Hollywood, packed with villains, heroes, and many people who fall somewhere in between. It is a story worth knowing, especially for women, because elements of this narrative keep on repeating. As Albert Einstein famously said, insanity is doing the same thing over and over again and expecting different results. Understanding and owning their reproductive histories is the only way for women to stay sane and gain control of their reproductive choices.

BOC (Before Oral Contraceptives)

Women have, of course, been controlling their fertility in one way or another since prehistory.[1] They've done so with varying success through the years, but nothing has ever rivaled the effectiveness of the twentieth-century methods. Some early contraceptive techniques had little or no basis in anything but superstition or erroneous ancient science. Sixth-century medical writer Aetios of Amida, for example, counseled women to use cat innards—they could choose to wear the liver on their left foot or the testicles in a tube around their neck—to ward off conception.[2] Medical historian Elizabeth B. Connell notes, "In the thirteenth century, Islamic women were advised to urinate in the urine of a wolf to avoid pregnancy."[3]

Other methods were a little more effective. The Bible's book of Genesis describes the withdrawal method, called coitus interruptus, in which a man pulls his penis out of the vagina prior to ejaculation. Abortion and infanticide were also common practices in many cultures at various points in history. There are prehistoric drawings in caves in France showing a man using an object to cover his penis while engaging in sex;[4] whether that item constitutes an early condom is still a matter of debate, but it is certain that ancient cultures, including the Greeks and Egyptians, used some form of penile barrier.[5] By the Middle Ages there is more evidence of early barrier methods, including the use of gum, alum, and animal dung to cover the genitals and the cervix.[6] Italian anatomist Gabriel Fallopius (who also provided key scientific advances regarding the female reproductive system) offers one of the first written descriptions of a condom: recommended for preventing syphilis rather than preventing pregnancy, it consisted of a linen sheath that had been presoaked in an herbal remedy.[7]

The potential effectiveness of chemical contraceptive agents, such as herbs, plants, barks, and metals, has been hotly debated by historians in the last several decades. John M. Riddle, historian and author of *Contra-*

ception and Abortion from the Ancient World to the Renaissance, translated written records of ancient contraceptive cocktails with the intention of discerning their chemical components and testing their efficacy. After reviewing a thousand years' worth of such data, Riddle concluded that many ancient methods of contraception probably not only worked, but worked well. He wrote that these methods—mostly botanical, but occasionally mineral and animal—were passed on by word of mouth by mostly nonprofessional people, so they were easily suppressed and eventually lost.[8]

We know that by the nineteenth century, all four major varieties of historic birth control—barrier, chemical, abstinence, and abortion—were being practiced in different forms in North America and Europe. Among other famous literary users, eighteenth-century Scottish journalist James Boswell wrote of "how he enjoyed prostitutes while 'clad in armour,' and Casanova told of his distaste for being shrouded in 'dead skin.'"[9] A modern version of the condom seems to have been invented in 1709 by one of Charles II of England's physicians, but condomlike items were manufactured by many different means and people. They were made from fabrics (such as silk), fish bladders, and of course, animal intestines.[10] Historian Andrea Tone writes, "The abundance of raw materials from slaughterhouses in Europe made condoms a staple export in cities like London, where a 1783 handbill advertising the wholesale business of one Mrs. Philips boasted of thirty-five years' experience supplying 'apothecaries, chymists, druggists . . . ambassadors, foreigners, gentlemen and captains of ships going abroad.'"[11]

Even through the mid-nineteenth century, most condoms that finished their journey in an American waste bin began it in a European slaughterhouse, although some enterprising American meat producers created lucrative side trades selling prophylactics. The processes for creating skin condoms varied and resulted in marked differences in their quality: low-quality skins were pasted or stitched together, creating a greater likelihood of flaws and gaps. Fine, beaten skins were known as "goldbeaters" because of the similarity of the technique used to produce them to that used in creating gold leaf. Other eighteenth-century inventions included the contraceptive sponge and syringe.[12]

New products emerged quickly on both sides of the Atlantic. In 1838, a

German inventor named Friedrich Adolph Wilde created the first modern cervical cap, and in 1842, German gynecologist W. P. J. Mensinga made the first diaphragm by placing a natural rubber sheet over a hard ring.[13] These European inventions sparked American inventors to follow suit. In 1846, an American manufacturer filed a patent for the first pessary (an item placed in the vagina often used to treat prolapsed uteruses but also sold as a "womb veil"). Marketed as "the wife's protector," this product by New Yorker John H. Beers was a wire loop covered with fabric.[14]

A huge technological advance for the entire world—not just the world of contraceptives—happened in 1839 when Connecticut inventor Charles Goodyear mistakenly dropped a mixture of rubber and sulfur on a hot stove. The result was a technique for processing rubber that he called "vulcanization" after the Roman god of fire. Among the countless other technologies that benefited from Goodyear's discovery were contraceptives. Mensinga remade his diaphragm, and many would-be entrepreneurs began making rubber condoms. As Andrea Tone puts it, "The rubber revolution in contraceptives had begun."[15] While there were various ways of making rubber condoms, they were all simple enough that "anyone could do it."[16]

Abortion, practiced throughout the eighteenth and nineteenth century, was another way that women chose to control how many children they had. While twenty-first century women think of birth control and abortion as separate things, women in previous centuries would have been less likely to see them as discrete. Abortion was legal in the United States until the mid-nineteenth century, and there is good evidence that women used this option generally up until the quickening (when fetal movement can be felt for the first time). Leslie J. Reagan writes, "In the 1840s and 1850s, abortion became commercialized and was increasingly used by married, white, native-born Protestant women of the middle and upper classes."[17] In other words, abortion was mainstream birth control with at least some cultural acceptance. Significantly, it was a long campaign on the part of the newly formed American Medical Association (AMA), begun in 1857, that ultimately led to the criminalization of the process. By the mid- to late-nineteenth century, several debates concerning fertility control had emerged. Most basically, of course, were fundamental issues regarding when and if pregnancy should be prevented—issues that we still grapple with today. Multiple factors such as age, marital status, class, and race imbue pregnancy prevention with different meanings for different people. While African American women were forced under slavery to reproduce as often as possible, social policy in the late-nineteenth and early-twentieth century shifted to discourage black women from having babies. As immigrants from southern and eastern Europe began to arrive in large numbers on American shores, those of Anglo-Saxon descent began to worry that they were being outnumbered. As a result, white women were encouraged to avoid birth control and produce as many children as possible. Babies were not equally valued, and therefore the reproductive options available to their potential mothers were not the same.

In the nineteenth century childbirth was dangerous, and for that reason some communities found the prevention of births acceptable. If a woman was seen as being in frail health, she might be more likely to opt for contraception than undergo the dangers of repeated births. A close second to the question of who should have children or prevent them was the issue of who should control contraception, men or women. In marketing a womb veil in the 1860s, Dr. Edward Bliss Foote promoted the device, saying, "It places conception entirely under the control of the wife, to whom it naturally belongs: for it is for her to say at what time and under what circumstances she will become the mother and the moral, religious, and physical instructress of offspring."[18] Unfortunately, such belief in the importance of female control of contraception and childbirth was not typical.

By the 1870s, there were a large assortment of available devices, including douching syringes, diaphragms, cervical caps, and condoms. Women and men could buy these items through the mail, in drugstores, and from other sources. At this point in time, contraception was a business almost anyone could get into. This meant that a lot of devices were available from a lot of places, but also that there was a tremendous amount of danger involved, somewhat like the natural medicine world today. Because there was limited regulation, it was difficult to tell the good products from the bad. And nothing was terribly good, especially considering the rampant misinformation about female biology—most prominently a belief that women ovulated during their periods, a mistake that led to many unwanted pregnancies.

The Criminalization of Contraception

In the second half of the nineteenth century, after the Civil War had ended, America underwent vast cultural changes. Cities offered young people opportunity and freedom, and single women began pouring into America's urban centers. Reproductive historian Rickie Solinger has chronicled the ways in which the city increasingly offered unmarried females unmatched potential for economic, vocational, and sexual independence, which made the new availability of fertility control important: "In short, the anonymity of the city gave women, married and unmarried, unprecedented need for and access to contraception and abortion . . . dangers of many kinds went with anonymity, but so did a new independence."[19]

Women's roles were shifting slowly but steadily, and forces with a stake in maintaining traditional power relationships began to mobilize against the social tide. In addition to shifting gender roles, there were big demographic changes in American life. Immigrants from southern and Eastern Europe were changing the ethnic composition of the United States in ways that threatened "native" populations, who were witnessing declining birth rates. Many powerful people of Anglo-Saxon descent decided that the only way to maintain the balance of power in the United States was to outbreed newcomers. Anxiety about the growing social freedom of women and the growing populations of immigrants (concerns that are resurfacing in conservative anti-immigrant rhetoric today) converged to create a cultural environment that was hostile to birth control. Solinger writes, "This crazy quilt of post–Civil War urban elements—thousands of young women separated from family authority and protection, libertarian and reform organizations espousing varieties of personal freedom, growing immigrant communities and other demographic trends . . . altogether stimulated a determined group of moral reformers to act in the interests of reproductive restraint. The goal was to save America."[20] These moralists saw getting rid of contraception as a way to "take back" American womanhood and protect the "racial health" of the country. As in so many points in American history, women's bodies became a place where those in power sought to influence social policy and enforce domination of one group over others.

One moralist, Anthony Comstock, a young Civil War veteran raised on a steady diet of strict Congregationalist Christianity, saw young girls as victims of an industrial behemoth that preyed on the weak. He wrote in 1876, "When the victims have been polluted in thought and imagination and thus prepared for the commission of lustful crime, the authors of their debasement present a variety of implements by the air of which they promise them the practice of licentiousness without its direful consequences."[21] Contraceptive entrepreneurs, in this figuration, created the problem of sexual licentiousness and then offered solutions to its physical but not its moral consequences.

In 1873 Comstock founded the New York Society for the Suppression of Vice (NYSSV), an organization that would become the major vehicle through which he promoted his social agendas. The NYSSV soon had sister associations in other major cities including Boston, Chicago, Philadelphia, and San Francisco. The same year he founded the NYSSV, Comstock drafted an anti-obscenity bill that he planned to take to Congress. His idea for curbing the sex industry was to prevent the mailing of items he deemed obscene between states. Womb veils and condoms, often sold by the same merchants as pornographic imagery or advertised in magazines alongside more salacious wares, were included among the forbidden items. Nearly half a century later, Margaret Sanger remembered this lesson of guilt by association and worked to draw a hard line between the sex trade and the birth control business.

When Comstock took his bill to Washington, it wasn't smooth sailing: some lawmakers objected that doctors should reserve the right to provide contraception at their discretion. However, perhaps in part due to the social censure that awaited anyone who objected to Comstock's bill (including unsubtle suggestions that those who opposed it had a financial stake in the trade or friends who did), the legislation passed. It was official; Congress had outlawed sending any "article of an immoral nature, or any drug or medicine, or any article whatever, for the prevention of conception."[22]

The decades that followed the passage of the Comstock Law saw a continuity of contraceptive sales during which a thriving birth control black market endured despite constant challenges. Whatever was being said in public, in private contraceptives were being used, and frequently this reality provided individuals, communities, and judges with opportunities for social activism.

Those jailed repeatedly for selling birth control were often acquitted or given slaps on the wrist that enraged Comstock, who continued to take the application of his law seriously and personally. Comstock understood that this was akin to legal nullification, and although it didn't constitute the norm, it was frequent enough that many repeat offenders readily returned to their profitable deviant ways. Many people with no economic interest in contraception privately and publicly opposed Comstock's uncompromising stand and saw it as out of touch with the realities of modern life. As Tone explains, "Although the frequent ridiculing of Comstock may help explain support for violators of the Comstock Law in general, it cannot account for the special leniency granted birth control offenders in particular. Rather those entrusted with enforcing contraceptive laws made choices that bespoke a tolerance of birth control and compassion toward those who sold it."[23]

Despite active resistance, the illegal status of birth control presented serious limitations for women and their partners. First, it created a world where regulation was impossible, where people of disparate qualifications could sell products of varying quality and safety. Second, it contributed to the increased classing of contraception: both contraception and abortion continued to be available for middle- and upper-class women who could afford to "buy secrecy."[24] Janet Farrell Brodie notes that most middle-class married women felt little to no impact from the Comstock Law and "had abortions and babies in the privacy of their own homes."[25] A third problem was that as long as the trafficking of birth control remained illegal, no scientific research could be performed on new methods.

Contraceptive Crusaders: Margaret Sanger, Marie Stopes, and the Battle for Legal Birth Control

Six years after the Comstock Law went into effect, Maggie Louise Higgens—Margaret Sanger—was born, the sixth child in a poor upstate New York family. There were forty-three years between the passage of Comstock's legislation and the opening of Sanger's first (illegal) birth control clinic in Brooklyn. Few historical figures are as complex and contradictory as Margaret Sanger. Was she the feminist crusader who marshaled socialist tactics in the service of gaining greater rights and opportunities for women? Or was she a proponent of negative eugenics who searched desperately for a drug that would curtail the growth of populations in "slums and jungles"?[26] Indeed, two distinct Sangers emerge from even a cursory look into the life of this legendary woman. Her beliefs and motives undoubtedly changed over the course of a long lifetime, but she could also be pragmatic and ideologically promiscuous in the service of her great cause.

Sanger's mother, Anne, was a devout Catholic who became pregnant eighteen times and birthed eleven children before eventually dying of cervical cancer. Ideology is, to some extent, biography, and this experience undoubtedly influenced young Margaret, who became a nurse, married, had a child, and began working in the slums of New York City. By her midthirties, Sanger was defying the Comstock Laws by distributing a pamphlet called "Family Limitation" and publishing a short-lived newspaper called *The Woman Rebel* (the first place in which she used the term she coined, "birth control"), which promoted, demanded, and educated readers about contraception. Early on, Sanger was unabashedly radical, and she saw the purpose of fertility control as creating new opportunities and freedoms for women. She looked to European models and ideas that borrowed from socialist principles.[27] By 1912, Sanger was already imagining a "magic pill" that could be used for contraceptive purposes, but it would be many years before this would become more than a dream.

Separated from her husband and newly exposed to many of the radical ways of thought circulating in early twentieth-century New York, Sanger set out in 1913 for Europe to learn about modern contraceptive techniques. A second trip in 1915 took her to Holland in the hopes of meeting pioneering doctor Aletta Jacobs, a great champion of the Mensinga diaphragm. Jacobs had started thinking about the value of a contraceptive system that was controlled by and carried the authority of the medical profession. She believed that only doctors could properly fit a diaphragm, and soon Sanger began to see the value of such logic. (In a satisfying irony, while Sanger was away, her estranged husband, William, was arrested by Anthony Comstock for distributing "Family Limitation." During the trial, Comstock caught pneumonia, which just a short while later killed him.)

In the fall of 1916, Sanger and her sister opened the first American birth control clinic in Brooklyn. Despite having more clients than they could handle, the two women were soon put out of business after a government raid. Sanger returned to the lessons she had learned from Jacobs, and just two years later she won a court case that allowed her to open a legal clinic that provided services under doctor supervision and for the treatment of gynecological problems only. It was the beginning of the end for contraceptive opponents. Sanger soon founded other clinics as well as the American Birth Control League, which would eventually become the Planned Parenthood Federation of America.

If there were two Margaret Sangers, there was only one Marie Carmichael Stopes. She was brash, egotistical, difficult, and an ardent and unapologetic eugenicist. Only a year younger than Sanger, Stopes was born in England in 1880. Unlike her American counterpart, both her parents were educated, and Stopes went on to become the youngest PhD in Britain.[28] She became interested in sexual health after her first marriage, when her husband experienced impotency; the two never consummated their union.

Shortly before her divorce, she attended a lecture given by Sanger at Fabian Hall in London.[29] The two had dinner that evening, and Sanger was impressed by Stopes's enthusiasm. A week later she provided Stopes with a cervical cap and some educational pamphlets on contraception. But their friendship was short lived, and in the years to come the two would become fiercely competitive. In 1918 Stopes wrote the popular and scandalous book *Married Love*, and by 1921, she and her new husband, Henry Verdon Roe, opened Britain's first clinic.

The relationship between the birth control movement and eugenic science is a murky yet enduring one. The idea for eugenic fertility control, dating from 1883, originated with Francis Galton, a cousin of Charles Darwin's. He believed that people of "superior stock" should be encouraged to reproduce, and other "inferior" people discouraged or prevented from doing so. It was based partially on a misinterpretation of Darwin, and partially on a reinterpretation of the work of English economist Thomas Malthus, who held that population growth would eventually outstrip the world's resources.

Two major schools of eugenics stem from Galton's original theory. Positive eugenics sought to encourage procreation in the "fit" members of society; in an American context this usually meant white, Protestant, native-born people. Negative eugenics tried to prevent or curtail births among "inferior" people—a category that originally included eastern and southern European immigrants, but quickly shifted to African Americans.

The relationship between birth control advocates and eugenics—and the alliances built between these two groups—went on to haunt both the feminist movement and the development of contraceptive science. Early birth control activists used two major strategies for making contraception respectable: they encouraged the medicalization of the process and products, and they took advantage of anxieties about the dangers of excess fertility in potentially destabilizing communities in society—in other words, the poor, and ethnic and racial minorities. Many people who were not compelled by concern for individual women and their rights were willing to accept birth control as a useful tool for maintaining the social status quo. Writing about Margaret Sanger, Rickie Solinger notes, "Sanger's appeal is classic because it divides the purpose of contraception into two: emancipation for women, and race betterment for society. Sanger did not apparently stop to consider whether these goals can coexist or if the second goal must, by definition, be gained only at the cost of giving up the first."[30]

But what effect, if any, did the eugenic ideals of clinic founders have on the women who sought their services? While Sanger increasingly accepted eugenic arguments about using fertility to control poverty and other social problems, she never deserted the opposite notion, namely that controlling fertility might provide a way out of poverty for many women. Dorothy Roberts notes that while Sanger "was motivated by genuine concern to improve the health of the poor mothers she served rather than a desire to eliminate their stock," she still relied on certain destructive principles, namely, "that social problems are caused by reproduction of the socially disadvantaged and that their child bearing should therefore be deterred."[31] Whether Sanger meant it or not, her embrace of these tenets damaged the birth control movement and created a space to abuse rather than enhance the rights of many women. As Roberts explains, "Sanger's shifting alliances reveal how critical political objectives are to determining the nature of reproductive technologies—whether they will be used for women's emancipation or oppression. As the movement veered from its radical, feminist origins toward a eugenic agenda, birth control became a tool to regulate the poor, immigrants, and Black Americans."[32]

In February 1930, Sanger opened one her famous clinics in Harlem. Perhaps because of concern in the African American community that her true intentions involved limiting their fertility for nefarious ends, patients declined to use the facility, and it closed just a few years after opening. The initial failure of the clinic contained lessons for future reproductive rights activists. After the first several years with an all-white staff, Sanger changed tacks and reopened the clinic with a black doctor, social worker, and nurses. The number of African American patients began to steadily increase. But despite acknowledging the desire of the community for health services provided by, as well as for, black women, Sanger was unwilling to truly cede control of the clinic to black leadership. Dorothy Roberts explains that Sanger, "like other whites in the birth control movement, saw the role of Black leaders and health professionals as facilitating their organizations' efforts among the Black population."[33] The women's movement in the second half of the twentieth century would face similar problems: while white activists desired the participation and support of black feminists, they struggled to share control and to reprioritize the movement as they understood it to truly accommodate diversity.

During the decades when eugenic thinking had the most impact on social policy, laws to allow the sterilization of those thought to be "unfit" proliferated. This trend began in 1907, when Indiana became the first state to pass a law allowing the sterilization of criminals and "imbeciles." Deciding which people fell into these categories was a responsibility entrusted to doctors and lawmakers. When several other states began to pass similar laws, some people pushed back with legal challenges. A truly dark moment for the American judicial system came in the 1920s with the case of a young Virginia woman named Carrie Buck. Buck, the daughter of a prostitute, was seventeen when she was raped and became pregnant as a result. Despite a horrible childhood in which she had been removed from her mother's care and placed in a foster home, Buck had managed to do well in school and was helpful with household duties in the home where she was placed. When she became pregnant her foster father immediately began legal proceedings to have the girl declared "feebleminded," a term used euphemistically and interchangeably with sexual promiscuity. After giving birth to a daughter while confined to a mental hospital, Buck was sterilized against her will. The resulting court cases eventually led to the Supreme Court upholding her sterilization. In one of the most regrettable and famous opinions he wrote, Justice Oliver Wendell Holmes concluded, "It is better for all the world, if instead of waiting to execute degenerate offspring for crime, or to let them starve for their imbecility, society can prevent those who are manifestly unfit from continuing their kind . . . Three generations of imbeciles is enough."[34]

In addition to sterilization laws, which disproportionately targeted African Americans and the poor, laws prohibiting interracial marriage had been passed in thirty states by 1940. While both measures would be repealed by the 1960s, as we will see later, sterilization abuse with racial and class dynamics continued through less legally sanctioned channels well into the 1980s.[35]

Condoms, Douches, and the Increasing Respectability of Birth Control in the 1920s and 1930s

If Margaret Sanger took the first tentative steps toward the legalization of female birth control, World War I accomplished the same task for men. Venereal disease—primarily syphilis and gonorrhea—had plagued the US military since its creation. In the nineteenth century, military leaders took a hard line against those infected with the illnesses, understanding them as evidence of a flawed character and not a larger epidemiological problem. Tone explains, "Enlisted soldiers were chronically under-diagnosed, and the afflicted were often treated punitively, as if their disease were secondary to their disgrace."[36]

By the start of the twentieth century, the military had seen dramatic rises in infection rates. Advances in science allowed doctors to test for venereal disease, and scientists worked on compounds that could prevent and treat them. By 1915, as Margaret Sanger was preparing to open her first clinic, the Navy had distributed and then banned the distribution of "preventative packs," containers of supposedly prophylactic ointment.

After America entered the war in April 1917, moral anxiety about unsanctioned sexuality was quickly trumped by practical concerns about the financial and human cost of preventable disease. A campaign mounted in 1917 sought to educate soldiers about the importance of self-restraint. However, not trusting too much to the boys' self-control, chemical prophylactics were reissued and soldiers' sexual activity was closely monitored. While the military never officially endorsed condom use, it is clear that manufacturers did a booming business during the war, and there is evidence that military doctors provided them secretly to interested parties. When soldiers, accustomed to resistance to condoms at home, were exposed to European society, where condoms were legal, many young men returned home to wives and girlfriends carrying contraband European rubbers.

In 1918, the same year that Judge Frederick Crane decided that Margaret Sanger could open her clinic for the "cure or prevention of disease," Congress voted to spend millions of dollars on studying and treating sexually transmitted diseases, a decision that opened the door for eventual increased use of condoms. Birth control was slowly being decriminalized, if only under the pretense of disease prevention. While this was a wonderful thing for American women and men, it meant that practically the only way women could prevent pregnancy was by playing the invalid or the victim. The only means to reproductive power was in the guise of weakness or illness.

It is important to mention that while concern about venereal disease during World War I allowed greater acceptance of contraceptive tools, it also led to shocking violations of women's civil rights. During the war more than fifteen thousand women—mostly poor, immigrant, or working class—were detained without charges on suspicion of having sexually transmitted diseases (STDs). Those who did were held for months and even years while they underwent treatment. The tendency to place the burden of preventing STDs—sometimes coercively—on women continues in the United States and other parts of the world to this day.

By the 1930s, the Great Depression had created a compelling and nonpathological need for family limitation. Even married, middle-class couples no longer necessarily had the means to support large families. Worrying about poor women having babies they couldn't support constituted a national pastime. Lest we think this tendency is past us, we need only look at the frenzy generated during our current economic crisis by

California mother Nadya Suleman, who had the audacity to have octuplets that she had no visible means of supporting. The social fury directed at Suleman went well beyond a normal response to a possibly unstable young woman who made a bad decision, and indeed, she became a symbol for members of society who refuse to fall in line in times of economic and social crisis and expect others to sacrifice for them.

In 1930, Mary Ware Dennett, a vocal advocate of birth control, won an important court case. When her sex education pamphlet, "The Sex Side of Life," was deemed obscene, she argued that the information she provided was accurate, clinical, and necessary. The court agreed with her, signaling that information about sexuality could now be circulated.

In 1936 two major court decisions effectively legalized birth control in the United States. *Youngs Rubber Corporation v. C. I. Lee & Co.* established the acceptability of transporting some forms of contraception for the purpose of treating and preventing disease, and *United States v. One Package of Japanese Pessaries* found more broadly that a doctor could prescribe contraception even when a patient wasn't sick or in danger of illness. Women no longer needed to pretend to be ill to get birth control, but they still had to go through doctors to obtain it. The medicalization of birth control was complete, and the AMA officially endorsed it as a legitimate part of a doctor's practice in 1937.

During this time, the Catholic Church emerged as a foe of legal birth control. The pope advocated the rhythm method and periodical sexual abstinence. Interestingly, the church also provided important anti-eugenicist arguments that every person, regardless of status or race, had the right to have children. The church would not mobilize so strongly against birth control again until the 1960s, with the legalization of the hormonal birth control pill.

Postwar America and the Development of the Birth Control Pill

World War II finished the work that World War I began: by the late 1940s, the majority of Americans used some form of contraception. Even as the placid suburbs of the 1950s contained the rumblings of second-wave feminism that would burst on the scene only a decade and a half later, the social politics of the postwar era set the stage for the development of one of the true great contraceptive innovations of all time: the birth control pill.

The story of hormonal birth control goes back to the turn of the century. Late nineteenth-century editions of *The Merck Manual* reveal that a coarse brown powder called Ovariin, made from the pulverized ovaries of cows, was being prescribed for menopausal symptoms and female complaints.[37] In 1889 a respected French scientist, Dr. Charles Edouard Brown Séquard, caught the attention of his colleagues when he announced that he had revived his aging body by injecting himself with extracts from guinea pig and dog testicles. The age of hormone exploration had begun, and doctors started imagining the possibilities these chemicals might possess. The various hormone developments between 1930 and 1960 are too numerous to mention individually, so I will attempt to highlight a few key discoveries here.

It took a few decades for the enthusiasm around hormones to turn to women's reproductive organs. It wasn't that doctors weren't eager to gain knowledge in this area; they simply didn't possess enough knowledge about women's bodies to know where to start. This changed in early 1919 when Ludwig Haberlandt, a professor of physiology at the University of Innsbruck, surgically implanted the ovaries of a pregnant rabbit into another rabbit, causing temporary sterility in the second animal.[38] In 1920, Edgar Allan, a Brown University student, successfully mapped the reproductive cycle of a mouse, including the monthly ripening of the egg and cellular changes. In 1929 the American biochemist Edward Doisy isolated and identified estrone, a type of estrogen, as well as two similar compounds in following years. The race was on to use this new knowledge to develop marketable drugs. As women's health pioneer Barbara Seaman wrote:

> Hormone research was hot, a frontier not just for science but for its Jekyll-and-Hyde counterpart, the development of new drugs for market. Easing the financial way for some researchers, drug manufacturers dreamed about new hormone product lines. They thought menopause, they thought menstruation. They thought beautiful skin, thicker hair,

more passionate sex. They thought of curing infertility, preventing miscarriages, and drying up breast milk in mothers
who preferred to bottle feed. Some of the more daring were
also thinking birth control.[39]

The first hormone drugs for women were biological, meaning they
were made from processing natural products, primarily urine. Early versions of Premarin—a drug that is still today, even after substantial
scientific evidence of its dangers, one of the best-selling drugs in America—were formulated from the urine of pregnant Canadian women. At
some point James Bertram Collip, one of the fathers of Premarin, realized
that this wasn't cost effective; he switched to the urine of pregnant horses,
which of course continues to be a main ingredient in the drug today
(PREgnant MARes urINe).

Soon after, in Nazi Germany, a chemist named Adolph Butendant
raced with colleagues to synthesize estrogen. Their first drug was urine
based, but eventually the team developed others, leading to the creation
of ethinyl estradiol, an estrogen approved a decade later that is still in
nearly nine out of ten birth control pills.

In 1938, a British scientist named Sir Edward Charles Dodds became
aware of the Germans' successes. Dodds was terrified that Hitler would
be able to use this new technology to terrible ends, including, of course,
sterilizing people he didn't like and making a huge sum of money in the
process. Dodds became determined to develop his own estrogen. The
good doctor, after a manic quest, succeeded in synthesizing diethylstilbestrol (DES), an estrogen that was significantly cheaper than the German
drug. To ensure, with finality, that the Germans would have no market
to corner, Dodds published his formula in the journal *Nature*.

At this point the genie was out of the bottle, and doctors, scientists,
and drugmakers all over the world raced to discover new uses for this
wonder product. Estrogen at that time was a drug in search of a disease.
No one really knew what it would do and what it wouldn't. What they
did know from the beginning was that it caused health problems, especially cancer, as Food and Drug Administration (FDA) documents and
medical journal articles from the era show.[40]

If synthetic estrogen was a European product, progestin (synthetic progesterone) was largely a North American one that came into existence, in part, under the guidance of refugee European scientists. Cholesterol was used to make the hormone in the 1930s because it was easily modified to make progesterone. The process through which this transformation occurred was both time consuming and expensive: it cost $1,000 to make one gram of progesterone during the 1930s.[41] By the end of the decade, drug companies were racing to find cheaper, quicker alternatives. Working with advances by Japanese scientists, American organic chemist Russell Marker traveled to Mexico to search for a plant and a process that would produce the sought-after hormone. Brilliant and volatile, Marker tested more than four hundred species of plants before determining that the Cabeza de Negro plant, a wild Mexican yam, yielded the highest amount of diosgenin, a substance that could be used to make progesterone.

Marker wanted to break the European monopoly on the production of sex hormones and saw his opportunity to do so. Unfortunately, he had just lost his funding from Parke-Davis, the drugmaker who had previously supported his work but who wasn't particularly interested in sex hormones. Marker decided to use his own money and joined with two other scientists to form Syntex, a pharmaceutical company, in 1944. Using his distinctive technique for processing progesterone, Syntex quickly became the largest international supplier of the hormone.

Quickly disenchanted when he felt that he wasn't receiving enough of the money from this enterprise, Marker left Syntex within a year of its founding, taking his formula with him. His former partners hired two European-born Jewish chemists to reconstruct Marker's work: George Rosenkrantz and Carl Djerassi. The scientists quickly explored new plants and possible techniques for making progesterone. In October 1951 Djerassi and a young student, Luis Miramontes, made a pure crystalline progestin product that they called norethisterone,[42] a substance five times stronger than any available alternative and powerful enough to potentially work as a contraceptive.

By then, Margaret Sanger, now in her seventies, returned to her dream of the "magic pill." To this end, she made an important match when she introduced Katherine Dexter McCormick, a wealthy heiress with a degree in science, to Gregory Pincus, a Massachusetts-based reproductive scientist. Both Pincus and McCormick were, in different ways, outsiders with painful pasts. Pincus was one of the most knowledgeable people in the world about the female egg. A Cornell graduate, he had originally worked as an assistant professor at Harvard, where he had created the first test tube rabbit embryo. This discovery was ahead of its time and stirred up a flurry of social fear about the ethical implications of such an advance. Instead of being lauded as an innovator, Pincus was characterized—sometimes in anti-Semitic terms—as a mad scientist.[43] After leaving Harvard, Pincus created his own laboratory, the Worcester Foundation for Experimental Biology, with colleagues.

Katherine McCormick had known Margaret Sanger since 1917, when she helped smuggle diaphragms into the United States. Katherine had married Stanley McCormick, heir to a large industrial fortune, the same year she became the second woman in history to graduate from MIT. Stanley was diagnosed a short while later with schizophrenia, and Katherine nursed him for decades. Sanger had been hoping to get money out of McCormick for many years, but while Stanley was alive, her funds went to schizophrenia research. After her husband's death, McCormick approached Sanger about getting involved in the birth control movement in a more significant way. Sanger jumped at the opportunity to nurse her pet project.

McCormick gave Pincus $150,000 and told him to find the miracle drug they were all waiting for. Pincus—"the egg man"—was joined by Chinese scientist Min Chueh Chang, a specialist in human sperm. Rounding out the team was Boston obstetrician and gynecologist Dr. John Rock, who had been conducting research on the effects of progesterone on fertility to try to help women who were struggling to conceive. He observed something he called the rebound effect—that while progesterone blocked ovulation during its administration, it seemed to trigger it once the hormone was withdrawn. Rock, an ardent Catholic (and a man who Margaret Sanger observed was as "handsome as a god") was a powerful ally who lent a certain mainstream legitimacy to what was otherwise the product of outsiders.

Lara V. Marks points out that women were involved throughout the development and testing of the Pill and were agents in its creation. Among the women she names are technician Anne Merrill, who conducted significant portions of the human and animal trials, and her assistant Mary Ellen Fitts Johnson.[44] These women initiated a tradition of active scientific participation in the making of the Pill that would be continued in the Puerto Rico trials by, among others, Dr. Edris Rice-Wray. Marks points out that the participation of these women provides a powerful counterargument to Pill critics who argue that it was a male product imposed on female bodies.

After small-scale investigations in Boston, Israel, and Japan, Pincus began to survey the globe for ideal locations to conduct the large-scale trials that would be required for FDA approval. It quickly became clear that such experiments would be impossible in the continental United States. Katherine McCormick, who continued to supply funds and active opinions, lamented to Sanger in 1955 that they needed a "cage" of ovulating females if they were to proceed.[45] The group eventually settled on Puerto Rico for several reasons. It was an island, which meant that it was more difficult for trial participants to disappear mid-experiment, and the territory was part of the United States, so doctors there were trained in "American style" medicine. Finally, the densely populated, largely impoverished community had an active need for and interest in family planning technology. Two main study locations were established. The first, in urban San Juan, was administered by Edris Rice-Wray. The second was in the more rural area of Humacao under the direction of another American woman, Dr. Adaline Satterthwaite.

There were problems with both locations. Many women dropped out, some because of side effects including nausea, dizziness, headaches, and vomiting. Others left when they read articles in Puerto Rican newspapers warning that the Pill was part of a eugenic plot to sterilize local women. Most seriously, two women died from mysterious causes that weren't conclusively tied to the Pill, but seemed likely a byproduct of hormone exposure.

Critics of the Pill would later point to serious problems with these trials as one piece of evidence that the drug was prematurely marketed to an eager population without adequate knowledge about safety. Writing over forty years later, Barbara Seaman noted, "How much Pincus wavered is evident in his papers, which are now available at the Library of Congress. They comprise approximately 44,000 items, filling 213 containers on 85.2 feet of shelf space. They reveal an awesome scientific and entrepreneurial brinkmanship, and make one wonder why Pincus didn't burn the evidence."[46] Among other scientific transgressions, Pincus falsified a control group after learning late in the trial that the FDA would require one, instructing recruiters to relabel "drop out" folders as controls.

Lara V. Marks defends Pincus and his cohorts, noting that scientific standards in the 1950s were vastly different from what they are today. She writes, "Any analysis of the Pill has to take into consideration the historical context in which it was developed. If the Pill is compared with other pharmaceutical products also coming on to the market at the time, those conducting the trials cannot be accused of negligence and supplying a questionable drug."[47] The Thalidomide tragedy in the 1960s would usher in more rigorous standards, and had such methods been applied to the Pill, it is possible that countless women could have been spared the "unanticipated" tragedies, including potentially fatal strokes and cardiovascular problems, that emerged in the decade following the Pill's approval.

Despite the problems it had encountered, the drug company G. D. Searle was given permission to market Enovid, the first Pill, for contraception in 1960. The world would never be the same.

The Big Round World and the Small Round Pill: Responses to Oral Contraception

When hormonal birth control hit the mass market in the 1960s, the most striking thing about it was how uncontroversial it was. Women embraced the Pill, and "between 1960 and 1962 the number of new prescriptions for the Enovid birth control pill increased tenfold, from 191,000 to 1,981,000."[48] While white women remained the largest consumers of oral contraceptives, women of all races and social groups utilized the new technology in growing numbers.

As Lara V. Marks argues, the story of the Pill is essentially a Cold War tale. Fear of rising populations in Communist and developing countries as well as poor and minority communities in the United States paved the way for more immediate acceptance of the drug's possible benefits. John Rock claimed that Communism and burgeoning world populations were "more than synchronous."[49] Critics of the increasing numbers of unwed mothers in the United States deployed military metaphors to make points about changing patterns of both black and white sexuality: the former were included in a sinister popular image, "the population bomb"; the latter were portrayed as dangerous agents of social change, part of the so-called sexual revolution. In the 1960s and 1970s these fears went a long way toward ensuring public acceptance of the Pill.

And of course, from women's perspective, the Pill offered freedoms they had never before enjoyed. Sexuality could be explored without restraint, family size could be limited, and extramarital affairs could be swept under the rug without a trace. For all these social actors—women, policy makers, and fear mongers alike—the Pill represented a potential solution.

In the mid 1960s, just as the Pill was becoming a household item, Barbara Seaman was working as a magazine columnist for *Bride* and *Ladies' Home Journal*. She began to receive disturbing letters from women and their families detailing complaints of Pill side effects that ranged from annoying to unacceptable to tragic. It was becoming clear that the Pill had been put on the market too early. Incensed by the implications of these women's experiences, Seaman was moved to research the Pill and write a book on her findings. In 1969, despite an injunction that nearly halted publication (and was based on accusations that later proved false), Seaman's book *The Doctors' Case Against the Pill* was published. In sharing the stories of women who had contacted her as well as the information she gleaned from top scientists working in the field, Seaman exposed the serious health implications associated with the Pill. Her book is generally credited, along with *Our Bodies, Ourselves*, with sparking the women's health movement.

Seaman's book caught the attention of Wisconsin senator Gaylord Nelson, who decided to hold hearings based around its findings. At the hearings, doctors testified for and against the Pill. Determined to have their voices heard, a group of young women who found themselves increasingly frustrated by the proceedings began a makeshift protest. Led by Alice Wolfson, a young Barnard College graduate, members of DC Women's Liberation shouted questions disrupting the hearings. "Why are ten million women being used as guinea pigs?" they demanded. The women were eventually removed from the hearings, but their protest caught the attention of the nation.

The combination of these incredible pieces of activism—Seaman's book and Wolfson's uprising—fostered the creation of the first patient package insert, the mandatory list of side effects that now comes with many prescriptions.[50] After studies confirmed the health dangers of the high-dose Pill, they were replaced by the low-dose Pill and eventually removed from the market in the 1980s.

While it has never regained the uncomplicated adoration it received in its early years, the Pill remains the most popular contraceptive for American women. By the 1990s, 80 percent of all American women born since 1945 had tried the Pill. Among other things, the Pill fundamentally changed the relationship between doctors and their patients, cementing the connection between contraception and the medical establishment. It also helped to give birth to—no pun intended—the concept of preventative medicine.

What lessons can women making contraceptive decisions learn from the history of birth control? For one thing, it is worth asking when, historically speaking, contraception has been tolerated and when it has been discouraged. Who was in power and what interests dictated policies about reproductive options? In what ways have women in diverse historical and social contexts resisted controls to their fertility? Most importantly, we must try to understand the patterns that run through histories of reproductive control and resistance as we try to understand the issues and controversies facing us today.

Chapter Two

A Pill Primer: Hormonal Contraception for the Twenty-first Century

When you make a thing, it is so complicated making it that it is bound to be ugly, but those that do it after you they don't have to worry about making it and they can make it pretty, and so everybody can like it when the others make it.
—Gertrude Stein, *The Autobiography of Alice B. Toklas*

Edris Rice-Wray had made up her mind: no one would ever be able to stay on this drug.

She was a faculty member at the Puerto Rico Medical School and medical director of the Puerto Rico Family Planning Association when Dr. Gregory Pincus asked her to assist him in enrolling eligible women to test the first contraceptive pill. Rice-Wray had been unaware that such a drug was in the works: "I thought about it and then I asked a lot of questions. I had to be sure it was safe, you know. I wasn't going to give them anything that wasn't all right."[1] Pincus assured her that it was perfectly safe. What he failed to mention was that it had been tested on a very small group of women for only four months. No one knew what would happen when women were given the drug for a longer period of time.

Enrolling women under age forty who had at least two children (to ensure that they were fertile), Rice-Wray began what would become one of the greatest experiments of the twentieth century. As she would recall later, getting women to sign on was no problem. Getting them to stick with the Pill regimen was another matter. Reasons for discontinuation were numerous and ranged from the social—some started to fear that hormonal contraception was an imperialist action to cut the Puerto Rican population—to the physical, as women began to experience multiple unpleasant effects. One young mother, Elsa Robles, began taking "Enovid" after the birth of her first child. She later recounted what happened: "I had horribly prolonged periods. Really long, sometimes they lasted almost a month. I was using so many sanitary pads—it really shook me up. It was like I was hemorrhaging. When I went out I was afraid to sit down in case I would bleed through."[2]

When Edris Rice-Wray wrapped up her part of Pincus's trial, she told him that from what she had observed, it just wasn't going to work; women would never knowingly subject themselves to these side effects. History would prove she was right about the Pill's dangers, but wrong about the willingness of female patients to endure them.

Half a century later, in the early winter of 2009, a young writer named Holly Grigg-Spall decided to go off the Pill after nearly ten years, multiple brands, and a particularly unpleasant interaction with one drug, Yaz. Grigg-Spall describes what changed her mind about the Pill: "At the end of 2008, I began to experience overwhelming anxiety, depression, debilitating brain fog and intense panic attacks which affected my work and relationship. For six months I thought I was losing my mind. After questioning every aspect of my life, and my sanity, I eventually discovered it was not me, but the birth control pill I was taking." Her moment of clarity came while sitting in a parking lot after a shopping trip with a friend, who had also been "feeling down lately, like nothing excited her anymore. She'd gotten more excited about leggings than anything else that month—including her long-term boyfriend. Her head felt like it was full of cotton wool, she couldn't think straight. She had no sex drive to speak of, but not just that, she had no drive at all." After sharing stories, Holly started to wonder if perhaps their birth control pills were part of the problem. Like so many women, Holly and her friend took the Pill every day without thinking of it as medicine or considering that it might impact their bodies in ways that went beyond preventing pregnancy. It took another year, but Grigg-Spall finally came off the Pill. All these years later, women like Grigg-Spall are learning through hard-won experience what Edris Rice-Wray saw from the beginning: that the choice to take the Pill is not always a simple one.

When I began learning about the Pill with Barbara Seaman at the end of 1999, women were marking its fortieth anniversary. The mood was decidedly celebratory, the moment was replete with widespread magazine and television coverage, and the message was clear: the creation of the Pill was a triumph for the feminist movement, and a huge step forward for women everywhere. In the midst of all of this good feeling, honest conversations about the Pill—about its history of safety concerns, its many risks and benefits—were noticeably absent.

A decade later, as we get ready to mark the fiftieth anniversary, little has changed. In twenty-first century American life it is taken as a given that the Pill is "safe." Pill hormone levels have been reduced since its birth, and life-threatening complications with the modern drug are purported to be rare. One hundred million women around the world are "on the Pill," and as a recent book on the subject posits, "100 million women can't be wrong."[3] But the lack of serious examination of the Pill has created an environment where women live with life-disrupting side effects for decades, unaware that a large consumer health movement has been asking questions about the dangers of hormonal contraception for fifty years.

As we approach this new anniversary, however, there are rumblings of discontent, signs of change. New chemicals and ways of distributing hormone drugs have led to a new batch of lawsuits. A new series of blood clots and strokes have replayed the avoidable tragedies of the 1960s and '70s, and once again, women have begun to ask whether or not the Pill should always be our first line of contraception. For the first time in many years, Pill prescription leveled out instead of growing in Canada.[4] Two Australian health writers, Jane Bennett and Alexandra Pope, published *The Pill: Are You Sure It's For You?*, a startling book that examines many of the potential health dangers of prolonged hormone use. And I have received e-mails from and had conversations with women around the country—women of different ages, races, and religions with different educational backgrounds and economic resources—detailing negative experiences with hormonal contraception that ranged from slightly annoying to life-threateningly serious. I am invigorated by this new engagement with contraceptive options and renewed willingness to question the Pill. All I can say is, "It's about time!"

I believe that the Pill represents something rare: a truly "new" thing in the world. It has changed women's lives unimaginably for the better. I also believe that we live in a culture that doesn't tolerate critical outlooks on hormonal contraception. If you ask questions, you must be a crazy conspiracy theorist, an opponent of "Western medicine," an unrepentant eccentric.

I am none of those things. I often take pharmaceuticals and am happy to take risks to reap drug benefits. My story is that of a skeptic who changed her mind, a person who took the Pill because, well, it's what you do, and who went on to believe that that sort of unquestioning allegiance is a mistake. Blindly worshiping at the church of the "magic bullet" is never the best thing for female consumers. If we are to truly value the gifts of hormonal contraception—and there are many—we must also be willing to ask tough questions about its risks, inconveniences, and unknowns. Many women will have no side effects at all with pill use, and there are many voices ready to educate women about the benefits of the Pill. On the other hand, women who struggle and have bad experiences lack strong, secular, feminist voices to illuminate their experiences.

When Barbara Seaman was writing in the 1960s, her goal was to warn women about a dangerous drug. My goal is to help women gain a more comprehensive and holistic knowledge of a drug that is generally safe. I also hope to give women who find that the Pill isn't right for them the confidence to stand up to a medical hegemony that insists that taking hormones is the only smart way to go. You need not believe that the Pill poses a serious threat to your health to simply not want to take it. It's your body, and your reasons are valid. While we can dream of a future with better, safer contraceptives, women are best served when they have good knowledge of those available to us today.

Hormonal Contraception Yesterday and Today

An Oberlin College graduate with a fondness for the poetry of Yeats, Barbara Seaman never intended to write about women's health; she wanted to pen song lyrics, or maybe novels. At first her weekly magazine column about sexual health was just an outlet to write and a way to pay the bills.

But as Seaman began receiving letters detailing the terrible side effects of the Pill, she realized her column was a serious tool that could be used to address women's concerns. Chronicling the drug's dangers in *The Doctors' Case Against the Pill* transformed her into a passionate crusader against the excesses of the pharmaceutical industry and the potential dangers of hormone drugs.

The original 1969 edition of *The Doctors' Case Against the Pill* outlined several potential problems that were being understudied and underreported. They included increased risk of blood clotting, stroke, cardiovascular disease, certain types of cancer, diabetes, sexual and mood side effects, gall bladder disease, weight gain, liver tumors, and reproductive tract infections with Pill use. Perhaps the best way to start asking questions about today's pills is to look back and compare them with yesterday's. Which concerns have been disproved, and which remain the same? Which problems have been alleviated in the five decades of chemical tinkering, and what new issues, unforeseen the 1960s, are we dealing with today?

What's In the Pill?

Before we begin talking about what can go right and wrong with the Pill, we must first be aware of what's inside it and how it works. The majority of oral contraceptive pills (OCPs) are made of a combination of synthetic estrogen and progestin hormones. Most contain an estrogen called ethynil estradiol at doses that vary from 50 to 20 mcg. Compare that to the world's first birth control pill, Enovid, which had 150 mcg of the synthetic estrogen mestranol.

As estrogen drugs have fallen under scrutiny in recent years, there has been a push to move patients toward using "natural" hormones. Qlaira, a new Pill introduced by Bayer-Schering—the company that brought us Yasmin and Yaz—uses a compound called estradiol valerate instead of ethynil estradiol. But if a hormone isn't made by your body, it isn't natural. As one writer on hormones explains, "It's like saying that a Twinkie is natural because it contains high fructose corn syrup."[5] At the end of the day, all chemicals are "natural," and this sort of language shouldn't be a determining factor in your decision to use hormonal contraception.

Progestins[6] are much more varied in dosage (although all are now well below the original Enovid load of 10 mg of norethynodrel), chemical structure, and safety profile than estrogens. They can be more and less progestational, estrogenic, and androgenic, depending on the formulation. Some progestins are older than others, and scientists often think of different compounds as falling into a first, second, third, and now fourth generation category. The problem with this breakdown is that no one understands exactly what constitutes a certain "generation." A less historically pleasing but more accurate way of thinking of today's progestins is to group them by chemical structure, but because studies and news articles continue to refer to "generations," I will explain which compounds generally fall into these groups.

First, the C-21 progestins (pregnanes) group includes medroxyprogesterone acetate (MDPA), the hormone used in the injectable contraceptive Depo-Provera. A second big group is the 19-nor testosterones. Older members of this group (sometimes called estranes) include norethistrone—the original progestin that Carl Djerassi struggled to make in his Mexican lab in the early 1950s—and norethynodrel, the progestin in Enovid. It also includes a number of compounds present in today's Pills, including norethindrone, norethindrone acetate, and ethynodiol diacetate.

Together these compounds are often called "first generation" progestins, although the last two compunds are sometimes called "second generation." Early female hormones were made by chemically altering the structure of other steroids, such as androgens (male hormones), which the body turns into estrogen and cholesterol. While the earlier progestins were miracle drugs in their way, they had a lot of unpleasant side effects, many of which were androgenic, such as skin problems and weight gain. Over the years, scientists have subtly tinkered with the formula, trying to maximize the benefits and minimize the problems. Today, most progestins are made from androgens and contain residual amounts of male steroid compounds, but have been engineered to curb earlier side effects.[7]

The second group of 19-nor testosterones makes up the majority of progestins in today's pills and include norgestrel, levonorgestrel, norgestimate, desogestrel, and gestodene. Norgestrel and levonorgestrel are often called "second generation progestins." Desogestrel, norgestimate and gestodene are frequently called "third generation progestins," and these newer compounds have been causing controversy in recent years as a result of serious side effects, as we will see later.

Further controversy surrounds a progestin made in a completely different way, drospirenone. This compound, used in the popular pill brands Yasmin and Yaz, is made from altering an antihypertensive compound instead of androgens. It is associated with higher potassium levels, making it a bad choice for women with kidney, liver, or adrenal problems. Sometimes called a "fourth generation progestin" or simply lumped in with other "third generation" compounds, drospirenone has also been associated with elevated blood clotting risk.

While pills with different progestins can be equally effective at preventing pregnancy, they have very distinct effects on each individual's body. Different pills are, to some extent, different types of drugs. This fact complicates both patient prescribing and the process of getting good data on oral contraceptive side effects. Most doctors experiment when it comes to choosing which brand of pills (and consequently which combination of hormones and doses) will work for individual women, but some doctors are coming to believe that testing hormone levels will help to predict who will do well on particular pills.

Combination pills (containing both estrogen and progestin) typically come in "monophasic," "biphasic," and "triphasic" formulations. A monophasic pill provides a steady dose of hormones throughout the month. A biphasic has two different doses of hormones, and a triphasic has three. Qlaira, Bayer-Schering's new pill, has four different hormone doses.

Pills that change hormone dose throughout the month do so because there is some thought that it more closely mimics the body's natural hormonal changes during a menstrual cycle. Studies have observed differences in the tendencies of these different pills to cause various side effects. Some women do better on monophasics and others prefer a pill with varying hormone doses. If a patient struggles on one type of pill, her doctor may suggest a switch to the other.

In addition to the differences in pills caused by various combinations of estrogen and progestin and differing hormone doses, many brand name pills are also available in generic form. These generics must be chemically similar enough to brand name versions to qualify as the same drug based on FDA's standards for generics. It is said that even small chemical differences can have a big effect on a person's body, and many women report that they feel different on generic birth control. Be aware that some states require specific instructions from a doctor for a pharmacy to provide a brand name product if a generic is available.

How Does It Work?

Pills work in three major ways. The female reproductive system is triggered when the hypothalamus (part of the brain) sends chemical messengers to the thyroid telling that gland to release hormones to the ovaries. Follicles in the ovaries slowly mature and release an egg, along with more hormones that eventually either nurture a pregnancy or lead to a period. The first way that birth control pills suspend this process is by blocking the surge of luteinizing hormone (LH) that would normally lead to ovulation. Sometimes ovulation happens anyway; no one is sure exactly why an egg will occasionally sneak through, but we do know that with lower-dose pills, it probably happens more often.

Second, pills lead to the thickening of cervical fluids. Over the course of a normal menstrual cycle, cervical fluids (sometimes called cervical mucus)—the moisture that starts at the gateway to the uterus—change. Around the time of ovulation, fluids become particularly hospitable to sperm in order to help them make the difficult journey through the cervix and uterus. When these fluids get too thick they can actually hinder, instead of helping, fragile sperm.

Third—and most controversially—the Pill can inhibit sperm and egg motility. That means that it becomes harder for sperm to swim up the fallopian tubes, and (this is the controversial part) it may become difficult for an egg that has been fertilized to implant in the uterine wall and begin to grow. Scientifically, a woman is not considered pregnant until a fertilized egg is implanted in her uterus, and the Pill does not affect eggs that have already been implanted. But some people believe that life begins with the fertilization of the egg, and since the Pill may affect a fertilized egg's ability to implant, some see it as an abortifacient.

In sum, the Pill works by stopping the production of an egg, blocking the sperm at the gate to the uterus, slowing sperm down as they move toward an egg, and if all else fails, preventing the egg from implanting. While this system is highly effective, the Pill isn't *quite* as good at preventing pregnancy as we are led to believe. We are used to seeing "typical use" failure rates for barrier methods—that means how often the contraceptive actually falters—but we see "ideal use" rates for hormonal contraception. However, even "typical use" failure for the Pill is quite good, and only six or seven women out of 100 who use the Pill as directed for a year will get pregnant, no matter what brand they use.

An important point to emphasize is that the Pill does not regulate a woman's menstrual cycle. In fact, it suspends the menstrual cycle and flattens a woman's natural hormone shifts. Doctors are often quick to rhapsodize about the potential health benefits of the Pill, but they are less willing to admit that there may be many health benefits to having normal menstrual cycles. We live in a culture that imagines that monthly cycles are useless outside of allowing pregnancy, a bad attitude that has resulted in a dearth of good research and information about this very basic part of female biology. Making the Pill the preferred contraceptive discourages women and health care providers from engaging with and learning from the menstrual cycle.

POPs

A newer and less frequently prescribed alternative to the standard pills are progestin-only pills (POPs). Originally marketed to menopausal women, these drugs—sometimes called "mini-pills"—have been shown to be useful for preventing pregnancy as well. They work slightly differently than pills containing estrogen, preventing ovulation only about 50 to 60 percent of the time.[8] They rely more heavily on other methods, such as thickening cervical mucus, to ultimately prevent pregnancy. It is even more important to take POPs at the same time each day than their combined counterparts; if you miss a pill by more than three hours, be sure to use back-up contraception until forty-eight hours after resuming pill use.[9]

POPs are thought to be more effective for breastfeeding women than for those in the general population (although this assumption is currently undergoing some revision, and some believe they are just as effective for all women).[10] Some researchers worry that breastfeeding babies whose mothers are on POPs receive some level of hormonal exposure through the milk, and thus are subject to the same side effects their mothers endure.[11] Others, such as the group Family Health International argue that "POPs do not affect the amount or quality of breastmilk," because "such small amounts enter the infant's system . . . no adverse effects on the health, growth or development of the infant have been found."[12]

Doctors and health groups are starting to look more closely at POPs because they seem to lack a lot of the unpleasant side effects of combined oral contraceptives (COCs) in trials; they don't cause as much nausea or as many headaches, and they may be better for mood problems. They also may be safer for women with high blood pressure or certain other cardiovascular risk factors (although it is worth asking why a barrier with spermicide wouldn't be better still for these women). More research and many more years of experience will be needed to confirm these benefits as well as to discover what dangers the drugs may hold. Still, they provide a promising new alternative to traditional oral contraceptives.

When Gregory Pincus first envisioned the Pill, he wanted it to be progestin-only. There were good reasons—including the tendency of Pincus's early Pill to cause erratic bleeding when unchecked—that the proto-POP was rejected. Today's POP still causes bleeding problems, and if you already have irregular or abnormal bleeding, or if you have breast or reproductive cancers or a history of these diseases, POPs are probably not right for you.

Risky Business: The Risks and Benefits of the Pill

I am out to lunch on a hot August day with a friend of mine who is a doctor. This young woman, in her early thirties, is a committed feminist and critical thinker. One thing that is not up for debate, as far as she is concerned, is the safety of the Pill. "Love the Pill!" she gushes over pizza and garlic knots, "Love it! I can't imagine advising patients to use anything else." When I cautiously tell her that I am writing about possible negative side effects, she scrunches her face disapprovingly: "Come on, Laura. This isn't the old Pill. And besides, it's the most studied drug in the world."

This last idea—that the Pill is our most studied drug—has become a mantra in recent years. Indeed, decades of experience and research have created an impressive body of studies and trials that help us understand these drugs.

The same thing was true, of course, for Hormone Treatments (HT) and Estrogen Treatments (ET) for menopause. In fact, ET and HT—drugs that are chemically similar to but lower in dose than the Pill—were approved for use in the United States twenty years before hormonal contraception. For decades women heard study after study insisting that taking estrogen or estrogen and progestin during the years prior to and immediately following menopause would offer a host of health benefits. Doctors assumed that prescribing these drugs to healthy patients was the most responsible thing to do.

Between 2001 and 2003, everything changed. The Women's Health Initiative, a massive fifteen-year trial that followed 161,808 women, became the first long-term, randomized double blinded clinical trial of HT and ET. When it got underway, doctors assumed it was a done deal; the study would only confirm what enormous amounts of prior science had shown: that taking the drugs was the healthiest thing that a mid-life woman could do. But the hormone trials came to early and screeching halts. The women taking HT and ET were having serious health problems: more heart disease, cancer, strokes, pulmonary embolisms, and blood clots than women taking placebos. These findings flew in the face of decades of research. It was a shock that sent doctors and their patients reeling. One of the reasons that the results of the WHI were so different than the findings of a staggering number of previous studies was because it was a different kind of study. Much of the prior research on hormones was based on small clinical trials, large observational trials, and meta-analysis—the same kinds of research that we have on the Pill.

The results of the WHI aren't applicable to young women and the Pill. The same hormones work very differently in women's bodies before and after menopause. Indeed many doctors believe that if the women being studied in the WHI had been younger, the results of the trial would have been very different. But the WHI does provide instruction for people of all ages about the limitations of observational research.

Unfortunately, we will never have a WHI for the Pill. This is for largely practical reasons: it is impossible to ask such a large group women to stay on the Pill for such a big portion of their fertile years. Ethical problems make placebo controlling pill trials difficult, and in the context of such a massive experiment, impossible. Even though the Pill is so studied, it has only been studied in certain ways.

HT and ET were on the market for sixty years before conventional wisdom about those medicines was overturned. There is still much that we don't know about the Pill, and because of limitations on the type of research we can do, much we may never know.

Taking Heart: Cardiovascular Side Effects of the Pill

One of the most terrifying aspects of the first generation of birth control pills was their tendency to cause blood clotting and strokes in young women. In 1969, Barbara Seaman documented the story of Julie Macauley, a mother of five who died at age twenty-nine from a pulmonary embolism. Macauley had been taking the Pill for less than a year when she began to have dizzy spells. After two brief hospitalizations, she died, leaving her devastated widower to care for their large family. Tom Macauley was stunned when the doctor treating his wife asked, "Was she taking birth control pills?"[13]

In the early years of the Pill, doctors often denied the increased cardiovascular risks of Pill use that were confirmed a decade later. Today's Pill is significantly safer, but some risk remains, especially for women over thirty-five, those who smoke, and patients with other health conditions that make such problems more likely. Women who don't fit these special precautions still have more blood clots, strokes, and heart attacks on the Pill, even if they are taking "low-dose" versions of the drug.[14]

As I was writing this book, I learned firsthand that cardiovascular risks are not totally a thing of the past. My childhood friend was hospitalized with multiple blood clots that led to a stroke. As she recovered from emergency surgery that left her unable to walk, write, read, or tie her shoelaces, her Columbia-trained neurosurgeon told her devastated parents that he suspected use of a menstrual suppression drug had contributed to the stroke. My friend wasn't taking a Pill for contraception; in fact, she did it because she had terribly painful periods and hoped to eliminate some of them.

I do not share this story to scare women away from the Pill—in fact, very few women who take hormonal contraceptives will experience a side effect this serious. Rather, I tell this story to highlight the fact that taking the Pill is never a simple choice; there is always risk involved. I believe denying or ignoring that such outcomes can happen makes it harder for the extremely small number of women who suffer them to receive proper care. My friend's care was delayed by assumptions among medical caregivers that she was inventing her symptoms.

As Dr. Richard P. Dickey notes, "Virtually all the excess mortality in OC [oral contraceptive] users is due to CVD [cardiovascular disease]."[15] In other words, if you are going to die from taking the Pill, it will be because of CVD. CVD can be caused by blood clotting in the vessel, such as deep vein thrombosis and pulmonary embolism; changes in the vessel wall, such as high blood pressure and isechemic heart disease; and problems that happen because of a combination of these factors, such a heart attack (myocardial infarction) and stroke.

Who Is Most at Risk?

With cardiovascular problems, certain preexisting conditions make oral contraceptive use more dangerous. These include high blood pressure, smoking, migraine headaches that are characterized by visual symptoms called auras, thrombophlebitis (an increased tendency to form blood clots), a family history of abnormal clotting, and obesity.[16]

While the Pill is a very studied drug, we have barely begun to scratch the surface on some very important safety issues. For example, how might the various Pills work differently in the bodies of women in different racial groups? Like age, race is a factor often left out or understudied in many drug trials. One recent article notes "studies of OCP [oral contraceptive pill] use have either not enrolled African American women or enrolled too few African American women to allow for the assessment of metabolic consequences of the OCP." After looking specifically at a population of black women taking the Pill, study authors concluded, "In African American women, OCP use is associated with an increase in markers of cardiovascular risks."[17] These warning signs included insulin resistance, glucose intolerance, and elevated triglycerides.[18] Risk/benefit analysis is always a tricky business, but it is made more difficult by science that doesn't acknowledge and study the particular benefits and drawbacks posed to specific communities.

Blood Clots

While blood clots remain a rare outcome for pill users, new progestins and new systems of distributing hormones have made this serious problem with the early pill something that women need to worry about again. Only thirty-two cases of thromboembolism (blood clots) per million women are seen between ages twenty to twenty-four, but this number goes up to forty-six cases between ages thirty and thirty-four, and fifty-nine cases between forty and forty-four.[19] Women who take the Pill face a threefold increase in the risk for this problem,[20] and it seems to be related to estrogen dosage,[21] with a risk around one to two cases per ten thousand women.[22]

Regardless of what pill you take, certain genetic factors (such a V Leiden mutation) and preexisting clotting problems make thromboembolism on the Pill more likely. If you have a family history of blood clotting or thrombosis, you may want to consider screening for such problems before starting oral contraceptive use.

There is growing evidence that certain newer third generation progestins may cause an increase in clotting more comparable with first generation pills. This possibility first made headlines in the mid 1990s when the Committee on Safety of Medicines (CSM) in the United Kingdom uncovered three unpublished studies that showed that clotting was more likely on OCs with third generation progestins gestodene and desogestrel.[23] These findings were controversial,[24] but they have been confirmed by further studies.[25] In 2007 the consumer group Public Citizen petitioned the FDA to pull pills with desogestrel,[26] but they remain on the market in the United States.[27]

In two 2009 studies Danish researchers again found that newer progestins were, in some cases, less safe than older ones, and that those with desogestrel, cyproterone, drospirenone, and gestodene caused more problems than those with levonorgestrel or norgestrel.[28] What this tells us is that newer isn't always better, and that much more research is needed before we can start to understand what the differences between these compounds mean.

Drospirenone, the progestin in Yasmin and Yaz, has fallen under particular scrutiny in recent years for its potential to cause blood clots. Approved in 2001 and 2006 respectively, Yasmin and Yaz became the top-selling pharmaceutical line for their maker, Bayer, and Yaz became the top selling birth control pill in the United States.[29] One twenty-one-year-old recently told me Yaz was the "classic" pill for college girls—but these pills may carry extra problems.

Serious troubles for Bayer began in October of 2008 when the FDA decided that ads for Yaz were misleading enough to require correction.

Exaggerations of the benefits—including claims that the drug could fix mild depression and acne—led to required mea culpas in advertisements that cost $20 million and showed a pretty young woman sheepishly admitting that viewers "may have seen some Yaz commercials recently that were not clear." In all, by the fall of 2009, seventy-four lawsuits had been brought against Bayer by women using either Yaz or Yasmin, many of whom had experienced blood clots. One of these, Anne Marie Eakins, developed blood clots in both lungs after taking Yaz to control PMS and skin problems.[30] The history teacher and mother of two survived, but lost part of her right lung. The literature on drospirenone reveals few differences from traditional oral contraceptives, but reviews on the progestin all conclude that a lot more research will be necessary to discretely understand it.[31]

The lesson of Yasmin and Yaz (and as we shall see, the contraceptive patch and ring) is that newer is not necessarily better; in fact, when it comes to pills, it is often wiser to stick with the drug you know. Hopefully consumers will not need more unexpected side-effects and avoidable tragedies to take this lesson to heart. Judy Norsigian, the tireless women's health activist who has worked with Our Bodies, Ourselves for over thirty years tells me, "It's so sad what has happened with some of the new contraceptives. It's all because the drug makers want new patents. So many of these adverse events were completely avoidable."[32]

High Blood Pressure

Hormonal contraceptives can sometimes cause a slight (often clinically insignificant) increase in blood pressure. The risk has gone down significantly since first generation Pills, which were six times more likely to cause women to develop high blood pressure.[33] Again, age, smoking, obesity, preexisting blood pressure issues, and family history impact the odds that hormonal contraception will raise your blood pressure. Antihypertensive medications and the Pill don't play well together: if you have preexisting blood pressure issues that you are controlling with medicine, you may want to consider a nonhormonal birth control.

Before starting the Pill, women should be screened for high blood pressure. If they have it, a serious conversation about risks and benefits is necessary, although some doctors argue that if high blood pressure is managed and the patient is young (under thirty-five), low-dose pill use may be possible.[34] Women with elevated risk should be encouraged to explore safer options, such as barriers, instead of OCs.

Heart Attacks

Very few young women have heart attacks whether or not they are on the Pill, but early studies found that using the drug increased this risk by two to four times.[35] Studies on whether the Pill increases the risk of heart attack for women with no cardiovascular risk factors have had mixed results, but it is known that[36] if you have other risk factors, such as high blood pressure or smoking, Pill use can increase your risk for myocardial infarction. Smoking makes it ten times more likely that a woman under thirty-five will suffer this outcome.[37] Keep in mind, of course, that we are talking about a very small risk.

A joint study between Virginia Commonwealth University and the Universite de Sherbrooke in Quebec found that women taking low dose pills had twice the risk for heart attacks when compared with non-users.[38] Some women were more at risk than others: women with diabetes and polycystic ovary syndrome (PCOS), for example, may be more likely to have this problem. John E. Nestler, one of the researchers conducting the study, noted that the Pill is often used as a treatment for PCOS (which, among other problems, causes irregular periods) despite the fact that the drugs may pose more health risks for this group[39]—a great example of how a medical problem may be masked, ignored, and even exacerbated by turning prematurely to hormonal contraceptives to manage it.

Stroke

The relationship between oral contraceptives and stroke (an interruption of blood flow to the brain) has been hotly debated since the 1960s, but most data confirms that Pill users have a twofold increase in risk when compared with non-users. Young women very rarely have strokes, though, so even this elevated risk is very small—perhaps 8 in 100,000 women.[40]

Smoking cigarettes raises the risk of having a stroke on OCs from twofold to eightfold, and being over thirty-five compounds this risk.[41] Women know that they shouldn't smoke, and many choose to lie about this lifestyle choice to doctors because they are embarrassed. In this way, though, doctors are often prevented from discouraging a group of people from Pill use who very obviously should choose another method.

Migraine headaches, particularly those that come with visual symptoms called auras, can indicate a significant increase in risk for stroke with the Pill.[42] A World Health Organization study found that women who had migraines and used OCs were eight times more likely to have a stroke than either women who had the headaches and didn't use oral contraception, or women who took the pill and didn't have headaches. They were sixteen times more likely to have a stroke than women who had neither migraines nor used the Pill.[43] For every rule there is an exception: Ann, a thirty-year-old lawyer in Boston, tells me that the only thing that reduces and manages her migraines is combined Pill use.[44] She swears she will never stop taking it, despite other annoying side effects, because it helps her get through the work day: "It used to be that anything would set off my headaches. If I got on an elevator and someone was wearing too much cologne, I knew I was in trouble. Now they're better. Not perfect, but better." These sorts of examples aside, if you are a woman with certain types of migraine headaches, you should think seriously about nonhormonal contraceptive methods.

Certain genetic mutations that cause blood clotting have been associated with increased stroke risk, including Factor V Leiden and MTHFR 677TT.[45] When women and their doctors fail to identify clotting problems, the results can be tragic. Deanne Stein was thirty-one, a non-smoker, and physically fit when her dermatologist put her on the Pill to help with skin trouble. The reporter for a local West Virginia television station had only been taking the pills for a short time when she had a stroke. It turned out that she had an undiagnosed clotting problem. Stein survived, but she now warns women to take the risks of oral contraceptives seriously: "I would never suggest a ban on the Pill. It is very beneficial for those women who can take them. But if you have any of the warning signs, it's just not worth the risk."[46]

Being seriously overweight, a problem that has been growing for many years in the United States, also puts women at risk for more strokes.[47] Studies estimate that women in this group are two to four times more likely to have a stroke while using hormonal contraception.

Some say that women should use the Pill despite cardiovascular risks because the risk of stroke during pregnancy is even greater—about 11 per 100,000,[48] compared with 8 per 100,000 who use the Pill. But, of course, this is a false comparison; it is not an either/or situation. A decision not to use the Pill does not necessarily mean a decision to undergo a pregnancy or forgo contraception.

Growing Confusion: Cancer and the Pill

The relationship between hormonal contraception and cancer is deeply confusing. The Pill seems to reduce the risk of certain cancers and raise the risk of others. While some associations are controversial, and in some cases the mechanism through which the Pill positively or negatively impacts cancer risk is still theoretical, it is worth trying to look generally at the more studied strains of the disease and OC use.

Uterine and Ovarian Cancer

Studies in recent years have shown that Pill use seems to provide protection against ovarian and endometrial cancers. Endometrial cancer is the most common reproductive cancer in American women, accounting for 6 percent of the total female cancers in the United States each year,[49] and ovarian cancer is the ninth most common. Just how much the Pill reduces the risk of these cancers is still up for debate,[50] but one meta-analysis estimated that women who don't take the Pill have a 2.4 percent risk of developing the disease through age seventy-four, and those who use OCs for twelve years have a 1.4 percent risk.[51] Another study thought the benefit would be greater, positing that eight years of use could prevent nearly 1,900 cases of the disease in the United States alone.[52] Still other studies insist that the benefit would be smaller: an estimate published in the British medical journal the *Lancet* reckoned that if 100,000 women between the ages of sixteen and thirty-five used the Pill, only ten lives would be saved. In any case, it is clear that the risk of cancer goes down somewhat with use, that longer use provides more protection, and that effects last beyond use, so even if you stop taking Pills you will have reduced risk.

An important point to make about disease statistics is that benefits and risks are often expressed relatively, not absolutely. That means they are expressed as percentages instead of real numbers. Relative risks are more interesting than absolute risks because they look dramatic. For example, let's say we are testing a drug on 200 women, 100 of whom are actually taking the drug, and 100 of whom are taking a placebo (sugar) pill. If two women in the placebo group get breast cancer and one woman taking the drug gets the same illness, I could write up my report and announce to the world that my pill cut the risk of breast cancer by 50 percent. Meta-analysis, another way of looking at data, has become popular in recent years. A meta-analysis pools data from many places over the course of many years to try and spot new health patterns or confirm older suspect ones. This way of analyzing data is important but flawed: it gives us valuable information, but often pulls together very different pieces of research to do so—studies that may or may not be relevant together. Always be willing to ask tough questions about a trial, even if you aren't a science person.

Ovarian cancer, while deadly, is relatively rare. It accounts for only 3 percent of cancers in the United States in women.[53] The Pill seems to offer the greatest protection in this type of cancer in women under twenty-five. The frequency of ovarian cancer is 14 percent less after a year of use and 50 to 60 percent less after five years. Meta-analysis has suggested that out of 100,000 women, pill use for five to eight years may prevent between 192[54] and 215 cancer deaths.[55]

A 2008 meta-analysis published in the *Lancet* sparked a cry for over-the-counter Pill access as a public health measure.[56] That reaction was certainly reductionary of the diverse health and economic concerns that must inform a decision about giving a drug "over-the-counter" status, but the results of the analysis were encouraging for pill users. It found that benefits from four to five years of use persisted (although lessened) up to thirty years after suspending hormones.[57] For women who used the Pill longer, greater benefits were seen: in the developed world, women who had used the drugs for ten years cut their risk from 1.2 cases per 100 people to 0.8 cases, and deaths declined from 0.7 per 100 to 0.5.[58]

Since most ovarian cancers in women occur after age sixty, and most people stop taking the Pill by age fifty, it is important to establish that the theorized benefit lasts for decades.[59] Many early users of the Pill have only recently reached their sixties and seventies, so much remains to be seen about the long-term benefits for ovarian cancer prevention.

In addition to ovarian cancer, OC use helps to reduce the likelihood that a woman will develop benign ovarian cysts. The reason for both cancer and cyst reduction is the same: since the Pill prevents ovulation, it creates far fewer opportunities for the problems that can happen when you ripen and release an egg.

Because low-dose pills and progestin-only pills are less likely to stop ovulation, they are also less effective in preventing cysts—in fact, POPs may actually increase the risk of developing function cysts—so if this is the problem you are trying to prevent, you are better off sticking with a slightly higher-dose, combined Pill.[60] But even if you have cysts, if they aren't causing pain and interfering with your life in any way, treatment with hormones, which come with their own risks, may not be the best option.

Colon Cancer

Colon cancer is the third most frequent variety of the disease among American women, and accounts for 536,662 new cases of cancer in women worldwide each year. It is possible that hormonal contraception curtails the production of bile acid, reducing the risk of this type of cancer.[61] A 2009 meta-analysis found that OC users reduced their risk of developing colon cancer by around 20 percent over never-users.[62] While the length of time which women took birth control pills for didn't seem to impact benefit, recent use did.

It is too soon to declare this meta-anlysis conclusive,[63] and improved screening, in combination with enhanced efforts to raise public awareness of this illness, remains the most important tool we can use to prevent colon cancer, which has declined 2.2 percent each year for over a decade.[64] Though it is rare, even young women can be afflicted with colon cancer: during the writing of this book my dear friend lost her partner (thirty-nine years of age) to the disease, and another family friend (age twenty-seven), continues to undergo chemotherapy and radiation. The effectiveness of the Pill as a preventative measure for colon cancer certainly deserves further study but isn't a reason to start OCs.

Cervical Cancer and STIs

Cervical cancer is a very different disease depending on who you are and where you live. For women in the developed world it has become a rare event, and deaths from the illness are relatively rare. This is due in part to advances in screening, such as Pap smears and human papilloma virus (HPV) tests, which allow the detection of the disease—which takes years to develop—in pre-cancerous and early stages. In the developing world, the story is different, and many women suffer and die from what is increasingly a preventable illness. As we will see when we look at Gardasil and advances in treating and preventing HPV, this is a disease that has been in the spotlight in the last decade as a series of truly new preventative methods have emerged.

Most cervical cancers are caused by HPV, which is transmitted primarily through sexual contact. HPV causes cellular changes that can lead, after years of unchecked development, to cancer.

There seems to be a small increase in the likelihood of developing cervical cancer with OC use. A 1995 meta-analysis estimated that 425 women between the ages of twenty and fifty-four who didn't use the Pill in every 100,000 got this cancer. For users of hormonal contraception, particularly those who took the drugs for eight years or more, an additional 125 women might be diagnosed with cervical cancer.[65] Considering how many women suffer from the illness each year, this is a very small number. Another large analysis reckoned that among women who used the Pill for five years, there would be an additional 67 cases per 100,000 women in the United States,[66] and still another trial put that number at 76 additional deaths per 100,000 women.[67]

It is difficult to theorize why cervical cancer and Pill use might be connected, but one possibility has nothing to do with how the drug works in the body. Pill users, as a group, may simply have more sexual partners than non-users, and it is even more possible that they neglect to use condoms, which, though not foolproof, indeed decrease transmission of HPV. Hormonal contraception may increase the chance of contracting HPV by causing something called cervical ectopy, which increases the surface of vulnerable cells on the cervix. Finally, it is possible that lower folic acid in the body—a potential result of taking the Pill—decreases the immune system's response to HPV and changes the cervical mucus in a way that makes women more vulnerable to infection.

The relationship between sexually transmitted infections and the Pill is a confusing one. Studies suggest that users have fewer cases of pelvic inflammatory disease (PID), but more incidence of chlamydia, an illness that can lead to PID. Pill users are more likely to engage in sexual activity that could lead to contracting chlamydia, but fewer Pill users' infections advance to PID at least in part because they are required to undergo yearly exams, which often include testing for STIs, in order to get prescriptions. It is also possible that the Pill somehow controls and tames chlamydia.

Whatever the effect of the Pill, it is important to use condoms if you have multiple partners. They should be the first line of defense against HPV, chlamydia, HIV, and all other STIs. Every woman who is sexually active should make sure to have regular Pap smears or some other variety of screening for HPV and pre-cancerous growths as well as for STIs.

Breast Cancer and Benign Breast Disease

There are few illnesses that inspire as much fear and emotion in women as breast cancer. It is the most frequent cancer in women in the United States, and most of us know someone who has dealt with the illness.

Since hormones were synthesized, scientists have been aware that they have the potential to cause breast cancers.[68] Charles Dodd, the British scientist who helped make diethylstilbestrol (DES), noticed that in the months after his male scientists started making and working with the compound, they began developing breasts. By 1940, the *Journal of the National Cancer Institute* was reporting that DES caused breast cancer in both male and female mice.[69]

Exactly what the risks of taking OCs are in terms of developing breast cancer remains controversial. What is certain is that very few *young* women get the disease: indeed, fewer than ten in every ten thousand under age thirty-five.[70] A re-analysis of data from fifty-four trials found a small increase in breast cancer risk with Pill use in those under age thirty-five.[71] This risk was greatest while using the drugs, and persisted for about ten years after use, eventually disappearing. Older formulations of the Pill were more risky, and recent trials of lower dose pills suggest that risks are now minimal.[72]

Some studies have suggested that while Pill users may be slightly more likely to get breast cancer, they are also more likely to be diagnosed at early stages when treatment is more possible (in particular, before the cancer has spread beyond the breast). As with PID, it seems possible this is due in part to more frequent visits to health care professionals, which are a required part of OC access.

The Women's Health Initiative (WHI) confirmed that menopausal women taking the hormone drug HT (a combination of estrogen and progestin similar to but less powerful than birth control pills) were at a 24 percent higher risk for breast cancer than those taking a placebo.[73] Women who took estrogen alone for the trial had lower rates of breast cancer than those who took a combination of estrogen and progestin, leading researchers to wonder if perhaps progestin is responsible for increased breast cancer risk in birth control pill users as well. The particular progestin used in the WHI—medroxyprogesterone acetate—has been implicated before in causing greater cancer risk.[74] As one author writes, "The previous assumption that progestin does not promote breast cancer development needs to be reexamined since a growing body of evidence indicates the opposite."[75]

The less-than-positive findings of WHI about hormone use inspired thousands to ditch their menopause drugs, and the results were fast and striking. In 2003, the year in which WHI halted its trials to much media fanfare, breast cancer dropped a stunning 7 percent.[76] Christina A. Clarke, leading a team of researchers writing in the *Journal of Clinical Oncology*, noted that the "drop was sustained in 2004, which tells us that the decline wasn't just a fluke."[77] Rates continued to decline in 2005, adding further fuel to the anti-HT fire. When I spoke to Jacques Rossouw, one of the lead scientists in the massive study, he told me, "The data for OC use and breast cancer are very mixed. I think a critical difference between OC use and HT use is that OCs substitute for the woman's endogenous hormones, so her total hormone exposure is only increased slightly in dose or duration, while postmenopausal HT increases the dose and duration of hormone exposure compared to menopause with no HT use."[78]

While HT and the Pill are different—and women take them at very different points in their lives—the increasing evidence that giving up hormones cuts breast cancer in older women poses some very important questions for younger ones. Because cancer can take so many years to develop, it can be tough to demonstrate causality. But if you have a family history of breast cancer,[79] or if you have had it in the past, you should ask your doctor if a nonhormonal alternative might be safer for you.

Women on the Pill are less likely to develop benign breast diseases, including fibradenoma and fibrocystic breast disease.[80] This benefit is only seen in current users. If you are among the small number of women who do develop fibrocystic breasts after starting Pill use, you may want to consider discontinuing use, as it could put you at an increased risk for breast cancer.

Many women develop swollen or painful breasts when they use the Pill, especially in the first several months of use. This problem can be addressed switching to a drug with lower estrogen potency and lower progestin content.[81] You may also want to try cutting caffeine, reducing salt intake, drinking plenty of water, and drinking diuretic herbal teas, such as rosehip.

Liver Cancer

The risk of liver cancer, a rare but almost inevitably fatal disease, is slightly increased with Pill use.[82] Since so few women develop this disease, it should not be a major consideration in your decision to take or avoid hormonal contraception. Taking the Pill raises your risk of developing benign liver tumors, too, but this condition is also infrequent, occurring in just 3 in every 100,000 users each year.[83] Using low dose pills probably alleviates this already slight risk. If you experience any growth in the liver, benign or otherwise, taking hormones can be very dangerous.

Jane Bennett and Alexandra Pope write, "Your liver is your largest internal organ and has a wider range of functions than any other organ in your body. Among other things it processes nutrients and detoxifies your blood . . . taking the Pill places considerable strain on your liver."[84] In particular, drospirenone, the progestin in Yaz and Yasmin, has been shown to potentially raise potassium levels in a way that may be dangerous, so women with kidney, liver, or adrenal problems shouldn't use these pills. Some doctors have advocated switching to an alternative distribution method—a hormonal device such as a contraceptive patch or vaginal ring—that delivers the drug directly in to the bloodstream.[85] As we will see, these newer methods may prove to be good options for some, but they currently carry their own risks of increased blood clotting and other problems.

All in Our Heads? Depression, Mood, and Libido

Like me, many women go off the Pill because they believe it causes unwelcome changes in mood and mental health. Since oral contraceptives first hit the market there have been women who claim that a small dose of hormones each day can cause big emotional problems, and today it is still one of the top reasons for discontinuing hormonal contraception.[86] Another group of women argue the opposite: that taking birth control pills helps to tame their premenstrual syndrome and stabilize emotional variability. Analyzing mood is tricky, particularly when we get into classifying what is "normal" and what isn't. Drugs that promise to end premenstrual fluctuations have been criticized by some feminists who argue that PMS is used as an excuse to dismiss women's legitimate concerns, sorrows, and complaints, and medical management of mood changes constitutes an effort to suppress noncompliance and unpleasantness in the female population.

On this issue, doctors are as divided as patients. When I spoke to Dr. Susan Rako, a Boston-based psychiatrist who has written passionately and persuasively against menstrual suppression drugs, she told me that the relationship between the Pill and depression has been "seriously overlooked."[87] Dr. Rako frequently treats young women who don't tell her they are taking oral contraceptives, and she sees it as an important piece of information for a doctor to have when treating mood symptoms.

The World Health Organization estimates that one in four women will become clinically depressed at some point in their lives, compared with one in six men.[88] Because women are more vulnerable to depression, it is particularly important to understand whether oral contraceptives could be playing a role in the problem. Over the years, doctors have studied different hormone concoctions to try to determine how the Pill might change moods. Decades and dozens of trials later, we still don't have good answers.

Some theorize that estrogen causes a deficiency of vitamin D, leading to other shifts in body chemistry, or that hormones pair with certain brain chemicals to suppress or alternately increase others. Other nutritional deficiencies, such as a decrease in B vitamins or increasing copper and decreasing zinc, may also play a role in making women feel blue.[89] Since pills work on the adrenal gland, some have theorized that adrenal fatigue and altered levels of cortisol (a hormone that is related to the body responding to stress) may be the reason that many people feel bad on hormonal contraception.

For women who feel better on the Pill, it is possible that positive mood changes happen because other health problems—terrible PMS, irregular bleeding, or extreme cramping, for example—are curtailed.

If we accept for a moment that the Pill does cause negative changes in mood for some women, it is unclear whether that shift is short term or long term. It is important to distinguish between depression—an illness that lasts for a long period of time and often requires treatment—and a mood swing, which is shorter and more prone to change. These are two very different conditions that may require different solutions and treatments, and it is possible the Pill contributes to or cures one and not the other.

Trying to predict which women will interact badly with birth control pills is impossible at this point, but some factors that might predispose a woman to Pill-instigated negative mood changes are coming into focus. If a woman has a history of depression, postpartum depression, or severe premenstrual mood changes, she may be more likely to have problems on the Pill. As you might expect, if women close to you in your family have had emotional problems on the Pill, you may be more likely to have them too, although of course older high-dose pills produced different problems than today's lower-dose ones. If you have trouble with vitamin B deficiency on the Pill, you may need to be careful about mood problems. Finally, women under twenty may be more likely to have negative mood or affect changes, while these problems seem to decrease in women over thirty.

There is no agreement about whether estrogen or progestin is more likely to cause mood problems, or what ratio of estrogen to progestin is best for reducing problems. Some studies have suggested that women who have a history of PMS before using the Pill do better with more progestin to estrogen, and those without a history of PMS fare better with a drug that has a lower progestin to estrogen ratio.[90] If this is true, then a history of PMS could be an important consideration in choosing a specific brand for women starting on oral contraceptives. One area ripe for future research is an examination of the way that cholesterol levels, known to be impacted by Pill use, can impact mood. Other open questions include understanding the roles individual hormone levels, family history, weight, and body fat distribution play in changing the way the Pill can make you feel.

Antidepressants have been suspected in the past of interacting with, and decreasing the effectiveness of, oral contraceptives. Herb-based oral antidepressants like St. John's Wort have been shown to interfere with the Pill in certain preparations and dosages but not in others.[91] While the Pill is safe to take with many drugs, be sure to tell your doctor if you are taking other medications. Women often fail to think of the Pill as a medicine, probably because we aren't sick when we take it. Giving your doctor a list of all the drugs you are taking, including the herbal ones, is a start to being safer.

Another thing pills have long been suspected of doing is hurting your sex drive. Many women choose the Pill because of its potential to create an ideal environment for sex, but these freedoms are sometimes undercut by the fact that while they can have sex without advance preparations, messes, and complication, they no longer want to. As with so many posited problems of the Pill, this one is hotly debated. Many doctors and scientists insist that there simply isn't good science to support the notion that pills kill libido, but generations of women have insisted that this is a potential pitfall of hormonal contraception.[92] Rebecca, a thirty-something Philadelphian, admits to suffering these side effects and says, "I don't know a woman who doesn't think it is real. The only people who don't think so are doctors."

Some doctors and scientists are starting to pay more attention to the problem. Dr. Lorraine Dennerstein, an Australian doctor at the University of Melbourne, has been studying women's health and sex for a long time. She notes, "About one third of women are having adverse effects on their sexuality by the oral contraceptive pill,"[93] adding, "it is rather strange that at the moment we have pharmaceutical companies spending absolutely millions of dollars to try to develop a pill that improves women's sexual interest or arousal. At the same time, we have freely available the oral contraceptive pill and other hormones which actually suppress women's sexual function."[94] (In fact, one drug maker, BioSanta, is planning to launch the "Pill Plus," a contraceptive that supplements with testosterone to try to curtail sexual problems, in 2011.)

Whenever female sexual problems fall under the social microscope, controversy is close behind. The 1990s saw the popularization of Viagra for erectile disfunction (ED) and the medicalization of men's sexual problems. The drug was a blockbuster, and by the end of the decade, a frantic search was on for a female version to treat was now called "female sexual dysfunction," or FSD. Since women's bodies have been medicalized for hundreds of years, the explosion of classifications for different problems of both desire and sexual function didn't constitute a new approach to female health, like it did with men. What did change, however, was the way that doctors thought about addressing sexual difficulties. For decades, the answers to women's sexual problems were thought to be psychological: if a woman didn't like sex, it must be because of a trauma, or a failure to mature emotionally, or some other problem that existed primarily in her head. Now, increasingly, it seemed possible that drugs could be administered when women expressed sexual dissatisfaction. In 1999, Dr. Irwin Goldstein helped organize a conference in Boston that vastly expanded (and some critics said invented) categories of sexual difficulty and disease. The conference also shot the gun to begin the race for "female Viagra."

In spite of Goldstein's hopes—paired with plenty of research and money—there are still no viable female libido drugs on the market. Researchers have begun to realize that, ultimately, we don't have a very good understanding of female sexuality, and women lack a clear marker (like an erection) to use as a gauge of sexual functioning.

In response to doctors like Goldstein, who insisted that all female sexual problems could be treated with drugs, a group of vocal critics led by NYU-based sexologist Leonore Teifer emerged to reemphasize the role of social and economic factors in female sexuality and to resist the further medicalization of female bodies. They insisted that it is nearly impossible to separate factors like gender inequity, social class, ethnicity, sexual orientation, socioeconomic factors, and experiences of sexual violence and shame from the biological parts that come together to make an orgasm. People—and in particular, women—aren't that simple.

Understanding that the relationship between bodies, cultures, and pharmaceuticals is rarely clear cut, how can we learn anything about the effect of oral contraceptives on sexual desire? Cynthia Graham, a Canadian scientist, first became interested in how the Pill impacts libido when she was a graduate student at McGill University studying the effect of taking birth control pills on severe PMS. She found that the Pill didn't seem to help PMS, but what it *did* do was cause sexual side effects for many of the women in the trial.

Graham tells me that part of the problem getting good data has to do with money—"it is very hard to get funding for this kind of research"[95]—and part of it is methodological. She believes that many studies in the past that failed to show potential sexual problems were flawed. They looked at long-term Pill users rather than those who were new to the drug. Because of this the group was self-selecting: women who had problems on the Pill got off before they were included in these studies. Another big obstacle has been cultural differences. When Graham worked on a large study that looked at women in both Scotland and the Philippines, problems encountered by the European women weren't evident in the Filipino population. Because sexuality is such an intersection of culture and biology, assuming that a trial in one population can tell us something about another is risky.

Today Graham is researching the extent to which libido problems lead women to get off the Pill (in which she looked specifically at new Pill users[96]) and the role of testosterone in diminished desire.[97] Her work is innovative in terms of design: she sometimes conducts placebo-controlled trials (difficult to do with the Pill, but possible if subjects are sterilized or have other protections against pregnancy and can take a sugar pill) and looks at hormone levels side by side with women's reports of their mood and sex changes. She believes that a small group of women's sex lives are indeed adversely affected by hormonal contraception, and the challenge for researchers is to understand which factors may make women more vulnerable to sexual problems with the Pill.

One theory about why the Pill might dampen sex drive is that taking it leads to lower levels of testosterone in the body. In 2004, drug maker Proctor & Gamble brought their testosterone-releasing patch to the FDA in hopes of making it the first approved drug to treat FSD. The bid failed, in part because P&G lacked long-term safety data,[98] but the idea that testosterone supplementation will boost libido in women persists. In studies of the Pill, women taking OCs did seem to have less testosterone, but there was no clear connection between having a low level of the hormone and diminished libido.[99] Other studies found that taking testosterone supplements didn't seem to improve sexual functioning for women taking the Pill who complained of problems.

Another theory on the link between the Pill and libido relates to the fact that desire peaks in the menstrual cycle with estrogen levels, right around the time that a woman ovulates. Because the Pill can flatten estrogen changes, some reason it could dampen desire. Others theorize that the *amount* of estrogen matters, and that perhaps having too much estrogen in a Pill might cause the problem—though no studies have conclusively shown this to be true.

Some believe that the type of progestin might be the culprit. Depot medroxyprogesterone acetate (DMPA), the progestin used in the injectable Depo-Provera, has fallen under suspicion because of its dramatic effects on male sexual function. While the drug has been used to treat aggression in male sexual offenders, evidence that it curtails desire in women isn't as strong,[100] and there are very few direct comparisons of the effects of different progestins on the sexuality of users.[101] Graham's study of women in Scotland and the Philippines found that while women on combined pills experienced a drop in desire, women on progestin-only pills experienced no sexual change.[102]

The relationship between changes in mood and shifts in libido remains unclear, but that doesn't mean you have to live with mood or sexual problems. I asked Graham what she would recommend to women experiencing libido decline, and she believes it is worth trying a switch to a different brand. She emphasizes, though, that there isn't a lot of empirical data on which to base this change—it's basically guesswork and experimentation. She also recommends keeping a journal to record what problems you have and when. And, as always, women in these circumstances may want to consider a switch to a barrier or other nonhormonal method.

The Pill may cause sexual problems beyond damaging libido: an unusual study recently examined how it could change women's sense of smell and alter some of their biological tools for mate selection. The "major histocompatibility complex," or MHC, is a region of genes that plays a role in the body's immune system. Some scientists theorize that women, picking up on subtle scent clues, tend to be attracted to men with genetically different MHC, strengthening their potential offspring's immune systems.[103] But when women take the Pill, the preference for difference changes, and they are attracted to people with similar MHC. This may be because hormonal contraception tricks the body into believing it is pregnant, influencing how companions are selected and prioritized, or because it dulls sensitivity to scent that peaks around ovulation in normally menstruating women. A study published in England in 2008 had female subjects smell the T-shirts of male subjects and rate the scent. Those who were taking hormonal birth control were more likely to rate the scents of genetically similar men as "pleasant and desirable."[104] A team of researchers at England's University of Sheffield found that because women on the Pill don't have the shifts of the monthly cycle, they may be disposed to pick mates who are less genetically suited to themselves.[105] Study author Virpi Lumma explains, "The ultimate outstanding evolutionary question concerns whether the use of oral contraceptives when making mating decisions can have long-term consequences on the ability of couples to reproduce."[106]

Some argue—convincingly—that evolutionary tools isolated in a lab don't have relevance in the complexity of real-world loves and relationships. And as we will see when we discuss menstrual suppression, it is dangerous to put too much stock in theories of what is "natural" for modern women based on imagining the sexual health of our primitive ancestors. As Alexandra Alvergne, another member of the Sheffield team, notes, "There are many obvious benefits of the Pill for women, but there is also the possibility that the Pill has psychological side effects that we are only just discovering. We need further studies to find out what these are."[107]

Inside and Out: Effects on Weight, Skin, Hair, Bones, and Organs

There are so many physical conditions that are known, believed, or suspected to be impacted by Pill use. A comprehensive list of each of these conditions would be long enough to comprise a book by itself. The ovaries impact metabolism, thyroid function, adrenaline levels, glucose regulation, uptake of vitamins, memory and concentration, brain waves, sleep patterns, energy levels, pain thresholds, balance, and even skin and hair texture. Given how many things the ovary effects, you can imagine that the results of suspending its functions can be far-reaching. Here are a few internal and external issues that have been tied to pharmaceutical birth control.

Weight, Metabolism, and Diabetes

While other potential side effects—like blood clots—may be more frightening, the possibility that the Pill causes weight gain has kept many women from selecting this method. Like sexual side effects, weight is both positively and negatively associated with OC use: some women gain weight on the Pill, others lose it. Older Pills with heavier hormone loads undoubtedly caused more variance, but some women still experience this unpleasant problem with modern drugs. In the case of women whose weight gain is the result of using progestin-heavy pills, which cause people to retain water at different points in the monthly regimen, a lower progestin dose or a different progestinal compound may help. For many, though, the problem is not so easily solved.

Weight gain is a symptom with much anecdotal evidence and little data to back it up.[108] A 2007 meta-analysis published in the Cochrane Library combined forty-four studies and found that most didn't suggest that the Pill caused women to put on extra pounds.[109] An article in the *New York Times*, echoing the sentiments of many doctors, explained, "Most women start birth control as teenagers and continue it through their twenties, a period when women naturally tend to gain weight . . . the link between the pill and weight gain is exaggerated at best."[110]

Other research disagrees, finding that all hormonal contraception, including POPS, can cause weight gain.[111] For women who experience this side effect, the impact on their lives can be dramatic and devastating. One woman in her midtwenties shared her experience with me: "When I went on the Pill in college, I put on a lot of weight—close to forty pounds. It totally changed my life and limited me in crucial ways. For some reason, I didn't consider that my birth control was causing my weight gain. When I finally went off the Pill I lost the weight. It made me so angry when I figured it out—I wish I had realized what was going on sooner."

One reason that taking the Pill might make you pack on pounds is that

OCs may change the way your body metabolizes carbohydrates. This can have more serious implications than just excess fat: it makes it more difficult for your body to use sugar and increases insulin resistance. When this happens you are at greater risk for type 2 diabetes and cardiovascular problems.

The documented interaction of Pills with diabetes is a very serious concern.[112] Hormones can negatively impact this dangerous condition in two ways: estrogen may increase glucose levels and decrease the body's response, and progestin can cause the body to produce too much insulin. In women who have never had diabetes, either gestationally or otherwise, and who have no family history of the disease, these changes in blood sugar are usually quite small. Women who have diabetes are a different matter, and major international bodies like the World Health Organization suggest that this group may want to consider alternative contraception. If diabetic women choose to stay on the Pill, their doctors should monitor any changes that occur with use.

The Pill may be slightly less effective for women who are overweight when they start taking it.[113] In their book *The Pill: Are You Sure It's For You?*, authors Jane Bennett and Alexandra Pope point out that the threshold at which Pills become less effective is lower than most women realize—you don't have to be seriously overweight to start having this problem.[114]

A recent study reported by the American Physiological Society studied how the Pill affects the ability of young women to gain muscle. A group of young women were placed on a ten-week workout regimen. Half of the girls were taking OCs and the other half were not. Scientists conducting the study monitored the workouts and at the end of the trial period measured hormone levels and muscle growth. The two groups gained muscle at different rates, and in different ways. Researchers concluded, "We were surprised at the magnitude of differences in muscle gains between the two groups, with the non-OC women gaining more than 60 percent greater muscle mass than their OC counterpart."[115]

It is evident that the Pill interacts with weight, fat, muscle, and metabolism, and women deserve better research and more answers before their concerns on this subject are written off by doctors and health care professionals as misperceptions and self-fulfilling prophecies.

Liver and Gallbladder

As we discussed earlier, the Pill can be hard on the liver, which metabolizes the hormones and sends them in to the bloodstream. Sometimes bigger liver-related problems can develop. Jaundice, a condition in which the skin and the whites of the eyes become yellow, happens when there is a high level of the bile pigment bilirubin in the blood. Its presence generally indicates a problem with the liver or gallbladder. It is thought that estrogen and progestin can have a toxic effect on the liver, causing or exacerbating this condition. If your pills make you turn yellow, it is likely a sign that they aren't right for your body. The condition goes away once pills are dropped.[116]

The American Diabetes Association notes that because the Pill can affect blood flow to the liver,[117] and this is already a concern for diabetic women, the Pill may also exacerbate existing risks for developing kidney disease.[118] This is another good reason for women with diabetes and blood sugar problems to consider alternative contraceptive methods.

The potential of pills to exacerbate gallbladder disease and gallstones has long been documented. This risk has declined with low-dose pills, and is very small,[119] although it may be higher on certain pills, like Yasmin and Yaz. If you have had gallstones, or have a family history of gallbladder surgery, take this under consideration when considering hormonal contraception.

Bones

Scientists have studied the relationship between estrogen and bone health for many years. Before the results of the Women's Health Initiative suggested greater health risks than benefits, postmenopausal women were routinely prescribed hormone and estrogen therapy to build bone mass and prevent fractures, goals the drugs have been proven to accomplish. Because of the effect of HT and ET on older women's bones, many have theorized that taking oral contraceptives would prove to be a boon for young skeletons, too, creating healthier bodies that would be less prone to break in old age.

Jerilynn C. Prior, a Canadian doctor with years of experience on women's reproductive health, argues that the benefits of young women taking estrogen for bone health aren't so clear. She explains, "A few years ago we showed that premenopausal Canadian women ages 25–45 who had used the Pill had lower bone density levels than women who had never used the Pill."[120] Another study found that women taking the Pill had more trouble achieving peak bone mass when compared with OC-free peers,[121] and two studies found that women taking the Pill had 20 percent more fractures then women not using hormonal contraception.[122] Significantly, even trials that find higher bone mass with OC use aren't able to show that it reduces fracture risk.[123]

With such inconsistent evidence, taking the Pill to build bone mass is not a good idea, especially when less invasive interventions (such as exercise, good nutrition, and taking calcium) are more effective. Concerns that the Pill may actually damage long-term bone health are serious enough to demand more research. As we will see later, particular forms of hormonal contraception, like Depo-Provera, have been shown to be detrimental to bone health, particularly for young women.

Bowels

Crohn's disease, an inflammatory bowel disorder, may be more common in Pill users. Women who have Crohn's disease are at an increased risk for blood clots, and if the illness is severe it may mean that pill use is not a good idea. When inflammatory bowel disease happens with OC use, stopping hormones seems to resolve it in most patients.

Menstrual Effects: Period Regulation, Spotting, and Fertility

One reductionary, but clear, way of talking about how OCs work is to say that they suspend a woman's monthly cycle. Women who go on the Pill often do so because they argue that it "regulates their period." In fact, women on hormonal contraception don't menstruate in the sense that other women do. The monthly bleeding, in this case, is more accurately called a "withdrawal bleed," and is the result of suddenly removing progestin from the body (which happens when women take the seven "sugar pills" included in birth control packs).

This has many consequences. A woman who goes on hormonal contraception because she is having bad or irregular periods eliminates the possibility that she can help detect what is going on through observing her cycle. Women who aren't on hormones can chart their cycles, and in many cases figure out what is causing their problem. Victoria, a woman in her early twenties with PCOS, shared her story with me: "I started on the Pill when I was very young. Years later, when I started to worry about hormones, I went off. I was surprised when my periods were irregular—very irregular. I only get one two or three times a year. At this point a doctor diagnosed PCOS. Because I want to have a baby in the next few years, I am very glad to know that I have this problem. Infertility is a symptom of the problem, and now I feel like I can start to do something about it. If I had stayed on the Pill I would never have known."[124]

Sometimes hormonal intervention may be a Godsend (for example, if you suffer from endometriosis, a condition that makes monthly bleeds excessively painful and difficult). In many cases, though, other solutions may be just as or more helpful.

Some argue, for example, that the Pill helps reduce iron deficiency anemia. Anemia is indeed a scourge in the developing world, where women struggle with parasites and other dangers that make them particularly prone to the problem. For these women, access to better sanitation and clean drinking water are much more imperative than access to hormones. Women in the United States and other developed nations don't suffer from the illness at such high rates, and are able to manage it in many cases with simpler solutions (for example, by taking iron supplements). And many women in the West may actually have too much iron in their bodies—a condition which, according to Dr. Susan Rako, a critic of menstrual suppression, can lead to high blood pressure and other cardiovascular problems.[125] Whether or not this is true, most American women do not need to take birth control pills to manage anemia.

The Pill is also said to help relieve painful menstrual cramping by cutting the level of prostaglandins—fatty acids that help control muscle contraction and inflammation—in menstrual fluid.[126] The small percentage of women who have such mind-numbing cramps that they are unable to function may indeed find that hormonal birth control is not just a relief, but an answer to prayers. But for women with milder cramps, taking the Pill to curb cramping is less of a medical decision and more of a lifestyle choice. Many find that taking a nonsteroidal, antiinflammatory drug such as ibuprofen can be just as effective against cramps as taking the Pill, since these mild painkillers also reduce prostaglandins.[127]

Another advantage of the Pill claimed by drug manufacturers is that it helps makes periods more regular. It is striking, then, that one of the top reasons women give for discontinuing pill use when they still need contraception is because of breakthrough bleeding and spotting.[128] Breakthrough bleeding and spotting probably happens because the synthetic hormones in pills don't properly stimulate the endometrium and its blood vessels after bleeding or maintain the endometrium until the end of the active pill cycle. Normal menstrual bleeding involves shedding a relatively thick lining. When you start hormonal contraception, the lining gets thinner, and while the body is adjusting, there can be unscheduled bleeding.

Of course certain gynecological conditions, such as endometriosis, can also cause bleeding, and practical problems like missing pills or having an interaction between the Pill and other medications can also contribute to the problem.

Women who take low dose pills with less than 20 mcg of estrogen are much more likely to have bleeding.[129] I developed spotting with two different low dose pills in situations that were years apart. Both times, the problem emerged after several months of use and got more pronounced with time. Bleeding that appears after six months of use may happen because of progressive endometrial atrophy, insensitivity, or resistance of the endometrium to the hormones, and an increase in the body's metabolism of hormones.

Importantly, bleeding can sometimes be a sign that a pill isn't working correctly, and backup contraception may be necessary.[130] It can also be a sign of a more serious health problem like pelvic inflammatory disease, spontaneous abortion, or ectopic pregnancy. Make sure that your doctor explores all the possible causes before simply switching your brand. The strategy your doctor uses will depend on when and how your bleeding happens (again, keeping a journal record of problems may make a significant difference in getting proper treatment).

The simplest things a patient can do to minimize the problem are to take her pills at the same time each day, be careful not to miss doses, and avoid lifestyle choices—particularly smoking—that can increase the likelihood of experiencing the problem. If you smoke you are 30 percent more likely to bleed in early cycles of taking the Pill and 84 percent more likely than non-smokers to have the problem after six months of use.[131]

If you are very young and your menstrual cycles are just getting started, or if you a perimenopausal, you should have a frank conversation with your doctor or health care provider before using OCs to treat your potentially unpredictable periods. Jerilynn Prior, a doctor at the Canadian Centre for Menstrual Cycle and Ovulation Research, explains that the "menstrual cycle can take many years to become established, even though regular periods commonly develop within a year or so of the first period."[132] Young girls often struggle with particularly painful and unpredictable periods. I can recall being woken at night as a girl by splitting cramps and wondering if I would be able to make it through the night without a hospital visit. Because girls (rightly) complain about these pains, doctors sometimes rush to put them on hormonal contraception for "cycle regulation." Prior doesn't think this is a very good idea, explaining, "because all forms of hormonal contraception are designed to disturb the brain control of ovulation, and this system needs to grow up in teenagers, we have concerns about anything disrupting that delicate and important process."[133]

A friend of mine who is a new doctor and who logs in many hours in a hospital clinic tells me that she believes that "cycle regulation" is often used euphemistically by teenagers and their doctors as a way to get contraception to young women who need it without parental disapproval. Because teen pregnancy is a serious problem, and many teenagers need birth control alternatives, I understand this reasoning, but still think caution is merited.

If the body is unpredictable and sometimes painful while it is winding up, reproductively speaking, in the first few years after menarche, these problems can also arise while it is winding down before menopause. A host of potentially unpleasant and life-disrupting side effects are associated with this time of life, including heavy and unpredictable bleeding, and many consider turning to the Pill for relief. But, as Jerilynn Prior notes, estrogen levels are often quite high during perimenopause, and when women gain weight during this time, they can get even higher. High estrogen levels compound the already elevated risks of cardiovascular problems that women experience with hormonal contraceptive use after age thirty-five. Adding the Pill could put women at an increased risk for blood clots, strokes, and heart attacks.[134] For these reasons, she recommends against using the Pill for contraception in this stage of life.

Fertility

It has always been difficult for patients and scientists to believe that taking hormones over time has no permanent effect on fertility. Dr. John Rock, who co-parented the pill into existence, was a fertility specialist who was originally interested in the ability of the progesterone to *increase* the likelihood of conception when withdrawn. In the 1960s and '70s, Pill critics worried that the opposite was true: that shutting off the ovaries for years or even decades would lead to sterilization in some women. The truth, it seems, is somewhere in the middle. The majority of women regain fertility after OC use in about one to three months,[135] a time frame that is similar to other contraceptive methods.[136] Remember, though, that your regained fertility after going off the pill will be similar to the average fertility of a woman your age who has never used hormonal contraception. So if you are forty when you go off the pill, you will not regain the fertility of a twenty-year-old.

For women over thirty, the process of regaining fertility can generally take longer, and one study suggested that it took half of the participating women a year or longer to get pregnant than women who were using barrier methods before trying to conceive.[137] Another study concludes, "A significant reduction in fecundity occurs after COC, IUD, or injectables, which is dependent on the duration of use."[138] There are two important points here: the first is that almost all women do regain fertility. The second is that for those over thirty and those who have been using the Pill for many years, it may take longer to do so.

For everyone who knows a woman with a horror story about failing to get pregnant after dropping OCs, there is someone who gets pregnant the first month that she doesn't take her pills. Both experiences are real, and highlight how much we still don't know about the effects of hormonal contraception on fertility.

Even if women aren't seeking pregnancy, they may be eager to know that normal cycles have resumed after Pill use stops. Women who had normal cycles before taking OCs will usually get a period within five weeks. It can take longer for women who were irregular before hormonal contraceptive, typically three months or more.[139] If your period doesn't come back within expected time frames, you should probably take a pregnancy test to make sure that that isn't the reason for your missing menses. If you are perimenopausal, you may not resume bleeding. Those who are perimenopausal should also be aware that high levels of LH during that time can cause false positives on a pregnancy test, so be sure to consult with your doctor if you experience this problem.

Getting Off the Pill

In the fall of 2009 I received an e-mail message from a friend of mine, Michelle. Michelle had been on the Pill for six years. At first she was happy, but in the past year had started to have problems. She started to spot and have more erratic bleeding. Her moods had gotten worse, and she said she just generally felt sort of sick all the time. "It's like having a perma-cold," she told me. After much thought, Michelle had decided she wanted to off the Pill. When she did, though, she started having other problems. Her skin broke out and she started feeling more easily run down. As Michelle described her problems giving up hormonal contraception, it got me thinking: In a society where such a high percentage of women take this powerful drug for years at a time, how many women have trouble giving up hormonal birth control?

Many women—myself included—have no problem giving up oral contraceptives. Others struggle. Jane Bennett and Alexandra Pope note that because the Pill affects nutritional balance, it is more important than ever to make sure that you are living a healthy lifestyle (including exercising, sleeping, and eating a nutritious diet) when you decide to ditch the Pill.[140] In addition, make sure to take a multivitamin and perhaps extra vitamin C. Ask your doctor about nutritional changes—such as cutting down on sugar and some carbohydrates—that may make the transition easier on your body. Periods may take several months to adjust, and may not immediately start occurring on a regular schedule. When periods do start coming, they may be heavier than previously experienced.

Remember to be patient and expect some shifts in how you feel. You may notice changes in your skin and hair, and changes in mood are normal. Giving up daily hormones is a massive change, and you need to be patient with your body as it adjusts. Be careful not to get immediately scared by changes and rush back to the doctor's office for a new prescription.

Some adjustments after giving up the Pill are psychological. Holly Grigg-Spall, who movingly describes her experience letting go of oral contraceptives in an excellent blog, Sweetening the Pill (http://www .sweeteningthepill.blogspot.com), tells me that since finally going off six months ago she has been jumpy with her new contraceptives. "When anything goes wrong, I run to get Emergency Contraception. I mean I've probably done that three times now. It's hard not to be scared."[141]

For women who are thinking of stopping hormonal contraception, there are a few practicalities to consider. Women on a combined Pill (with estrogen and progestin) and those using the contraceptive patch and ring can stop taking their pills at any point (bleeding within a few days of stopping pills is to be expected).[142] Women may find it easiest, however, to wait until the end of a pill pack to stop taking their pills. If you are using progestin-only pills, you should wait until the end of a pack. In all cases, use backup contraception to be on the safe side. If you have been getting Depo-Provera shots, simply stop going for your regular injection. Hormonal IUDs should be removed just before a period is expected while other implants can be removed by a doctor at any time.[143]

Parting Thoughts on the Pill

When Barbara Seaman took on the Pill and its safety problems, she made the point that these medical hazards didn't exist in a vacuum. The dangers of the Pill were permitted to exist, and they were hidden and exacerbated by unequal power relationships. This started when doctors testing the Pill decided to do so on poor Puerto Rican women in part because it was a population that didn't have as many medical ethical and legal protections. It was made worse by pharmaceutical companies who valued profits over the health of people using their products. It continued in a society where women were prescribed the Pill by doctors who treated them like children and often suggested that side effects were "all in their heads." And it was perpetuated by male partners who were happy to let women bear the burden of contraception in every organ of their bodies.

These injustices weren't separable from the medical facts of the Pill. In fact, the physical dangers and social problems created and compounded each other. "Fixing" the Pill meant working to alter inequalities in power between those promoting and those consuming the drug.

Today, much has changed, but more than we would like remains the same. It is still important to be conscious of social factors that can both make the drug itself more dangerous and limit the ability of women to use it in safest and most effective way possible.

Think about these two things. 1) The Pill is one of the most-studied drugs in the world. 2) There has never been a long-term, randomized, double-blinded trial of Pill use on the scale of the Women's Health Initiative. What this means is that we have a *lot* of information on hormonal contraception, but not the best, most conclusive kind of research. It is impossible to perform such a trial for many reasons. The most basic is that it would be impossible to enlist a large group of women willing to remain on contraception for a large portion of their reproductive years.

Pill use is dictated by life. Relationships end, children are born, things change. This does not good science make. What we have for the most part, then, are observational trials, meta-analyses and shorter, smaller placebo-controlled studies. The limitations of oral contraceptive research mean that there are certain questions that will, at least for the foreseeable future, remain open.

The Pill offers many benefits to women, but it is far from perfect. If you are one of the millions who use oral contraceptives, be a smart consumer. Keep a journal of any side effects, problems, benefits, or other bodily changes. Don't be afraid to tell your doctor if you are having problems, and don't let anyone tell you that the things you are experiencing are "all in your head." Likewise, if you are happy with the Pill, don't let anyone make you feel bad or unnecessarily scared to use a drug that has been such a useful tool for so many women. For those of us who use and love hormonal birth control, and for those of us who have had bad experiences and don't like it, let's work to understand, respect, and empower choices that are different from our own.

In the next chapters, we will look more specifically at different types of hormonal and nonhormonal contraception and ask how our experiences, risks, and potential benefits change with age, biological development, race, ethnicity, economic background, and geographic location. Birth control pills, like all available contraceptive methods, are not "one size fits all." Let's begin asking the complicated question of how we may find the best fit for us.

Chapter Three

Hidden in Plain Sight: Nonhormonal Contraceptive Options

I know everyone says "out with the old, in with the new." But after six years on hormones and one on a diaphragm, all I can say is "in with the old."

—Amy, age 27

This story is a mystery and we are the detectives. We have been called to investigate a disappearance: a once ubiquitous, very useful birth control option has vanished, and it is time to get it back. We must unravel the case of the disappearing diaphragm.

In today's contraceptive landscape, female-controlled barriers are almost completely absent. Other nonhormonal methods such as IUDs are growing in popularity, but they account for a tiny fraction of total usage in the United States. The vast majority of young couples today use two methods of birth control: the Pill and condoms. Older couples (over thirty-five) opt in significant numbers for either tubal ligation or vasectomy. Given that many women find they are unable—or unwilling—to use hormones to control fertility, and many more will grow dissatisfied with the Pill and its cousins as they age, it is striking that alternative methods are so underutilized. While condoms are without peer for STI prevention, it is worth asking about women-controlled contraceptive options that don't involve taking drugs. Are methods like diaphragms really obsolete, or have they been too quickly pushed aside because, among other reasons, they aren't significant moneymakers when compared with pharmaceutical methods? Why have diaphragms disappeared, and is their disappearance really the best thing for women?

Barriers to Knowledge: Vanishing Diaphragms and Cervical Caps

When Wilhelm Peter Johan Mensinga, a German gynecologist, created the first modern diaphragm in 1842, it was an invention that slowly and quietly shook the world. The mid-nineteenth century saw an outpouring of contraceptive creativity in Germany that included not only Mensinga's creation, but an early modern cervical cap as well. Mensinga was a vocal advocate of contraception, which he said was useful for political as well as medical reasons.

What distinguished Mensinga's product from the others was its consistency and reliability. Science had finally begun to play a role in assessing how well a contraceptive functioned. The doctor conducted small informal tests on a dozen patients from various social groups. Contraceptive Historian Robert Jütte notes, "Mensinga's work thus marks the beginning of an era of comparatively 'reliable' knowledge about contraception that is substantiated by both statistics and case histories. From this point, it is not far to the clinical studies of the 1950s."[1] In choosing to compare the success of working-, middle-, and upper-class women, Mensinga was already acknowledging an issue that continues to surround the diaphragm (and many other contraceptives) to this day: the extent to which economic status and lifestyle factors play a role in the appeal, efficiency, and usefulness of a method. Mensinga insisted, in contrast to later commentators, that even women with limited access to education and sanitation could successfully choose a diaphragm.

Following in Mensinga's footsteps, other inventors and entrepreneurs, including many Americans, rushed to develop diaphragms and cervical caps. Edward Bliss Foote was one of these enterprising people, and after graduating from the Pennsylvania Medical College, he created his own version of the cervical cap called the "womb veil." He marketed the device in a book, *Medical Common Sense*, which he published in 1864. The device cost six dollars and, Foote enthused, it put "conception entirely under the control of the wife, to whom it naturally belongs."[2]

The issue of female control is still a complicated one. Indeed, being responsible for the procurement and proper use of birth control affords women a measure of power, even as it puts responsibility for the outcome more fully on female shoulders. Potential burdens of this kind of control include financial issues of paying for sometimes-expensive methods, legal dangers in obtaining controversial methods, and physical and medical complaints that can result from using various options. These two sides of the same coin—control and burden—account for deeply divided opinions among women. While some insist, like Sanger, that female-controlled methods are the only way to go, others wonder why there is no pill for men and argue that such diverse responsibilities placed on women constitute another method of controlling female bodies.

In the late nineteenth and early twentieth century, though, any ability to prevent pregnancy represented an irresistible alternative for couples. Especially in a time before modern birthing science, the prospect of repeated childbirth and the ensuing health hazards quickly nullified other concerns.

By the dawn of the twentieth century, increasing numbers of women in the United States and abroad were opting for the diaphragm. Margaret Sanger's long, vexed love affair with the device began at this time. She became intrigued by the Mensinga diaphragm in 1915, when Dutch doctor Aletta Jacobs championed the device. But when Sanger was ready to open her Brownsville clinic in 1916, no American manufacturer had started making anything like the reliable Mensinga product. Because birth control was still illegal in the United States, as was bringing the devices in to the country from Europe, Sanger opted instead to offer the Mizpah, an American-made cervical cap marketed primarily for treating prolapsed uteruses. It had the added advantage of being "one size fits all" and therefore not requiring a doctor's fitting.

This changed a few short years later when Sanger and her second husband, James Slee, created the Holland-Rantos Company, the first corporation in America to make and sell birth control devices—mostly diaphragms—solely to doctors and the medical profession. Women who wanted the devices would have to have a fitting at the doctor's office. Putting devices in the hands of doctors disassociated birth control from vice and made its distribution seem like a medical, not a moral, issue. Sanger realized that in order to change American perceptions about contraception, the practice would need to be married to medicine.

Andrea Tone notes, "By the 1930s, thanks largely to Sanger, the diaphragm and jelly had become the most frequently prescribed form of

birth control in America."[3] But although diaphragms were the most prescribed method of birth control in the mid-twentieth century, at no time
did the majority of American women use them. Indeed, use was limited
to a small number of women who were heavily middle class and white.
This was probably due, at least in part, to the reliance of the method on
access to medical professionals to properly fit them. The problem wasn't
that poor or uneducated women couldn't use the method; it was that they
lacked access to it.

By this point, Sanger was already starting to look for something better. Her feminist position on family planning was beginning to twist
toward eugenics. Frustrated with the low rate of diaphragm use in low-
income communities, she started to believe that the method was too
sophisticated for poor women, especially women from parts of the world
that, as population control advocates argued, posed a threat to the American way of life. The notion that the majority of women couldn't handle
the responsibility of inserting a barrier method began to set the stage for
the advent of the Pill. From the beginning, the emphasis of the Pill was
not on respecting female autonomy, but rather on offsetting women's
incompetence.

Within a decade of the legalization of hormonal contraception, women
were forsaking barriers in dramatic numbers for both the Pill and the new
IUDs. The diaphragm and the cervical cap experienced a renaissance in
the 1970s and 1980s as information about the dangers of the Pill and IUDs
began to proliferate, and after the 1970s Dalkon Shield scandal—when
that IUD was found to cause severe internal injuries—use of diaphragms
and cervical caps in America climbed to account for 6 percent of all American contraceptive use. But the damage had been done, and the barrier
never regained its former place as a prominent player on the contraceptive
playing field.

As the years passed and safety concerns about other forms of contraception decreased, the diaphragm began to slowly disappear. Between 1988
and 1995, use fell by two thirds, making up only 2 percent of total American birth control use. That number continued to decline, and today only
.3 percent of Americans use a diaphragm, making it less popular than Natural Family Planning, the method of choice for .4 percent of birth control
users.[4] The percentage of women who choose cervical caps is too small to

count discretely. A blogger on the popular site Feministing.com describes a conversation with an older coworker: "She couldn't believe that I didn't know any woman my age who use a diaphragm. Most are on the Pill, I told her."[5] Indeed, the closest contact most women under forty have had with the diaphragm is watching the television show *Sex and the City*, in which the main character, Carrie Bradshaw, uses the device.

The reasons for this vanishing act are numerous. The safety of the Pill and the IUD have improved substantially, and in this age of HIV/AIDS, many couples opt for condom use. But not all of the reasons are practical. Birth control pills and other hormonal methods have made tremendous amounts of money for their manufacturers; a diaphragm, by comparison, only generates a small amount of income. Compare the Pill, which costs between $30 and $80 each month, with a diaphragm, which has a one-time cost of around $60 and lasts up to two years (although many doctors recommend being refit each year just to be on the safe side). There are additional costs for spermicidal jelly. Pharmaceutical giants pour enormous sums into advertising the Pill, using powerful television and print media images to promote oral contraceptive use. Ubiquitous commercials showing stylish, hip, ambitious, urban women continue to promote a certain idea of what makes an ideal contraceptive. At the same time, the use of older devices has been painted in unflattering cultural colors. The Pill is a Porsche, the diaphragm a Model T. It isn't just about pregnancy prevention anymore, it's about lifestyle choice. For the woman who has everything, taking the hot new brand of pills is akin to a designer bag, a killer job, or an elegant apartment.

In schools, sexual education programs inform students that while diaphragms are an option, it's best not take risks. The Pill "works" better, although in this case, of course, the only marker of efficacy is a lack of pregnancy, and the other side effects of hormonal contraception are ignored. From a teenage perspective, this set of priorities makes sense. But misinformation about the diaphragm eliminates it as a potential option for those who want to explore nonhormonal contraceptive possibilities.

Education is not the only factor holding back barrier use: access is increasingly a serious problem. Traditional cervical caps are not currently available in the United States. Diaphragms are becoming more challenging to find by the day. I spoke to one young woman who had to visit three different doctors before she found one that would fit her with a diaphragm, and she went to four pharmacies before she located one that would stock the item. Many practitioners aren't trained to fit the devices properly or have limited experience doing so. Anyone can write a prescription for a pill, but it takes skill to choose the right size for a barrier. In addition, physician education—often funded by pharmaceutical companies—has stressed pill use to the point where (and I can speak from multiple first-hand experiences) health care providers are hostile to the idea of diaphragm use and encourage women to try many brands of oral contraceptives before exploring other options. I attended a reproductive health conference with graduate school–age women, where I listened to a presentation on contraceptive access. The young educator passed around samples of the various options so we could see them up close. As the diaphragm wound its way through the rows, I heard one woman giggle and say to her friend, "My God, it's *huge*." "I know," the other said, "it's so eighties."

I believe it is worthwhile to work to overcome negative preconceptions and revive this old girl, this remnant of contraceptive past lives, as an active, available option for today's women. In a country with record rates of uninsured people, and particularly many uninsured young women, it is worth asking why we would dismiss such a cost-effective, easily reversible birth control method. Barriers are the most effective woman-controlled, nonhormonal option besides a copper IUD and tubal ligation. As women age, the risks associated with hormonal contraception rise, particularly after age thirty-five. With so many vital pieces of knowledge about long-term hormone use remaining inconclusive, it would be a mistake to turn this easy, proficient option into a dinosaur before its time.

The Real Story behind Barriers

A major perception of young women about diaphragms is that they are messy and difficult to use. I believed this before I tried one, and I was shocked to find that the diaphragm is simple to prepare and insert.

A diaphragm is a rubber cup with a bendable ring that holds its shape. To use it, a woman fills the device with a tablespoon or two of spermicidal jelly, folds it in half, and inserts it into her vagina, checking to make sure that the dome is covering her cervix (the small, firm, knobby protrusion located between the uterus and the vaginal cavity). After intercourse, a woman must wait six hours before removing the device. Repeated intercourse is possible without taking the diaphragm out; one need only insert more spermicide into the vagina.

I mastered the technique after about two weeks of practice; at first I struggled to find the right angle and to feel secure that it was in properly. After that warm-up period, use could not have been easier. It takes about the same amount of time to insert a diaphragm that it does to put on a male condom, but because it is inserted before intercourse—sometimes hours ahead of time—it doesn't interrupt the mood or the moment in the same way that male barriers can. Inserting a diaphragm is slightly more complicated than popping a pill, but diaphragms free you of the need to think about birth control until you plan to have intercourse.

Diaphragms, like all birth control options, have drawbacks and contraindications. Women who have just given birth shouldn't use them for a couple months and should be refitted after the birth of each child (although use while breastfeeding is fine after six weeks have passed). Women who have had recently had cervical surgery or undergone an abortion should likewise choose other methods. Those who have never had sex or are new to intercourse may have trouble inserting the device. People with an allergy to latex or spermicide, or people who are predisposed to urinary tract infections and toxic shock syndrome are not good candidates for this option. When women are menstruating they should use alternative contraception, probably a condom. Women should learn to recognize the movement of their diaphragm, so that in the rare instance it is dislodged or moved during sex, they will know quickly enough to act and prevent method failure or consider emergency contraception if necessary. Diaphragms are not a good choice for women who lack frequent access to sanitary facilities. They should be washed after removal with soap and water and inspected frequently for holes and tears.

When HIV/AIDS became an international health concern, researchers hoped that diaphragms could provide some level of protection against the infection. They reasoned that since the cervix is particularly vulnerable to infection, blocking it might provide a shield to disease. The MIRA (Methods for Improving Reproductive Health in Africa), a joint scientific study involving the University of California, San Francisco, and the Medical Research Council of South Africa, set out to test the usefulness of offering patients a diaphragm along with condoms. The results, published in the *Lancet*, found that the device didn't offer statistically significant protection above that provided by condoms alone.[6] Condoms (male and female) are still the only barriers shown to provide HIV protection. The study was not designed to test whether diaphragms provided more protection against STIs than no barrier at all, and that remains an open question.

The cervical cap is a small, shot glass–sized silicone or latex plug that fits using suction over the cervix. It is significantly smaller than a diaphragm. The FemCap, the only available FDA-approved version of this device, resembles a tiny clear plastic sailor's hat. FemCap isn't fit like a diaphragm. Rather, it is available in three sizes: one for women who have given birth, one for women who have been pregnant but haven't given birth, and one for women who have never been pregnant. As with a diaphragm, the cup is filled with spermicide before inserting. It is utilized by squeezing the cap's rim, inserting the device into the vagina, and placing it directly over the cervix. Once inserted, the user should gently touch the cap to ensure that it is firmly suctioned in place. Eight hours after sex, the cap can be removed by pulling to release suction. The same side effects and cautions that apply to diaphragms apply to this method, with the additional disadvantage that the device is more frequently felt by—and thus a source of discomfort to—partners.

What is the reality of barrier efficacy? Is it simply less safe to rely on a diaphragm? That more pregnancies occur in barrier users than in women on the Pill cannot be denied. But when efficacy statistics are presented, particularly to young people, the ideal success rates for the Pill sometimes appear alongside the typical rates for barrier methods. Most women are well aware that ideally, the Pill works in the first year of use 99.7 percent of the time. Fewer women know that the typical use statistic for the Pill is much lower, with a success rate of only 91.3 percent.[7] So for every hundred women who take the Pill for a year, between one and eight or nine of them will become pregnant. The diaphragm, when used correctly, works 94 percent of the time, with a typical use success rate of 84 percent. For every hundred women who use a diaphragm for a year, between six and sixteen will become pregnant. Compare this with a male condom, which typically works about 82 percent of the time. What this means is that while not perfect, the diaphragm is an extremely effective contraceptive method.

Efficacy for the cervical cap is, unfortunately, lower than either a diaphragm or condom. For women who have never given birth, the ideal success rate is 91 percent, while the typical use success rate is 84 percent—similar to the diaphragm rates. But for women who have given birth, the usefulness of the method declines precipitously, failing somewhere between 26 and 32 percent of the time. This brings up a "chicken-and-egg" problem: a traditional cervical cap requires a precise fitting, and it is difficult to say whether more demand for the method would also create a demand for more skilled practitioners to provide and fit it, ultimately improving the device's success rate. FemCap's efficacy may be slightly higher, but good discrete data on the device is hard to find.

Barriers aren't for everyone, but they are a sensible, welcome choice for many. So much of this discussion has to do with how our perceptions of what is burdensome are formed. For me, remembering to take a pill every day and dealing with the bleeding that resulted when I forgot was burdensome. I spoke to one woman in her early thirties who had three unwanted pregnancies (and abortions) while taking the Pill because she simply couldn't remember to take it routinely. Coping with mood swings is burdensome. For some, dealing with the increased possibility of urinary tract or vaginal infections is burdensome. For others, the idea of having to touch intimate parts of their body is burdensome. Each woman is unique, but unfortunately our contraceptive world treats women as if they are the same. The conversation should not involve arguing that one option is better than another. In fact, that is exactly the problem. What *is* necessary is that women and health care providers become open to the idea that considering an array of options, and embracing the necessary experimentation to discover which works best for each individual, is the best approach to contraceptive health.

Condoms for Her and Him

Most people growing up in the era of AIDS have at least some awareness of male condoms. Today's prophylactics have little in common with their thick, fragile forerunners. A trip into most American drugstores provides a contraceptive buyer with multiple condom options, each promising thinner, sleeker, more sensitive products. Much less attention is given to the female condom, which, considering the disappointing results of tests of diaphragms for HIV/AIDS prevention, remains the only female-controlled contraceptive that can also reliably stop the spread of STIs.

Introduced in the early 1990s, the female condom is a seven-inch-long polyurethane device with a flexible ring on either end. It is held in place by one ring that sits over the cervix while the other stays outside the vagina, providing partial coverage to the vaginal lips.

While it made excellent media fodder following its release and marketing, the female condom never caught on with most women and remains more of a curiosity than a health safety tool. People saw the device as cumbersome, a larger, less sensitive version of the male condom. It is said to make strange noises during sex, and to feel, as one male user frankly put it, "like making love in a garbage bag." They can reduce sensitivity for some women and even curtail orgasm. A twenty-eight-year-old law student told me that she and her boyfriend tried a female condom on a whim because they were sitting alongside male ones in the student health service center. "I actually didn't know he was inside me—that's how little I could feel," she explains. Some women disagree, arguing that the two rings actually enhance sex, providing clitoral and cervical stimulation.

Another factor in women's reluctance to adopt the option is a lack of education. Susie Hoffman, an assistant professor of clinical epidemiology at Columbia University, notes, "In the United States there has been strong bias against it . . . but if presented the right way, many women do like it."[8]

One serious drawback of the method is cost: female condoms are far more expensive than their male alternatives. On a recent trip to my closest pharmacy, I checked to see if the items were available. There was one brand of female condom, priced at a whopping $18 for three. The Web site Drugstore.com offers them for slightly less, at $14.99 for five. Since female condoms can't be reused, this makes them cost prohibitive for many women.

The imperative of finding new ways of preventing the spread of STIs has led to a recent product remodeling that seeks to address some of the flaws of the original model.[9] Polyurethane has been replaced with synthetic rubber to reduce costs, and the design has been altered slightly to reduce the embarrassing and irritating squishing noises. Educators stress that the new design feels more natural. Manufacturers estimate that the cost of each condom can be reduced to $0.60 a piece for international distribution, which is still high when compared with the male condom at $0.04.

Yet there are advantages to using the female condom. It has efficacy comparable with male condoms, between 79 and 95 percent. This female-controlled method has sparked international interest, particularly in Africa, where thirty thousand women in Zimbabwe signed a petition calling for access to the devices and ten thousand people have been trained in Ghana to teach women how to use them.[10]

The male condom is the king of contraceptives. It dates to prehistory and functions on the simplest possible principle: put something between the vagina and the penis to prevent the transmission of sperm. Condoms are the only form of reversible birth control for men (other than pulling out), and they are easily available across the country at almost any drugstore.

Before sex, a condom is rolled onto the erect penis. If a man is uncircumcised, he may want to pull back the foreskin before doing so. With one hand, the top half inch of the condom is pinched to push out air and make room for semen. The other hand rolls the thin tube (usually made of latex, but occasionally another material like polyurethane or animal skin is used) down to the base of the penis. A tight band holds the device in place. After intercourse the male partner should withdraw before he loses his erection, being sure to hold the condom in place while doing so to prevent slippage. Condoms can't be reused, so they should be thrown out after sex. Partners should be careful to avoid direct contact between male and female genitals after taking off the device because the penis might still have sperm on it. Contrary to some teenage beliefs, condoms should only be used one at a time—not doubled up—to prevent breaks and tears.

Condoms are a method with great efficacy variation. With perfect use they can be as much as 98 percent effective at preventing pregnancy, but with actual use failure is closer to 17 percent. This means that how you use condoms makes a big difference in determining whether they will prevent pregnancy. Practice makes perfect, but using lubricant to prevent tearing and storing condoms in a temperate dry place also help. Avoiding heat not only maintains the structural integrity of the device, but it prevents spermicide (present on many condoms) from losing effectiveness. Most condoms will last from two to three years with proper storage, but you should always look at a condom when putting it on to make sure that it doesn't have any obvious holes or tears. Avoid oil-based lubricants and other chemicals that can cause the material of the condom to break down.

Spermicidal Options: Films, Jellies, and Sponges

Contraceptive sponges have been used since ancient times. Modern versions were extremely popular in the nineteenth century. Famous free thinker and contraceptive advocate Annie Bessant recommended an early version in her self-published 1879 guidebook, *Law of Population*.[11] But the sponge, like the diaphragm, fell out of favor with the advent of the ubiquitous Pill.

The Today Sponge is a famous but infrequently used contraceptive that is most well known for being the method of choice of Elaine Benes, a fictional character on the wildly popular 1990s television show *Seinfeld*. When the sponge was pulled from the market in 1994, Elaine lamented the loss and hoarded her remaining supply for partners deemed "sponge worthy." The first withdrawal of Today—America's only contraceptive sponge—happened because of a problem with the FDA. The company that made the sponge, owned by the larger drugmaker Wyeth, was found to have problems with its manufacturing plant that the parent company deemed too expensive to fix. Instead, they opted to stop making the product.

Another company, Allendale Pharmaceutical, acquired the name and the rights to the product, and eleven years later reintroduced it to the market after rebranding the item and launching a massive advertising campaign. The Today Sponge was now marketed with imagery worthy of a "chick lit" bestseller, complete with pink packaging and a flirty cartoon spokeswoman. By December 2008, Synova, the company that eventually bought Allendale, had gone into bankruptcy, and the product was again pulled from shelves. In the past year, the sponge has once again become available. Only time will tell if this reemergence is permanent or simply the next chapter in the tumultuous history of sponge availability.

The Today Sponge is a small plastic foam object about two inches in length with a loop on one side for removal from the vagina. To use it, a woman wets the sponge with at least two tablespoons of water, and, folding it away from the loop, inserts it as far into the vaginal cavity as it will go. Users should check to make sure that the cervix is covered. The device works by covering the cervix and also releasing nonoxynol 9, a spermicide that is activated when the device is wet. The sponge can remain in the body for up to thirty hours, during which time intercourse can happen repeatedly. It must remain in for six hours after the last intercourse.

Like cervical caps, the sponge works much less effectively if you have had a child. For those who haven't given birth, the failure rate is somewhere between 9 and 16 percent. For those who have delivered a child, the failure rate climbs to between 20 and 32 percent. Those who are allergic to sulfa drugs (a preservative used in the product contains this chemical); women who have recently had a baby, an abortion, or miscarriage; and those prone to toxic shock syndrome shouldn't use this method. The sponge shouldn't be used while a woman is menstruating. If the device breaks apart, or if a woman is unable to remove it, she should see her doctor.

Other spermicidal options, such as contraceptive film, foam, cream, and jelly, should be used as partner contraceptives, in combination with another method (such as a condom or diaphragm). Used alone, their failure rate is very high. The most common spermicide (which works by immobilizing and, as the name suggests, killing sperm) is nonoxynol 9. Many women (and men) have allergies to this chemical, and if you find that you are one of them, you should seek other options. Nonoxynol 9 can be a vaginal irritant, causing micro-tears that make it easier for viruses and pathogens to enter the bloodstream. For this reason, health educators recommend that people at high risk for sexually transmitted infections avoid nonoxynol 9, making sure to use condoms without nonoxynol 9. Generally, spermicides are inserted into the vagina about ten minutes before intercourse and remain effective for about an hour.

Writing the Next Chapter: Today's Intrauterine Devices (IUDs)

When I mention that I am writing a book on birth control, the Planned Parenthood health educator with whom I am speaking brightens. "Are you going to mention IUDs?" she asks. "You really should—they're hot right now." It's a funny idea that this contraceptive, which has been around for decades and frequently received less attention than either hormones or barrier options, is suddenly back in the limelight. In fact, health organizations, including the Alan Guttmacher Institute and Planned Parenthood, have recently reemphasized the usefulness of intrauterine devices by raising their profile in educator and clinical training. Today's IUDs—one of which is nonhormonal and one of which is a hybrid with a hormonal piece—still live under the shadow of disgrace and distrust cast by older, more dangerous devices. Whether today's version is indeed better remains to be seen, but most women's health experts are cautiously optimistic.

While modern IUDs are a relatively new invention, the idea that putting something in the uterus could block pregnancy is an old one. Renowned gynecologist William Parker writes that in ancient times, "nomadic people placed stones in the uteruses of their camels to prevent pregnancy during long journeys."[12] It is likely that the technology was employed in humans as well during this time.

Modern IUDs appeared on the scene in the nineteenth and early twentieth century. By the mid-nineteenth century, there were over 123 designs listed in the *Transaction of the National Medical Association*, and one doctor complained that other physicians were recklessly "filling . . . the vagina with such traps making a Chinese toy-shop out of it."[13] Early versions were pen-shaped items made from metal and rubber. The devices gained an early acceptance from doctors that other methods—namely diaphragms—lacked.

Some early models were a subcategory of other so-called pessaries, used to treat multiple gynecological problems. Usually, a pessary was a device that was inserted into the vagina for either bladder support or contraception, like a diaphragm. In the case of the stem pessary, a device was inserted partially into the uterus with a connecting stem holding it in place at the cervix. This early device wasn't very effective, and worse, frequently caused uterine infection and inflammation. Still, women used the option, and German case histories gathered during the First World War include the story of a thirty-year-old Bavarian woman who requested a uterine "splint" after the birth of her second child.[14] Other designs used silkworm thread modeled in the shape of a ring.

The Grafenberg ring, created by German gynecologist Ernst Grafenberg in the 1920s, was a coil made of silkworm thread with a silver or gold ring was the first commercially manufactured IUD. Grafenberg was initially encouraged by low pregnancy rates of women using his contraceptive. It wasn't perfect: it was large, so insertion was either excruciatingly painful or required anesthesia. Despite this, he tested it on two thousand women without serious safety problems,[15] including the risk of uterine perforation that had characterized earlier stem models. After many women later became sick and some died, however, both the German government and the doctor himself (who would soon seek refuge from the Nazis in the United States) disowned the ring.[16] The technology hung on in Japan, where doctors altered both design and materials, increasing its safety.

While European and Japanese women embraced this new birth control option, American doctors continued to insist that it was dangerous. In the 1920s, J. Whitridge Williams, an obstetrician at Johns Hopkins Medical School and a critic of the device, carried his watch on a chain alongside a gold IUD ring that he claimed to have extracted from the placenta of a baby he delivered, using this as evidence that the method didn't work and was a dangerous "fad" method of contraception.[17]

American scientists gradually began to think about developing and improving IUDs after the Second World War. Several technological advances encouraged this: the creation of malleable plastic allowed the production of IUDs that could be inserted without cervical dilation and anesthetic, and the antibiotics used to treat possible infections became more readily available. All of this meant that IUDs could be made and put in more cheaply, and that medical complications could be treated before serious and life-threatening problems developed. The first of this "new generation"[18] of devices was created by New York gynecologist Lazar Margulies. This nonring, plastic item had a short life, in part because the long string that protruded from the cervix and assured female patients of its presence caused problems for male sexual partners.

Still, it was a brave new world, and by the 1960s the IUD, along with the Pill, entered the American consciousness in a major way. The two options, pharmaceutical and mechanical, had a lot in common, most notably the fact that they were both doctor-controlled methods that required medical supervision for their usage. The stories of the Pill and the IUD are historically aligned and intertwined, even as they are divergent. The Pill was—and is—a star on the rise. It has had ups and downs but remains today the top reversible option for American women. The IUD has proved less alluring, and while both pill and device have suffered safety black eyes, the latter has been less resilient at bouncing back in the public consciousness.

The IUD had supporters as it rose to prominence in the 1960s. The powerful Population Council, for one, liked the long-term effectiveness of the "coil." Council members worried, among other things, about burgeoning fertility around the world and its potential to foster the growth of Communism. They also worried about the growing populations in America's low-income communities and wondered whether women who lacked education and basic financial resources could be relied upon to consistently take pills. The idea of a device that could be inserted and left, without maintenance, for several years seemed impossibly appealing. By the late 1960s, the Council was not only funding research on the technology, but had sent over 6 million devices to developing nations,[19] along with knowledge about how to manufacture them.

Domestically, the IUD was initially marketed, unsurprisingly, to women at public clinics. These women were disproportionately low income, and many were nonwhite. Even as the option grew in popularity among middle-class white women, doctors continued to discourage its use in those populations, advocating it only for poor women or for those who had finished bearing children.

By the end of the 1960s, another group of people were starting to think that the IUD provided a better alternative to the Pill: women's health activists. Bolstered by alarming safety problems with the Pill, members of the women's movement concerned with health issues wondered if perhaps this "new, safe" option provided the modern alternative to dangerous drugs. In her groundbreaking book, *The Doctors' Case Against the Pill*, Barbara Seaman warned that although IUDs had problems—including infection and uterine perforation—the serious problems seemed limited to older devices, and newer ones were safe. Decades later, when I asked her if she had any regrets about her long career, Seaman hesitated before responding, "Yes . . . I wish I had been more cautious on IUDs."[20]

As concerns about the Pill grew, women dumped the drug in large numbers. Many looked for an alternative, and by 1971, they turned to the Dalkon Shield.

At this time, FDA lacked the ability to regulate devices. This meant that the IUD market was an open one, with numerous devices of varying safety, materials, and efficacy flooding the population. An image of twentieth-century options reveals an array of products that visually run the range from squiggles to pine tree–shaped towers to candy cane–like swirls, and even bat-shaped coils.

Historian Andrea Tone has pointed out that, in keeping with military metaphors common in discussions of population control in the 1960s and 1970s (think "population bomb"), images of conflict were frequently used to tout the effectiveness of IUDs: "'aggressive, battle-hungry IUDs invade, irritate, infect, and finally subdue the ultimately powerless uteri.' Toughness, visual and medical, was valued, and device makers struggled to make their versions look intimidating."[21] The Dalkon Shield got its name, in part, because it looked like a policeman's badge.

Just as the bad safety information was emerging about the Pill—and the Nelson pill hearings, along with Seaman's book, were taking it public in a big way—a gynecologist and vocal pill critic named Hugh Davis was publicizing the results of his testing of the new device, which he claimed had an efficacy rate on par with oral contraceptives. Only later, after the Shield proved tragic for many women, was it revealed that Davis secretly held a financial stake in the product and that he conducted methodologically compromised tests on it. On the face of things, the Dalkon Shield seemed to be the answer to women's—and manufacturers'—prayers. In 1970 a company called A. H. Robins paid three quarters of a million dollars for the chance to make it, outbidding formidable challengers like Upjohn. Despite the fact that later trials had shown Davis's pregnancy prevention estimates to be overly optimistic, the company went ahead with manufacturing and marketing the IUD.

It was a perfect storm: an inventor who hid his involvement and conducted faulty trials, a manufacturer who knowingly published false information about its product, a new design that was undertested and marketed to a hungry population.

Andrea Tone points out that the Shield had two major design flaws. The first was actually an innovation to prevent the uterus from expelling it as a foreign object. To prevent this problem, the Shield added prongs that blocked expulsion from the uterus, but also blocked doctors from easily inserting and removing the IUD. The second was the use of a fiber on the string that encouraged the growth of infection. This latter problem occurred despite the fact that manufacturers were warned of the danger. FDA veteran and women's health advocate Susan Wood notes, "It was a bad design, plain and simple. And a lot of women suffered because of it."[22]

In a tragic case of people valuing marketing over science, more IUD users and their doctors chose the Shield than all other devices combined—over 2.2 million in the United States and 1.5 million internationally. Of those, close to 700,000 had been bought by global aid organizations for international use.

The problems began right away. Doctors noticed that women having the Shield inserted had terrible pain and even trauma. The item's brochure promised that it could be put in with minimal pain, but on the ground, doctors saw a different set of experiences. The dangers didn't end there, and at least eighteen women died from complications that included septic abortion. Other serious problems were infection, pelvic inflammatory disease, and infertility.

A tidal wave of complaint letters and the threat of a damning medical journal article led the manufacturer to send letters to doctors admitting possible problems. Once the lawsuits began and horrific stories started making the papers—one woman told of a brain damaged baby born with the Shield—A. H. Robins took off the gloves and began to get down and dirty, claiming that promiscuity on the part of users led to problems. At the same time, they began quietly advising doctors to take the devices out of patients. Despite shocking stories of its dangers, the Dalkon Shield died a slow death. It took only four years for the device to rise to the top of the market and for its problems to lead its maker to stop marketing in the United States. It took ten more years of lawsuits, negative medical information, and media reports chipping away at A. H. Robins before the company finally filed for bankruptcy in 1985. In all, 8 percent of women who used the Dalkon Shield—around 325,000 people—filed claims against the maker. Among other results of the debacle, the FDA gained the ability to regulate devices as well as drugs.[23]

The IUD Today

Modern IUDs are still, to a large extent, tainted by this history. Even as massive organizations like the Guttmacher Institute tout their usefulness, women remain suspicious. As a younger generation of women with no memory of the disasters of the 1970s and early 1980s make choices about birth control, this is changing—but slowly. One study interviewed thousands of women over the phone about their knowledge about IUDs. Researchers found that women lacked awareness of and information about the option when compared with other possibilities—the Pill, condoms, and so on—and also felt that it was unsafe.[24]

While women worldwide have embraced IUDs in large numbers,[25] Americans have not. Doctors and female patients were slow to accept the technology and never chose it in numbers anywhere near those in other parts of the globe. By the 1970s, it is estimated that 10 million women were using IUDs. Today that number may be as high as 160 million. Despite this, the Guttmacher Institute reckons that only 2 percent of American women make the IUD their contraceptive of choice.[26]

The modern IUD is a small device, often plastic and T-shaped, that is inserted into a woman's uterus. Once in the womb, the object causes mild irritation—usually not enough to allow real infection, but sufficient for inhibiting sperm mobility. Today there are two available FDA-approved IUD methods. The first, ParaGard, is a copper-releasing IUD. Copper has long been associated with contraception. In ancient Greece, one well-known potion for pregnancy prevention involved diluting copper ore with water and taking the concoction orally.[27] It is thought that copper encourages the cells in the uterus to produce a compound that kills sperm.[28] While introducing metals into the body is usually a dangerous enterprise, and copper is toxic, the amount of the metal in ParaGard is so small that it isn't considered dangerous. The device can cause heavy periods and increased cramping, particularly during the first few months of use. Some estimate that it increases menstrual flow by 50 to 75 percent.[29]

Newer nonhormonal models that are approved in Europe but not in the United States may decrease this problem by altering the T-shape design. But the new models may pose unique problems, such as higher expulsion rates (which occurs in some women when the body identifies the IUD as a foreign object and ejects it from the uterus).

The second American option, Mirena, is a hybrid device that works like traditional versions but also releases small amounts of the progestin levonorgestrel. Because it uses progestin, it is not a nonhormonal method. In this case the hormone works to thicken cervical mucus (which makes pregnancy more difficult) and partially inhibits ovulation. The amount of progestin is very small, and there is debate among scientists and doctors as to whether it works systemically (in the entire body) or remains local. Because of the hormonal component, some scientists refer to Mirena as an "IUS" or "Intrauterine System." Some health advocates argue that Mirena is a wolf in sheep's clothing—not really an IUD, but rather a hormonal implant similar to the disgraced Norplant. What is certain is that the two types of IUDs are erroneously lumped together in conversation when their profiles—and often the patients for whom they would be appropriate—are different.

Both hormonal and nonhormonal IUDs can cause bleeding trouble. Mirena can cause irregular bleeding, and some women have the device removed for this reason. On the other hand, Dr. Jerilynn Prior of Canada's Centre for Menstrual Cycle and Ovulation Research (CeMCOR) recommends the device for treating severe and disruptive perimenopausal bleeding, the erratic and often disruptive flow that can happen in the months and years before periods stop.[30] Because women in perimenopause still need contraception, this is one population that might benefit from choosing Mirena, although of course the results of the Women's Health Initiative suggest that any hormonal option must be carefully considered in aging women, particularly for long-term use. As with other menstrual suppression drugs, while bleeding patterns are likely to become irregular when use is initiated, complete period cessation is a frequent outcome for many women. Bayer, which makes Mirena, estimates that 20 percent of women will stop bleeding after a year of use.[31]

Because Mirena uses such low doses of hormones, ovarian action is only partially suppressed. While this means that ovulation is unlikely to occur, it also means that ovarian cysts and ruptured follicles are more common. Women who have gynecological issues like fibroids or endometriosis should probably choose another option.

Both devices, ParaGard and Mirena, are very effective at preventing pregnancy. Data shows that for every thousand women who use the non-hormonal option each year, ten will become pregnant—that's a failure rate of 1 percent (although "ideal" effectiveness is higher, with a failure rate of .3 percent).[32] Mirena is even more effective, and out of a thousand women who use the device for a year, only two will have pregnancies,[33] a failure rate of .1 percent to .2 percent. It seems strange to discuss "ideal" and "actual" use statistics for a method that, in theory, shouldn't be subject to patient fallibility in the way that options like the Pill are. The gaps between theoretical efficacy and what actually happens probably exist in part because of provider mistakes while inserting the devices. It is worth asking if such a device can claim an "ideal" efficacy, or if that is simply rhetorical and misleading in this context. There really isn't much that a woman can do to make her device "work" better except check the string that protrudes from the cervix occasionally to ensure that the IUD is still there.

Some couples feel this string during sex and sometimes find it unpleasant. Women who use IUDs are less likely to have an ectopic pregnancy—which happens when a fertilized egg starts growing outside the uterus—than women who don't use contraceptives, but if they do get pregnant, that conception is more likely to be ectopic.[34] This is a life-threatening condition that requires immediate medical attention.

Method failure is extremely rare, but for women who experience it, the results can be at best difficult and at worst horrific. The chance of pregnancy occurring is increased when the device becomes embedded or with the occurrence of accidental uterine perforation that happens while it is being put into the body. When a woman becomes pregnant while using an IUD (non-ectopically), she is at a much higher risk of miscarriage than she would be without the IUD. The device is usually removed because it can cause an array of problems including sepsis and premature labor. As worrying, particularly with Mirena, are the potential effects of the IUD on a growing fetus. The potentially tragic influence of estrogen on developing fetuses has been known since the 1960s and '70s. Diethylstilbestrol (DES), an estrogen drug, was prescribed from 1938 to 1971 to prevent miscarriage. The Centers for Disease Control estimates that between 5 and 10 million people were exposed, in utero, to a drug that proved not to prevent pregnancy loss and instead caused devastating problems—including increased cancer and reproductive abnormalities—in exposed offspring.[35] As the case of women taking the hormone diethylstilbestrol (DES) during pregnancy tragically demonstrated, prolonged exposure to hormones in the womb can have a dangerous outcome, potentially causing cancers and reproductive abnormalities. Even Mirena's manufacturer admits that "long-term effects on the offspring are unknown" but that congenital abnormalities—including a "slight masculinization of the external genitalia of the female fetus"[36]—has been seen in the small number of births that have happened under these conditions.

The majority of experts think IUDs are safe for all ages, but doctors are cautious about recommending them to younger women. Any form of IUD is rarely the first or even second contraceptive to be offered to young patients. In a Guttmacher-funded report, Adam Sonfield notes that even in European countries where IUDs are actually used in higher numbers, doctors are slow to consider them as a first option for younger women.[37] Commercials for both the IUD and the IUS recommend it for women who have "completed their families." Young women who want an IUD may encounter doctors who are unwilling to insert the device, though this is changing as more doctors have come to believe that the devices are generally safe.

Women who don't think that they want more children but aren't sure may find that the IUD provides a good alternative to sterilization. It has the same benefits—high long-term efficacy and limited time investment—but unlike tubal ligation, is easily reversible for most women. For those contemplating children imminently, however, the IUD may not be the best choice. The device doesn't adversely affect fertility in most women, but from a cost perspective, it is a method whose benefits are best seen when women can use it for longer periods of time.

Doctors' and manufacturers' reluctance to recommend IUDs to young women also hearkens back to the Dalkon Shield disaster. Because many young women suffered infertility as a result of using that model, and device makers suffered financial ruin as a result, those marketing IUDs are slow to encourage younger women to try their wares even as large public health organizations insist they are safe for all ages. Safety studies have suggested that for the most part, modern IUDs don't directly cause pelvic inflammatory disease (PID)—a general term for serious infection of the reproductive organs that can lead to complications such as infertility—although it can happen in some instances. PID is most commonly caused by an untreated sexually transmitted infection. While it is very rare for a modern IUD to initiate PID, it can exacerbate the problems when the PID already exists because of an STI.

When I asked Cynthia Pearson, director of the National Women's Health Network, about IUDs for younger women, she told me that her organization "never really got over its skepticism of the IUD's association with infection. I try to read the new studies as they come out and it seems to me that there still is a real, albeit small, risk of infection in the immediate aftermath of the insertion."[38] She added that this risk doesn't seem to last in the long term, which she notes is "an improvement since the old days."

The problem, Pearson notes, is that when big family planning groups advocate for the IUD, they stress that complications that develop have to do with individual behavior, not a problem with a doctor's supervision or the device itself. Blaming women's health problems on their sexual choices is a dangerous, but not uncommon, way of framing contraceptive conversations. Pearson stresses that while, in theory, doctors could screen out women at greater risk for problems, "they never DO screen out everyone with 'risk factors' because no one can say with perfect foresight what they'll be doing and who they'll be with in the future."[39] Because of the risks of infection, however small, women at high risk for STIs should closely consider this problem before choosing the option. This is particularly true if patients already have an STI before inserting the device, or if they contract the problem soon after. Women considering an IUD (and all women for that matter) should first be tested for sexually transmitted infections, including chlamydia and gonorrhea, leading causes of PID.

Another concern for younger women considering the IUD is that they are more prone to device expulsion (as are women who have never had a baby), and with Mirena, young women are more likely to have ovarian cysts. One major advantage of the IUD is cost. A 2009 study in the journal *Contraception* found that the ParaGard copper IUD and the Mirena option represent the most cost-effective methods of birth control available to American women.[40] In a country where nearly one in three people between the ages of nineteen and twenty-six are uninsured and countless others go without health care, this fact has increased the appeal of the option for some younger women. This cost analysis assumes that a woman will leave the device in for many years; for those looking for shorter-term birth control, it doesn't have this benefit.

Many women find cost to be more prohibitive when it comes to the nonhormonal IUD, because it is less accessible and not always covered by insurance. Tatiana, a twenty-six-year-old Latina woman who works as a computer specialist in the Washington, DC, area, had suffered with birth control pills that adversely affected her mood and threw her into depression. Unfortunately, when Tatiana reviewed her insurance policy, she found that it would cover Mirena, but not ParaGard. In order to obtain the latter option, she would need to pay out of pocket—money that, even with a good job, she didn't have.

In addition to insurance hurdles limiting the accessibility of ParaGard, some women find that doctors and nurses pressure them to choose Mirena. One twenty-two-year-old woman describes her experience:

> I did research online before going in for my consultation, and was very excited about the copper wire IUD. I really liked that it has no hormones, and it's 99.9 percent effective and good for up to ten years.
>
> When I went to my gynecologist for my consultation/insertion, the nurse who showed me in had brought in Mirena, the IUD with progesterone, as opposed to ParaGard, the copper wire that I'd been leaning toward. She seemed to assume I would go with Mirena, as did my gynecologist, to the point that I wondered if they had some sort of financial deal with the company. I was only looking for information and it was very hard to get; without presenting me with any statistics or comparative data to comfort me (I was nervous) the nurse basically said that if I wanted ParaGard, then fine, and I should sign a piece of paper to

certify that I had read the ParaGard brochure even though I hadn't, and got rather put out when I asked if I could see the brochure first. "Are you really going to read it?" she said. She brought it and I read the whole thing. Although this was a very scary gynecologist visit, I am *extremely* happy with my IUD and very glad I did research on my own so that I knew that the ParaGard was a better fit for me than the Mirena.[41]

As with many forms of contraception, there is controversy surrounding IUDs that plays out in complicated and frightening ways. It has been speculated that an IUD works in part by preventing the implantation of a fertilized egg to the uterine wall, a situation that some feel constitutes abortion. It has not been proven that IUDs work in this way—and whether a fertilized, unimplanted egg constitutes a fetus is another matter entirely (this idea is inconsistent with most scientific definitions of pregnancy)—but because some pro-life activists consider the method a form of abortion, certain health care providers are reluctant or unwilling to provide it. A story that made headlines in the early months of 2009 serves as a cautionary tale about the intersection of personal belief, public health, and the danger of so-called conscience rules. An Albuquerque, New Mexico–based nurse, Sylvia Olona, is currently facing a lawsuit from a patient who claims the health care provider pulled out her IUD when she came in seeking care.[42] The nurse claims that the device was removed by accident, but a review of past incidences revealed something more sinister. Olona had "accidentally" removed several IUDs from patients and was outspokenly opposed to the devices. As she attempted to comfort the frantic young woman, Olona assured her that it was all for the best—the thing was really just an abortion waiting to happen—she had actually done her a favor. Once the IUD was out, the nurse refused to insert a new one. Under broader conscience rules established in the last gasps of the Bush administration, such refusals may be legally protected (although of course the unwarranted removal does not enjoy such shelter). While the Obama administration has worked to undo some of this last-minute damage, the ability of providers to refuse various services continues to pose a threat to reproductive rights. Even the most infrequently used methods of contraception place women at the center of cultural and political controversy.

Female and Male Sterilization

No methods of birth control are so broadly practiced and so little discussed in American life as female and male sterilization. Most people are shocked to discover that sterilization (when we count women and men together) is the most popular method of contraception in the United States. As of 2002, 27 percent of American women using contraception and 9.2 percent of American men were sterilized. Perhaps one reason we don't talk more about this very common set of procedures is because of this tends to be the birth control option of people who have had as many children as they want, people who on average are older. But this is changing somewhat as younger couples, for a variety of reasons, increasingly choose to remain child-free. Jeanne, thirty-six, told me about her partner's decision to undergo a vasectomy in his late twenties: "I never wanted kids, and Mitch feels the same way. I was going to have my tubes tied and he said, 'No, vasectomy is less invasive, it's more reversible—I'll do it.' I thought, 'Wow, this guy is a keeper.'" Mitch had trouble finding a doctor who was willing to perform the surgery on a young man without any children. They finally did, and both have been happy with the decision despite living in a world where friends are increasingly focused on babies and children. "I'm in my midthirties now," Jeanne tells me, "and I keep waiting to get blindsided by this desire for kids. But it hasn't happened yet."

Tubal ligation is the most common form of nonreversible birth control in America. This outpatient procedure involves cutting, burning, or blocking the fallopian tubes with clips or bands so that eggs are unable to travel to the uterus. Even though the body continues to ovulate after the surgery, the eggs have no way to travel downward and the sperm aren't able to venture upward. Doctors can perform a tubal ligation in a doctor's office, clinic, or hospital using either local or general anesthetic. Usually, this is a laparoscopic surgery, meaning that gas is used to inflate the abdomen, and the procedure is performed using a tiny telescope-like instrument inserted into the body through cuts at the navel and above the pelvic bone. The advantage of laparoscopic surgery is that it is less invasive and patients can recover more quickly.

After surgery, a woman will need to rest for two to three days, but the procedure is immediately effective. It is still a good idea to wait at least a week before trying to have sex to make sure that the body has had time to heal. Tubal ligation is 99.5 percent effective for pregnancy prevention, though there is a small chance of ectopic pregnancy. It is possible to reverse the surgery in some cases, but women undergoing sterilization should think of it as a permanent decision. In the cases where it is reversed, the risk of ectopic pregnancy increases.

Because it is a permanent decision, it is important for women to think more carefully and dynamically about this choice than they would about reversible methods. Possible life changes (a breakup with a partner, a spousal death, or the death of a child, among others) should be considered before opting for surgery.

Women who have tubal ligations have few side effects, but abnormal bleeding and bladder infections are two possible problems. Some women say that they experience a condition called "post-tubal sterilization syndrome." While this is controversial, and some doctors deny that it exists, many women insist that they experience symptoms such as irregular and painful periods, midcycle bleeding, and even loss of periods. Hormone levels are generally minimally affected. The surgery is expensive, but it can be cost effective over time.

In 2002 the FDA approved a procedure called Essure, which works like tubal ligation but doesn't involve surgery. With Essure, a doctor places tiny "microinserts" into the fallopian tubes by going through the vagina, cervix, and uterus rather than making surgical cuts. The procedure, like IUD insertion, requires only local anesthetic. During the three months following insertion, body tissue grows around the microinserts to eventually block the fallopian tubes. This process takes time, so Essure isn't immediately effective and other birth control is necessary in the meantime. After three months, a doctor tests to make sure that the fallopian tubes are fully blocked. The procedure isn't reversible, and because it is new, there is a lot we don't know about potential problems and side effects. Still, it promises another option for women who want nonreversible birth control.

There are other less common forms of female sterilization, including hysterectomy (where either the uterus or both the uterus and ovaries are removed), but this much more invasive surgery with far-reaching health implications and dangers is usually performed because of other serious health problems.

Vasectomy, the most common form of male sterilization, is even less invasive than tubal ligation. In this procedure, which is generally performed under local anesthetic in about fifteen minutes, the doctor makes a small cut in the skin of the scrotum. The vasa deferentia (tubes that carry sperm) become visible and the doctor cuts them. Once these passageways are severed, sperm have no way to enter the ejaculate. A man will still produce semen; it simply won't have sperm in it. The procedure is 99.9 percent effective, although in rare instances the tubes may repair themselves and unplanned pregnancy may result.

After a vasectomy, a man will typically rest at the doctor's office before going home (faintness is a typical side effect of the surgery). Once home, he should rest from work for two days and avoid strenuous labor for at least a week. Sexual activity should also be delayed for about a week or two while the body is healing. Men don't become sterile immediately after having the procedure. Sperm maturation is a slow process, and at first some sperm remain in the ejaculate and in various stages of viability. After about ten to thirty ejaculations, doctors will typically perform follow-up tests to make sure that ejaculate has negative sperm counts.

Vasectomy isn't just less invasive than tubal ligation, it is also more reversible. In about 70 percent of cases, the severed sperm tubes can be repaired. This doesn't mean that pregnancy will definitely be possible; in fact, it becomes much less likely. Because of this, people opting for vasectomy should consider that it may well be permanent and treat the decision as a final one.

Sterilization in America has a shocking and difficult history of being implemented through coercive and violent means. This history lays bare the ways that control over reproduction is used to reinforce power relationships and as a site for social engineering. Historian Dorothy Roberts traces the history of sterilization abuse in America back to the treatment of slaves, noting that castration was used as a punishment for African American men accused of various crimes, sexual and otherwise.[43] Mandatory sterilization of criminals became a popular tool of social control in the late nineteenth and early twentieth century. Forced sterilization under eugenic laws resulted in thousands of people being stripped of reproductive and human rights during the first half of the twentieth century.

It is easy to distance ourselves from these bodily violations committed so many years ago. Slavery and even the now-discredited pseudoscience of the early twentieth century can seem impossibly distant from our own lives, particularly for those of us who have spent almost as much of our lives in the new century as in the one that came before. And yet, when it comes to sterilization abuse, to paraphrase William Faulkner, the past isn't over; it isn't even past. Even in the 1960s, when "the last nail was barely in the coffin of eugenic theory,"[44] a new type of coercive sterilization began to be institutionalized. Ironically, as desegregation allowed African Americans and other people of color new access to health care in public facilities, it created a novel way for doctors and lawmakers to impose racist social policy on the bodies of women. In the 1970s, sterilization was one of the fastest growing methods of contraception. Between 1970 and 1980, the number of women who were sterilized rose from 200,000 to over 700,000. Working through public health care, including the Medicaid program, many doctors worked to bully, threaten, and pressure women of color and poor women into giving up their fertility.

Sometimes authorities threatened to withhold welfare and other forms of economic relief until women agreed to be sterilized. Other times, doctors threatened to refuse services, such the delivery of babies, until mothers agreed to undergo ligation or hysterectomy. Some doctors simply performed the procedure without permission after a birth or other medical intervention. This was done for a number of reasons: sometimes the woman already had several children and her doctor decided she shouldn't have any more; other doctors did it to give medical residents surgical practice; some felt that the women in their care weren't intelligent enough to use reversible birth control; and, of course, some were driven by ideas about quelling social unrest by reducing the population of poor and nonwhite people.

Dorothy Roberts notes that in the South, hysterectomies were often called "Mississippi appendectomies,"[45] and she tells the story of Minnie Lee and Mary Alice Relf, the children of illiterate farm workers in Montgomery, Alabama, who were sterilized in 1973 at the ages of fourteen and twelve. Mrs. Relf, who couldn't sign her name, consented to her daughters' participation in a trial of Depo-Provera by signing an *X*. She did this at the urging of nurses from a federally funded hospital in the area. After the Depo-Provera trials ended because of concerns about the drug's potential to cause cancer, the two girls were sterilized instead.

Legal action to try to achieve some justice for the Relf sisters exposed how rampant and racially based sterilization abuses were: legal documents for the case, tried in the 1970s, estimate that between 100,000 and 150,000 poor women were sterilized each year under the auspices of federally funded health care programs. Of these women, almost half were black.[46] African American women in the South were not the only victims of these sorts of abuses: American Indian women were also subjected to programs of coercive sterilization. During the 1970s as many as 25 percent of women on reservations underwent some sort of nonreversible procedure. And in Puerto Rico, the site of the Pill trials, a massive campaign to sterilize women led to as many as one third of women between fifteen and forty undergoing "la operación" by 1968. In the early 1970s, a group of Latina women brought a legal case in Los Angeles against a hospital that had sterilized them without giving informed consent: the women had been given information and consent forms they couldn't understand. In addition, some were told that the surgery was reversible.[47]

Helen Rodriguez-Trias, the Puerto Rican doctor and heroine of the women's health movement, was one of the women who led the battle to end these atrocities. The Committee to End Sterilization Abuse (CESA) organized in the mid-1970s for reform and for the establishment of guidelines to protect Medicaid patients and other women receiving reproductive health care through public funds. Among CESA's recommendations were provisions to insist on a thirty-day waiting period before a procedure could be performed, extensive information and education in the patient's native language, and a requirement of written consent on the part of the patient.

In the late 1970s, women's groups led mostly by white activists fought to ensure that women who wanted sterilizations could get them. For white women the problem was different: very few doctors would agree to perform the procedure on a white middle-class patient unless "her age multiplied by the number of children she had equaled 120."[48] So a woman in this group who had no children wouldn't be a candidate for the surgery regardless of her age, marital status, or desires.

The result of these two different sets of experiences led to a clash between white and nonwhite feminists that in many ways articulated the racial tensions underlying the second wave women's movement.

Rodriguez-Trias later explained, "We were unprepared for the ferocity of the opposition to our guidelines." She added that while the feminist movement was "very diverse . . . the more public positions articulated by the movement didn't concern the experiences or concerns of women of color or poor women."[49] Mainstream groups led by white feminists such as Planned Parenthood and the National Abortion Rights Action League (NARAL) refused to support CESA's objectives and even actively opposed them in some instances. Despite this, in 1978 CESA's guidelines became government policy. Today, though health care policies have undergone massive reforms, African American women are much more likely to be sterilized than white women, even though they comprise a smaller part of the total population. While progress has been made to reduce race- and class-based reproductive abuses, much work remains.

Final Thoughts on Nonhormonal Methods

So, in the end, who killed the diaphragm and the other nonhormonal methods of birth control? Well, I suppose you could say it was the magic bullet. Or at least the idea of a magic bullet—the notion that hormonal options could be made to work for every woman. This happened despite extensive clinical and anecdotal experience to the contrary. In some ways it was an inside job: the same medical communities that used the diaphragm as a vehicle to professionalize contraception were quick to disown the method when persuasive, pharmaceutically funded information suggested that hormonal methods were the only way to go. Perhaps, though, reports of the diaphragm's death have been greatly exaggerated. I, for one, hope that that is the case. In a world without enough contraceptive options it would be a tragedy to unnecessarily eliminate a unique and historically useful one.

It is significant that the IUD—the only nonhormonal method getting attention from large public health and medical groups—happens to be a long-term method whose use is totally dependent on medical practitioners. Methods that allow women more freedom to choose when and how they will be used should be encouraged and made accessible.

Women want to look to the future when it comes to birth control, but new technology isn't always quick to arrive. When it *does* arrive we find that newer isn't always better, and from a medical safety perspective, sticking with older time-tested methods can be a smarter way to go. While we embrace new ideas and hope for better options, let us not forget the wellspring of knowledge that past technologies hold.

Chapter Four

By Any Other Name: Alternative Distribution Methods and Hormonal Contraception

With the Pill turning fifty, now is the perfect time to reflect on the birth control innovations this queen of contraception has inspired. Recently I interviewed college-age women at a small school in the northeastern United States about their experiences with birth control, starting with a seemingly simple question: how has contraception changed over the past fifty years? Many of the young respondents who shared their stories with me had similar answers, telling me that contraception has undergone substantial changes in recent decades. There are new methods coming out every day, they said—look at the vaginal ring, the contraceptive patch, injectable and implantable birth control, and even a chewable pill.

Thanks to successful drug company marketing, it can be easy to believe that the past twenty-five years have seen an enormous number of new contraceptive options hit the market, including Depo-Provera, Norplant, NuvaRing, Ortho Evra (the birth control patch), Mirena (the hormonal IUD), low-dose pills, and of course, menstrual suppression drugs.

It is important to realize that while these are all alternative distribution methods—meaning they help drugs reach your body in different ways—they are also all forms of hormonal contraception, using the same estrogen and progestin that have made up the Pill since its creation. So what are the unique advantages and disadvantages that might encourage a woman to choose one of these younger methods over the older daily Pill? How do issues of age, race, and class motivate these Pill alternatives, and in what ways must we understand them as "new" from a safety perspective?

In this chapter I examine similarities and differences between alternative hormonal contraceptive methods and the Pill. I also address the question of why the new developments in contraception have been almost exclusively hormonal, essentially a simple repackaging and remarketing of the same oral contraceptive drug. If the original Pill constituted a true fertility control innovation, why have the past fifty years brought simply "me too" drugs, and what has happened to prospects for truly new methods?

False Starts and Uncertain Futures: Norplant and Long-Lasting Contraceptive Implants

Ironically, it is the failure of one method—the Dalkon Shield IUD—that has seriously hampered the development of new ones. When infection, infertility, and other health problems caused by the Shield led thousands of women to participate in legal actions against the device's manufacturer, liability insurance for contraceptives shot to astronomical heights. Many drug companies decided they had had enough and got out of the birth control business altogether, with many more simply curtailing involvement to marketing existing drugs. It simply didn't make economic sense to spend time and valuable research and development dollars chasing new methods.

The birth control pill changed American medicine. It showed that it was possible to successfully market a preventative pill to a healthy person, potentially for decades of continuous use. This caused seismic changes in the pharmaceutical industry, and today, disease-free midlife patients are often counseled to consider long-term drugs for cholesterol, mood, pain, and menopause management and as interventions in bone and sexual health. Drug companies have realized they don't have to stick with contraception: there are untold horizons for preventative medicine and plenty of new drugs—for men as well as women—to pursue.

Financially speaking, it has been hard to improve on the profitable Pill. A drug that doesn't need to be taken monthly would almost certainly represent a less lucrative option for manufacturers, so there has been no real incentive for contraceptive innovation.

Population control groups and some sexual health organizations have been on the opposite side of the issue. International groups interested in contraception have been highly motivated to find methods that require less stringent patient adherence and less repeat involvement in fertility control. Some argue that women with limited access to health care are less likely to stick with a method that requires repeatedly procuring pills each month (or even every couple months). Others suspicious of long-acting methods that take some measure of reproductive control out of women's hands have pointed out that these devices have been disproportionately and sometimes coercively pushed on poor women in developing nations and low-income women in the United States.

The idea of a long-acting contraceptive implant has been a serious possibility since the 1960s, and over ten hormonal compounds have been tested over the years as possible candidates. The idea is simple: hormones are placed in flexible and nonbiodegradable tubes and inserted under the skin, where they gradually release enough of the compounds to prevent pregnancy. All of the implants to hit the American market so far have been progestin-only methods.

Given the cost of insurance required to be in the birth control business, the only entities that can afford to be players in research and development are drugmakers and large organizations, and the former are simply not very interested in doing so.

But large nonprofit groups, such as the Population Council, have both the resources and the interest in making new methods. Norplant, the first of all the alternative distribution methods to be approved in the United States, was developed by the Population Council and first used for contraception around the world in the 1980s in part with the help of $15 million dollars in American and foreign aid.[1] The international introduction of Norplant was not always a pretty story: Indonesia, one of the first countries to adopt the device, promoted and even forced its use in many ways, including withholding paychecks from women who didn't agree to insertion and requiring Norplant use as a condition of certain types of employment.[2] A program in Peru in the 1980s administered by the United States Agency for International Development (USAID) offered only Norplant and sterilization to the patients it serviced. In Bangladesh a massive program targeted poor women with the device. In all cases, the emphasis was on making sure that women had the device put in and little attention was given to how they would get it out if they changed their minds about it. This meant both that doctors weren't adequately trained in removal and that women often lacked the resources to access the doctors. Nonetheless, declining birth rates in test populations led to the view that Norplant was a successful and promising method of birth control.

The Population Council wanted to market the device to American women, but they lacked the funds, so they eventually partnered with Wyeth Ayerst, one of the few pharmaceutical companies left standing in the field of contraceptive development by the end of the 1980s. Norplant[3] was made of six 2.4 mm silicone tubes, each containing 36 mg of levonorgestrel, a progestin. A doctor implanting the device would make a 3 to 5 mm incision in a patient's upper forearm and insert the tubes in a "fan-like pattern."[4] By 1990, it hit the American market. The option enjoyed a very short honeymoon before the problems that continue to plague it today came to be understood by American women.

The first problem Norplant encountered wasn't really its fault. By 1992, enormous controversy and media attention were swirling around the terrible problems suffered by women with silicone breast implants. Historian Andrea Tone notes, "When silicone gel breast implants began to be taken off the market in 1992, Norplant fell under suspicion because its rods were made of silicone (although not silicone gel)."[5] The result was that implantation of new Norplant devices, which was as high as eight hundred per day in 1990, plummeted to less than sixty by 1995.

Other safety problems more substantively tied to the Norplant device began to rear their heads. Many women had unpredictable bleeding and scarring at the insertion site. There were other side effects, including weight gain, arm pain, and mood changes, but bleeding remained the most upsetting for many patients. If women had bleeding problems (and other symptoms) on oral contraceptives, they could simply stop taking the drug. But Norplant was less forgiving: once a woman had the device implanted, it was expensive and painful to take out.

Summer, now a thirty-something waitress in Salt Lake City, UT, was in her early twenties when she had Norplant put in. At the time she was an on-again, off-again student at the University of Utah and was waiting tables part time to put herself through school. She'd been in a relationship for several years that had ended when she had a reluctant abortion after becoming pregnant while on the Pill. Hoping never to be in a situation like that again, Summer decided to try Norplant. Two years later, she was desperate to get the device out of her arm. It had caused lots of problems, the worst of which was shooting pains in her arm that made carrying trays and accomplishing the other tasks required for her work difficult. More pressingly, she was married to another man and ready to start a family. Unfortunately, she lacked the financial resources to remove the Norplant tubes. "I ended up taking twice the shifts, letting other things go," Summer told me. "I was just desperate to save the money for removal."[6]

Many women found themselves in similar situations, particularly low-income women and those in developing nations. In the summer of 2001, I met a young doctor from Nepal at a conference related to the massive United Nations Beijing + 5 gathering. She shared her story with me. Trained by an international population control group, she inserted hundreds of Norplant devices. She was undertrained to do so, and the providers of the implants never suggested that there could be side effects. When her patients started experiencing problems, she was equally ill equipped for removal, and some patients had scarring. Others were simply unable to make the long journey back to the clinic. As she told the story to me and a small group of women's health activists, tears came to her eyes. "No one told me there would be problems like that—I would never have used it, and I certainly wouldn't have put it into so many women."

Other international health workers and their patients found it to be a useful method. Abigail Fee, a young Harvard student, was living and conducting research among the Ewe women of Ho, Ghana, in West Africa. She became accustomed to women who came to the clinic where she was working bemoaning the fact that they could no longer get Norplant. Social stigma made it difficult for many women to get contraceptives and therefore necessary that women conceal their use. A long-term method was, in this context, ideal, and they were willing to put up with the side effects.

These two examples illustrate the difficulty of assessing risks and benefits in the diverse contexts in which women (and their doctors) make contraceptive decisions. None of this is simple, and calling a drug "bad" or "good" is too easy. Different birth control options are good for certain people, bad for others, and mixed for the majority of women. What is less debatable, in the case of Norplant, is that doctors and health care providers should have been better informed about its potential risks and problems.

Another problem for Norplant was the perception that it was a shiny new engine of social control waiting and ready to coercively manage the fertility of low-income and nonwhite women. These concerns were well founded: the initial terms of the Norplant debate in America focused on its usefulness for curtailing births in poor communities. Indeed, within two days of the drug's approval, the *Philadelphia Inquirer* ran an editorial entitled "Poverty and Norplant: Can Contraception Reduce the Under class?"[7] In making its argument for creating "incentive" programs that would bribe women to have the device inserted in exchange for benefits or food, the article singled out women of color and "black poverty"[8] as problems that the new birth control might be able to curtail. While activists decried the blatant racism and classism of these arguments, state legislatures scrambled to put together bills proposing just such tactics. In all, thirteen states created two dozen bills that some activists argued would have used Norplant "for social engineering purposes, making the use of Norplant a condition of receiving welfare payments or enticing women on welfare to use Norplant through financial incentives."[9] Due in no small part to the constant efforts of African American women's health activists, none of these proposals was put in to place, although many less obvious means of pressuring poor women to have the device inserted did happen.

An official program to use the drug coercively did enter into public practice: female prisoners convicted of sexual crimes were offered a choice between Norplant and prison, and forced to undergo insertion as a condition of release.[10] While such practices were gradually made illegal, both proposed and enacted plans for eugenic uses of Norplant served to highlight that a painful national history of forced sterilization of poor, disabled, and minority women was not as far in the past as many believed.

Sheldon Segal of the Population Council was quick to react to accusations of racism by insisting that none of these uses of Norplant were proposed or designed by its maker; he also insisted that the buck for such abuses stopped with the lawmakers and judges who saw such unsavory potential in the six little tubes: "It was developed to improve reproductive freedom, not to restrict it,"[11] he wrote in the *New York Times*. Others noted that the way in which Norplant was developed—with a focus on limiting pregnancy, as opposed to making more complicated forms of reproductive autonomy the goal—undermined this claim. Author and law professor Dorothy Roberts became one of the most outspoken voices in favor of examining racial and class contexts of Norplant. In chronicling the launch of the contraceptive, Roberts notes, "What appeared to be an expensive contraceptive marketed to affluent women through private physicians soon became the focus of government programs for poor women. Lawmakers across the country have proposed and implemented schemes not only to make Norplant available to women on welfare but to pressure them to use the device as well."[12] These programs included offering free insertion—but not removal—of the device to low-income women and to teenagers predominantly in schools with low-income and nonwhite students. There were also reports of doctors pressuring patients to try the insert. Such "provider coercion" remained largely anecdotal,[13] but it further tarnished an already singed image, bringing Norplant closer to recall.

Many public health researchers pointed out that while concern about forced uses of the device "might well have served to reduce the magnitude of the problem by creating an atmosphere of vigilance,"[14] it also branded a potentially useful contraceptive. Researchers from Columbia University's Mailman School of Public Health conducted a study of two thousand low-income women, many of whom were using Norplant as their primary contraceptive. After conducting a series of interviews, they found that only three claimed to have been unduly pressured by physicians to undergo insertion.[15] While it is important to mention that this trial received some financial support from Wyeth Ayerst, the maker of the device, Jadelle, also called Norplant II, it is also worth recognizing a crucial point it makes: just because a poor woman chooses a long-acting contraceptive doesn't mean she was forced to do so. In fact, many studies indicate that women from diverse social and economic backgrounds were excited by the prospect of a new birth control option.

What the Columbia researchers failed to unpack were the reasons that long-acting contraceptives inspired such resistance and anger from many women, particularly in communities of color. Like it or not, a device that a woman cannot insert or remove herself and that renders her unable to conceive for several years, takes immediate agency over a woman's fertility out of her hands. The mere existence of such a method creates potential for abuse, and in America we have a documented history of using contraceptive technology in unjust and coercive ways. If women like Dorothy Roberts hadn't been so vocal in their criticisms of Norplant, it could very easily have taken up where forced sterilization left off. The very act of placing Norplant in the context of other technologies used as agents of social engineering probably prevented it from becoming one.

This is not to say that women aren't the losers when a birth control option is pulled from the market: indeed, greater contraceptive variety is a good thing for women, assuming they are given accurate safety information, and the removal of Norplant from the market narrowed an already slim field. Recognizing the potential for terrible mismanagement, however, is crucial to ensuring that such options remain in the service of individual women and not government bodies, empowered social groups, or even the medical community. The extent to which improper coercion went on behind physicians' doors remains unknown, but it does seem that a disproportionate number of young, nonwhite, and low-income women received the method during its short tenure.

The problems with Norplant had as much to do with rapid and under-informed marketing and with concerns about social pressures as it did with the unacceptability of the device for many women. It is hard to know what might have been if the time had been taken to properly train doctors, assess side effects, and educate patients.

But it was not to be, and Norplant became a pharmaceutical cautionary tale, a sort of "that's what you get" for other drugmakers already wary of contraceptive research and development. Hundreds of women experiencing various side effects filed lawsuits against Wyeth Ayerst—so many that other drugmakers dubbed the situation "Norplant Syndrome."[16] Even when a second-generation version of the device, Jadelle, also called Norplant II, was approved by the FDA in the late 1990s, manufacturers began to reconsider the advisability of marketing Norplant at all. In 2000, the rumblings became official, and Norplant was withdrawn from the market completely.

As Andrea Tone notes, the controversy highlighted an ongoing debate about "what defines the threshold between acceptable risk and product liability."[17] In other words, to what extent should a product maker ensure that a new product be risk-free, and to what extent are patients who seek new methods already agreeing to be part of an experiment? When are drug companies being irresponsible, and when are patients being unrealistic about the risks of contraception in general, and new birth control devices in particular? Barbara Seaman used to advise people not to "be the first kid on your block to take a new drug," but of course, if we are to have any knowledge about medicines, someone must eventually be willing to try them. Making sure that those who do aren't disproportionately low-income women or populations who have been disempowered in other ways is an important part of the project of responsibly developing new drugs. The decision to be part of a medical experiment can be a noble one, but it should always be a choice. The Norplant example shows that while institutionalized versions of this type of medical discrimination—such as the formal testing of the original birth control pill on poor Puerto Rican women—are far less common, less formal incarnations of this dynamic still make certain populations of women more vulnerable to the risks inherent in any new drug.[18] That said, women in all situations should be allowed to decide if they are willing to be at risk for certain dangers to receive certain benefits. Adults should have the option of taking a drug even if it carries risks as long as they are fully informed about their options and have true access to them.

Sadly, today, in part due to the Norplant fallout, drugmakers have retreated even further from contraceptive research. It was a mediocre drug that might have gotten better and which was still a welcome choice for many women. It was a potential health hazard whose rapid introduction and removal from the market ultimately means fewer birth control options, both because of its withdrawal and because of the limits it imposed on future contraceptive research.

Jadell, a later version of Norplant, is composed of two rods, both longer than the original Norplant's six. Each contains 75 mg of levonorgestrel, which is released in the body at a rate of 80 µg per day in the first month of use. This gradually reduces over time to 25 to 30 µg by the end of nine months. It can remain in the body up to five years. Although Jadell is approved in the United States, it has never been marketed here. It is available in other countries but is still relatively uncommon. There is no reason to believe that the side effects of the new device would be very different from those of the older one.[19]

The only implant currently available on the American market is

Implanon, a device that lasts for three years. It is made by Organon, a Dutch drugmaker that is now a division of European pharmaceutical giant Schering-Plough (currently in the process of merging with Merck). Organon also markets the contraceptive ring. Implanon was approved in the United States in 2006 after the Norplant debacle. It is made up of one 4 cm rod containing 68 mg of the progestin etonogestrel (also the progestin used in NuvaRing). It is inserted in the nondominant arm and is invisible when placed under the skin, though it can be felt by lightly pressing on the area over it. A doctor who has been trained by the device's manufacturer should insert it approximately five days after a menstrual bleed begins. It must be removed within three years or a patient is at higher risk for infertility or ectopic pregnancy.

The effectiveness of Implanon is on par with the Pill: less than one woman per hundred (.38) will become pregnant using it in the first year of use. Like oral contraceptives, it works by suppressing ovulation and changing cervical fluids. Implantation and removal are relatively simple; on average, it takes less than a minute to put it in and three and a half to five minutes to take it out.[20] A small group of women may experience more trouble with removal, either because the rod has become displaced or because it breaks while it is being taken out. Because it has only one rod, these problems are less likely to occur, but doctors can opt to use ultrasound to locate the device before attempting to remove it to minimize the likelihood of problems if they are anticipated[21] (meaning the doctor can already tell that the device isn't where it's supposed to be). While Implanon seems to be better than Norplant when it comes to insertion and removal, users still have some of the same problems with unpredictable bleeding.[22] Authors reviewing eleven clinical trials concluded, "Implanon use is associated with an unpredictable bleeding pattern which includes amenorrhea, frequent, and/or prolonged bleeding." So while you could have normal or lighter than normal bleeding with this method, you could also have either no bleeding or prolonged bleeding.[23] This side effect is the reason that 36 percent of women in clinical trials discontinued the method.[24] Other side effects are similar to the Pill: headaches (15.3 percent), weight gain (11.8 percent), acne (11.4 percent), breast pain (10.2 percent), mood changes (5.7 percent), and decreased libido (2.3 percent).[25] The manufacturers caution that few very overweight women were included in the trials of Implanon and efficacy for this group is uncertain.

Today, a patient can also choose Mirena, a hormonal IUD that many women's health activists argue is actually a contraceptive implant. Like Implanon, it is active for several years (in this case up to five years) and contains progestin only. Mirena, which I discussed at greater length alongside the copper IUD earlier, is most decidedly a hormonal method and an alternative distribution system with all the risks and benefits of these drugs.

Still Standing? Depo-Provera and Injectable Contraceptives

Elsimar Coutinho wasn't ready to go back to Brazil just yet. The young doctor had been enjoying an exciting fellowship in New York City through the Rockefeller Institute. Coutinho's adventures in the United States began in 1959, just as the Pill was spreading through the American market. Among other things, he met Dr. George Corner, one of the "discoverers" of progesterone, and worked with other bright lights in the field of hormone science.[26] Before going home, Coutinho visited Upjohn, the pharmaceutical company in Kalamazoo, Michigan, where he learned about a new progestin, medroxyprogesterone acetate (MPA). When he finally arrived back at his medical school in Bahia, he began working with this compound, testing its usefulness for the prevention of premature delivery or spontaneous abortion. To Coutinho's credit, he stuck with the evidence and admitted that the drug didn't prevent miscarriages, something that may have prevented another DES-style tragedy of dangerous fetal exposure to hormones. What he found during his trials, though, was that even six months after ceasing MPA injections, patients still hadn't started ovulating again. As he would note years later, "The study serendipitously led to the discovery of the first long-acting injectable contraceptive."[27]

The contraceptive shot, which came to be called Depo-Provera, would have a rocky road to approval in the United States. Unsuccessful attempts were made by Upjohn to bring the drug to market in 1973 and 1975. Women's health and consumer groups, such as Public Citizen, lobbied strongly against prematurely approving a drug that they felt had too many open health questions. Animal studies had shown higher cancer risks as well as slower than normal return to fertility after discontinuing use. Another deeply troubling feature of Depo-Provera was the fact that despite its health uncertainties, it had been tested on women in developing nations for ten years and low-income African American women in Atlanta, Georgia, for eleven.[28] These tests were conducted long before issues about the injection's potential to cause cancer, stroke, and permanent sterility had been resolved. In 1992 the FDA finally took the plunge and made Depo-Provera available to American women for birth control (it had been used off label for many years). It is currently available in more than eighty countries and has been used by over 90 million women.[29] Since 2005, a lower-dose subcutaneous[30] version, Depo-SubQ Provera, has also been available.

Women who opt for Depo-Provera receive an injection of 150 mg of MPA every three months at their health care provider's office, usually before the eighth day of a menstrual cycle. Pregnancy rates are low on Depo, with less than one pregnancy (.3) per hundred women in a year of use. Depo shares side effects and risks with the Pill, including a small increase in cancer risks. Like the Pill, Depo can cause headaches, skin changes, fluid retention, breast tenderness, and libido and mood changes. As with oral contraception, patients with migraines, cardiovascular complications, and trouble with depression should discuss with their doctor whether this contraceptive is the right choice for them.

Depo-Provera also comes with its own unique risks, which are thought to be due to the administration of excess progestin and not enough estrogen in the body or perhaps to the particular progestin used. The worst of these risks is that its use, particularly over long periods of time, leads to bone loss. While the reason for this isn't certain, it seems likely that it is the result of not having enough estrogen in the body working on the bones.[31] As evidence of this serious problem emerged in the years after approval, it prompted great concern. Young women, especially those still in their teens and early twenties, are a population particularly drawn to injectables because of both ease of use and the ease with which use can be concealed. This is also an age that is crucial for laying down bone mass to prevent skeletal problems, such as osteoporosis, later in life. As young women were opting for the shot in the hopes of hiding birth control use from parents, their own skin was concealing an equally distressing fact:

thinning bones. In November 2004 the FDA placed a "black box" warning on Depo. In an accompanying "talk paper," the agency noted that while the "contraceptive injection has been used as birth control for decades throughout the world and remains a safe and effective contraceptive," it was also becoming clear that "prolonged use of the drug may result in significant loss of bone density, and that the loss is greater the longer the drug is administered." They added ominously, "this bone density loss may not be completely reversible after discontinuation of the drug."[32] Because of this, the FDA warned in the black box that "Depo-Provera Contraceptive Injection/depo-subQ Provera should be used as a long-term birth control method (i.e., longer than two years) only if other birth control methods are inadequate."

Studies in teenage girls have shown bone loss in the hip, femoral neck, and lumbar spine[33]—areas of concern as women age (a hip fracture can be disabling and even fatal for an older person). The real fear is that as young girls fail to attain high bone mass at certain ages, it will put them at greater risk for serious fracture when they are postmenopausal (a time when bone thinning accelerates). It seems that while women experience more density loss during the first years of treatment, they lose more over time and are less likely to regain bone after many years of use. If you already have lowered bone density or osteoporosis, or if you have a family history of these conditions, it should inform your decision about using Depo-Provera. The same is true if you use other chemicals that can reduce bone mass, such as drinking excessively, smoking, or taking corticosteroids and anticonvulsant drugs.

In recent years, many doctors and health professionals have argued that the risk of Depo-Provera to bones has been overstated. The problem, these people explain, is that while no one is disputing that the drug causes loss of bone density,[34] what is up for debate is the recoverability of that mass. Some data suggests that information on bones isn't as bad as was originally feared, especially when it comes to building back bone after giving up Depo. According to these sources, the mass is regainable. A review article in the journal *Contraception* studied the bone mineral densities (BMD) of postmenopausal women after they had stopped using Depo, the BMD of premenopausal women after they had stopped, and the BMD of teenagers after they had stopped. The postmenopausal women had bone densities on par with nonusers and didn't have significantly increased fracture rates.[35] Both premenopausal women and teenagers showed partial to full recovery of losses after discontinuing use of Depo.[36]

While the FDA has recommended limiting use of Depo-Provera to two years, other organizations disagree.[37] The World Health Organization (which helped to develop the drug), the American Society for Adolescent Medicine, and the Society of Obstetricians and Gynecologists of Canada have argued that women between the ages of eighteen and forty-five should use the method for as long as they want, as long as they are counseled on maintaining good bone health (for example, getting calcium and vitamin D and engaging in weight-bearing exercise).

Much more research in this area is needed before a conclusion can be made, but it would be worthwhile to conduct more studies on whether women regain bone mass after going off the shots. It is distressing that so many health professionals continue to champion this method for teenagers and twenty-somethings while this very serious question remains unresolved. Women face dramatically different sets of choices that impact their readiness to engage in a certain method's set of risks, but it is hard to argue that if faced with equally effective methods (Depo and the Pill), women wouldn't choose the one with a better safety profile. Of course, studies show that teenagers don't always do very well with the Pill (let alone barriers). They forget to take it and get confused about accounting for missed pills, and they have trouble getting new packs. These realities of women's lives must figure into the balance.

This gets to the heart of some serious (and not easily answered) questions about what constitutes good contraceptive health. While pregnancy prevention is indeed an important outcome to consider, it must always be measured against other problems that may be equally serious. The problem with Depo is that the population who might want its distinct advantages—very young women—is the one most affected by one of its serious problems: bone loss. So while near perfect pregnancy prevention and less day-to-day responsibility in attaining it may be most important to a woman in her teens or early twenties, this is precisely the moment when her choice can be damaging.

With young women in particular, health care professionals have a tendency to set up an all-or-nothing scenario in which the risks of a contraceptive are cast favorably against the health problems that proliferate with pregnancy. This is a faulty comparison, since there are many available birth control methods to choose from. It is certainly true that teenagers are particularly vulnerable to the negative effects of unplanned pregnancy. But it is imperative to balance efforts to find reliable but side effect–prone contraceptives with efforts to empower young women to use healthier available methods correctly. If regular oral contraceptives prove less dangerous (yet more prone to user failure) than alternative distribution methods, then perhaps we should work to help young women use the Pill correctly rather than assuming educational efforts will get us nowhere and asking young women to bear the additional health burdens.

Other side effects that seem more pronounced in Depo-Provera than a typical combined oral contraceptive pill are irregular bleeding and weight gain. In a way, this injectable is the first menstrual suppression drug. Like later pills such as Seasonale, Depo-Provera creates unpredictable bleeding that resolves for many (but not all) patients with continued use. As with menstrual suppressants, most women will have some spotting or bleeding in the first month after receiving as injection, and many women (50 percent) will have breakthrough bleeding in early cycles. This declines during the first year of use, and after twenty-four months, 68 percent of women will have ceased to bleed.[38] With Depo-SubQ, more women continue to experience bleeding or spotting over the course of the first year of use. Like other menstrual suppressants, it is a good idea to take a pregnancy test each month to ensure that you aren't pregnant. While pregnancy is unlikely, continued exposure to hormones can harm a developing fetus, so it's good to be on the safe side.

Many women using Depo-Provera gain some weight on the drug.[39] Reports vary, but users probably put on an average of 5 pounds in their first year of use, and this amount goes up to 8 pounds after two years and 13.8 pounds after three years.[40] Weight gain with Depo-SubQ was slightly lower, but essentially the same.[41] Who is likely to gain weight remains an open question. Authors of one study note, "It is a concern that women who were not obese at the start of the study were twice as likely to become obese over the next three years if they selected DMPA over NH (non-hormonal) contraception."[42] Others believe obese women are more vulnerable to experience weight gain with this method, especially during the first year of use.[43] While scientists continue to explore which women will put on weight, they have found that those who do are increasing fat in the body, not just retaining fluids.[44] Women who switch to nonhormonal methods lose some of the weight, while those who switch to the Pill may continue to gain a very small amount.[45]

Women using Depo seem to gain more weight than those using other hormonal contraceptives, including traditional oral contraceptives and implants.[46] The latter is important because it seems to point to the particular progestin, rather than progestin-only contraception, as the cause of this particular problem. Since it remains difficult to predict who will have weight gain, researchers at the University of Texas argue that closely monitoring changes in pounds over the first six months of use can help to curtail this problem.[47]

It is possible that progestin-only contraception is better for women with cardiac problems, but more research is needed on this subject.[48] Most women take slightly longer to return to fertility after stopping their shots, and there have been anecdotal reports of permanent loss of ovulation,[49] but most women will resume fertility within ten months.[50] Because many of the problems associated with Depo-Provera are attributed, in one way or another, to progestin, there is some thought that adding estrogen to the injection might lessen some of its side effects. A 2008 *Cochrane Database of Systematic Reviews* review found that combination injectables had smaller rates of discontinuation of use due to side effects.[51] Estrogen/progestin combination shots might have the potential to mitigate the bone problem seen in the progestin-only formula, as well as improving irregular bleeding patterns, although this remains uncertain.

Another important thing to mention about MPA: it is part of a drug called Prempro that was included in the estrogen and progestin arm of the massive Women's Health Initiative trial. Prempro also contains Premarin, an equine estrogen not found in birth control pills. When the trial was prematurely halted in 2002, it was because patients taking Prempro had more heart attacks, breast cancer, strokes, pulmonary embolisms, and blood clots than women taking a placebo. The older age of the participants in the WHI trial undoubtedly makes a big difference in how hormones worked in their bodies, but the results of this valuable study raise a lot of questions about how our knowledge of hormone drugs is still evolving in profound ways.

Skin-Deep: The Contraceptive Patch and the Vaginal Ring

Twenty-first century alternative distribution methods have provided hope for drugmakers burned by the struggles of nearly thirty years of trying to develop nonpill hormonal contraceptives. Transdermal contraception and vaginal contraception require less patient adherence than "once-a-day" pills, and they are relatively expensive—and therefore profitable for drugmakers. Like Depo-Provera or Norplant, these devices don't require the patient to monitor them every day. Like the Pill, they must be replaced at significant cost each month. And unlike Depo-Provera or Implanon, patients apply and remove these methods themselves.

In the 1990s, the success of antismoking medicines popularized the idea that you could take pharmaceuticals through a skin patch. Ortho Evra, first approved by the FDA in 2002, is currently the only available transdermal contraceptive. With this method, a patient receives three patches each month. Starting no later than the fifth day of the menstrual cycle,[52] she applies one of the patches to her buttock, lower abdomen, upper arm, or upper torso (notably the breast is left out because of concerns about cancer). Studies have found no difference in the speed or concentration with which the hormones are absorbed based on where on the body the patch is placed.[53] The patch is made of three layers: a flesh-colored film that protects the chemical and adhesive parts, a sticky layer that also contains the active hormones (a total of 750 µg of ethinyl estradiol and 6,000 µg of norelgestromin, a progestin, with 20 µg of ethinyl estradiol and 150 µg of norelgestromin released daily),[54] and a backing that is removed before application.[55] This item is surprisingly resilient: the patch can be worn in the shower, swimming pool, and steam room. You can't douse it in lotion, and you must try to keep the area free from toiletries and cosmetic products, particularly those with oil bases. At the end of seven days, the patch is removed and another applied immediately in its place. The patch is left off every fourth week so that the patient has withdrawal bleeding, after which the cycle repeats again. It is very important to make sure that the patch stays on: hormones won't be properly absorbed in the body if the patch becomes partially or completely detached. Only about 5 percent of patches come loose,[56] but if this happens, replace it immediately. If you forget to switch your patch, it is reassuring to know that many doctors believe it is more forgiving of dosing errors that the Pill, so even if mistakes are made, you are less likely to get pregnant,[57] but obviously you shouldn't rely on this.

It is very common to have a skin reaction to the patch: one study found that 14 percent of women experienced this side effect,[58] while another suggested it might be as high as 20 percent.[59]

Transdermal contraception prevents pregnancy with about the same efficacy as the birth control pill, although recent studies suggest it may be slightly less effective in obese women.[60] Side effects are similar to those found with traditional OCs, but patch users have more breast tenderness (especially in the first months of use) and nausea.[61] On the positive side, patch users had less irregular bleeding than those on the Pill.[62] Even though women profess greater satisfaction with transdermal methods than with oral contraception, they tend to go off the patch just as often, and early discontinuation is higher.

After approval of the patch, hopes were high that it might prove safer than older hormonal alternatives. But it turns out that despite lower dosing, women absorb higher concentrations of estrogen with the patch than with the Pill—as much as 60 percent more. In the late fall of 2005, the FDA responded to this emerging information by issuing an update warning that using Ortho Evra could cause greater estrogen exposure and possibly more blood clots.[63] Two early studies found conflicting results: one concluded that use of the patch didn't actually increase blood clotting,[64] while another found that it caused a twofold increase in risk.[65] The first study, which found no increased risk, was conducted by the Boston Collaborative Drug Surveillance Program (BCDSP) in cooperation with Johnson & Johnson, the drugmaker. Despite the mixed results, the FDA changed Ortho Evra's label to let patients know that they might have a higher risk of blood clotting with the patch. In 2008, the FDA revised the label again when a later study by BCDSP also found more blood clots with Ortho Evra than with birth control pills.[66] All told, it is estimated that as many as forty women died between 2002 and 2006 using the patch before FDA labeling reflected an increased danger.[67]

Uncertainty about the patch has mounted since 2005, with prescriptions dropping from 9.9 million in 2004 to 2.7 million in 2007. The consumer advocacy group Public Citizen has petitioned the FDA to remove the device from the market, citing blood-clotting dangers. Sidney Wolfe, the tireless face of that organization, added fuel to the fire by noting that patient lawsuits led to the discovery of two unpublished studies from 2001 that indicate that the manufacturer, Johnson & Johnson, was aware of the clotting problem before the patch received an FDA green light.[68] The Web site for Ortho Evra now leads visitors to a stern warning about the possible side effects, and the future of the method is in many ways uncertain.[69]

As the patch struggles, the NuvaRing seems to be taking off. In my research I spoke to dozens of women who had used or were using the ring with varying degrees of satisfaction. The ring may have many of the same health concerns as the patch, but this remains to be shown as clearly in a laboratory. Because of this, despite individual reports of similar health problems, the ring has benefited from the patch's disgrace: it may be in this case that "no news is good news" for drugmakers and very dangerous for consumers.

A combined estrogen/progestin contraceptive, the vaginal ring is a small 54 mm round tube made of a polymer. Each month, a patient inserts the ring into the vagina and leaves it for three weeks. On the fourth week, the device is removed and a withdrawal bleed occurs. The ring has 11,700 µg of etonogestrel (a progestin) and 2,700 µg of ethinyl estradiol, which it releases at a constant rate of 120 µg of etonogestrel and 15 µg of ethinyl estradiol per day over the course of a cycle.[70] NuvaRing users may take out the ring for up to three hours for sex or other activities to prevent displacement.[71]

While more data is needed, research at this point holds that the ring doesn't cause more blood clotting than traditional pills. According to one study, patients who switched from the patch to the ring have improved markers for thrombosis, meaning they seem less disposed to get a blood clot.[72] Despite this, it is estimated that the FDA has had over three hundred reported serious events associated with (although not conclusively caused by) ring use, including strokes, blood clots, and even some deaths. In 2007, Jackie Bozicev, a thirty-two-year-old mother of a two-year-old son, collapsed after taking a shower.[73] She was rushed to the hospital where she was declared dead. An autopsy determined that the cause was a blood clot that traveled from her pelvic area to her lungs.[74] Bozicev's widower, Rob, also in his thirties, couldn't believe his young wife had suffered this fate and was even more shocked to learn that the cause of the clot might be her birth control. Reading this tragic story, it is hard not to remember the story of Julie Macauley, the young mother who died on the early Pill, told so movingly by Barbara Seaman in the original 1969 *The Doctors' Case Against the Pill*. It is harder still to believe that so many years later we are still relearning some of the same lessons of the dangers of the original Pill.

It isn't clear why either the patch or the ring might be less safe than pills. It could be because of the way the hormones are absorbed into the body or because they use third generation progestins that have been associated with greater clotting risk. While we wait for better information, over one hundred lawsuits claiming injury from the NuvaRing go forward,[75] and women continue to use the method, unaware that it may pose greater clotting risk.

Women deserve to have all the information before they make a choice that could come with increased health risks, but arguing that we should learn more about these dangers is not calling for the ring to be pulled from the market. One ring user told me just how well the device works for her. A twenty-something artist living in Brooklyn, Lin had always used pills but had never been able to take them as reliably as necessary. The result was two unplanned pregnancies followed by two abortions. A switch to the ring has given her a sense of control over her fertility and solved her problems with remembering to take the drug. For teenagers who need hormonal contraception that doesn't need to be taken every day, perhaps the ring provides a good alternative to Depo-Provera.

Ring users have less nausea, depression, and weight gain than pill users, but more breast tenderness. Local problems, such as vaginal infections, leukorrhea (thick discharge that can indicate problems in the vagina), and itching in the vaginal area are more common for ring users. Unlike a diaphragm, the ring doesn't need to be fitted to an individual or placed over the cervix. It can, however, fall out as a result of sex, tampon removal, or straining.[76] Most of the time, women are aware when this happens and can put the ring back in, but once in a while they aren't so lucky. One young graduate student from Washington, DC, shares her story: "I had a bad experience with the NuvaRing. I did not realize that it had fallen out. By the time I realized what had happened and switched to the Pill, it was too late to remedy the problem. This story ends in an abortion."[77] There are also very rare instances of the ring being displaced in the body; in one unusual instance, a twenty-five-year-old nurse put in her ring and experienced burning urinary symptoms within a day. At the end of the three-week period she went to remove the device, only to discover it wasn't there. An ultrasound revealed that the device was in her bladder and was the source of her urinary infection.[78] This sort of problem is exceedingly rare; expulsion of the ring is a far more common problem. Most women find the ring easy to both insert and remove.[79]

Bleeding on the ring, like the patch, seems to be more regular than what women experience on the traditional Pill,[80] although the data is confusing. Because some women use the ring "off label" for extended use—that is, for menstrual suppression—it is important to remember that irregular bleeding is a reality of hormonally eliminating monthly bleeds, regardless of the way in which you take those compounds. While the ring may cause predictable bleeding when you take it out for a monthly bleed, this isn't true when you are using the method continuously.

New methods can bring benefits, but they can also be unpredictable. Faye, a recently married woman in her thirties, switched to the ring five years ago. She had been with the man who is now her husband for several years and was having trouble on the Pill. Always the first of her friends to try something new, she decided to give the ring a try: "It was all right at first, but within two months it killed my sex drive. I mean killed it dead. I'd never just not wanted to have sex before, and I realized after a few months that the only thing different in my life was my birth control."[81] Faye went back to the Pill, despite other complications, and has found that things have returned to normal in the bedroom. Some studies show that women experience an increase in libido with the ring as compared to the Pill,[82] but when it comes to hormones and new ways of taking them in, everyone's body is different.

Some women—particularly younger folks—find that the ring can interfere with intercourse in a more immediate way. Some people's partners can feel the device during sex, and a smaller group found that they or their partners dislike the sensation. One study found that "interference with intercourse" was the main reason women gave for stating that they disliked the method.[83] This was less likely to be a problem in older women and with continued use of the method.

Looking to the Future

While, clinically speaking, much remains to be seen about the safety of these methods, new contraceptive products are always exciting. Even as we temper our enthusiasm for recent "innovations" by realizing that they carry both some of the old problems of hormonal contraceptives as well as their own distinctive issues and a lack of long-term safety data, each new product gives us the hope that it will be a better way to manage our fertility. I invite you to start asking some hard questions about contraceptive innovation. Why have there been so few truly new methods? And what possibilities exist in the future for making a product worthy of the adjective "novel"?

Women face the unfortunate reality that protecting our safety often comes at the cost of discouraging drug and device innovation. How can we strike a balance between making sure that patients aren't unnecessarily endangered by their birth control and ensuring that women have numerous and growing options? Finally, years of experience have taught us that trying something new usually means risking unanticipated side effects and dangers. Each woman must decide for herself the extent to which her need for something different outweighs her concerns about trying an untested method.

Chapter Five

Of Tides and Phases: Menstruation and Birth Control

Menstruation may not be important in itself, but it is highly symbolic of femaleness, and the ways in which people deal with it show us a lot about how women are viewed.
—Sophie Laws

It may seem obvious to suggest that any conversation about contraception should necessarily involve one about women's monthly hormonal cycle. After all, every birth control system, whether it involves popping a pill or charting your temperature, is based on understanding when and how ovulation happens and figuring out how to prevent conception.

Although we use the phrase "birth control," and certainly we hope our chosen methods *prevent* pregnancy, what we are really controlling and manipulating is the monthly menstrual cycle. A woman should understand *how* her method works, in the long term and short term, in addition to understanding *how well* it works. Your doctor can give you statistics about efficacy in ten minutes: for example, the Pill is 99.9 percent effective. But comprehensively knowing how and what the Pill does is a process that involves true body knowledge.

Our contraceptive choices are largely informed by the cultural ideas we internalize about periods at young ages and the bodily metaphors we become conversant in when we are practically children. Early in our lives, most women receive some sort of information about what goes on in our bodies each month that causes us to bleed. The information is usually more or less scientific, and we receive it when we are relatively young (somewhere between ages ten and fifteen). For most of us, it stops there, and we have little reason over the years to go back and refresh or complicate the very basic details we learned in middle school health class or perhaps from a parent.

We'll soon get into the reasons for the spectacular silence surrounding one of the most basic female bodily processes, but first, for those of us who are more than a few years from health class, let's remember together what makes up a monthly cycle.

When a female baby is born, she already has all the cells that will eventually become her eggs. This is different from men, who continuously produce new sperm throughout their lives. Women are born with all the necessary pieces to make a baby already in place in their bodies. In total, there are probably around 450,000 of these cells (although of course every person is different). That number decreases with age.

When a biologically female person begins to mature sexually, periods begin. It happens because enough hormones are running through the body to encourage the hypothalamus, a tiny gland in the brain, to begin a complicated chemical reaction that will eventually result in menstrual bleeding. Women are used to being told that perceptions about our bodies are "all in our heads," but in the case of menstruation, it really does begin "up here" rather than "down there."

The hypothalamus sits just above the brain stem and helps to coordinate bodily processes including hunger, thirst, libido, and sleepiness. At some point, it sends out a chemical message to the pituitary gland, a pea-sized protrusion immediately below the hypothalamus at the base of the brain. Like colleagues developing a new project together, the pituitary takes the initial idea sent by hypothalamus and expands on it, producing two chemicals, follicle-stimulating hormone (FSH) and leutinizing hormone (LH). At first the body makes much more FSH than LH. This hormone works on the ovarian follicles like water on seeds, causing several to begin sprouting—but only one will actually grow into a full-fledged egg. As the follicles grow and ripen, they release estrogen, which begins to thicken the lining of the uterus.

There are a lot of reasons for this thickening, including, of course, creating a space for a potential pregnancy. Rising estrogen levels cause other changes. First, they alter the cervical fluids (sometimes called cervical mucus), making them thicker and able to keep sperm alive for longer periods of time. Second, they send a message back to the hypothalamus, which, again in concert with the pituitary, leads to the release of a gush of LH.

Until this point, several follicles have been ripening and readying to make an egg. For reasons that aren't entirely understood, when the surge of LH reaches the ovaries, it causes one (and rarely, two) follicles to race ahead of the others and burst, producing an egg. The tiny egg will live only a short time—around twenty-four hours—and is carried along the fallopian tube by tiny hairlike projections called cilia.

During the egg's journey, and even after it has either been fertilized or died, the follicle it burst out of is still working. The ruptured follicle, now called a corpus luteum (yellow body), continues to manufacture estrogen and primarily progesterone. Progesterone functions both to protect a potential pregnancy and to let the body know not to produce any more eggs. It also raises the body temperature, which remains high until menstruation, and if you're controlling pregnancy with the fertility awareness method (which we'll talk more about soon), it lets you know that ovulation has occurred.

If fertilization and implantation don't happen, the arteries in the lining close off, preventing blood flow to its surface. The blood in the lining pools and gathers and eventually bursts forth, carrying the endometrial lining with it, and a woman gets her period. This generally occurs around fourteen days after a woman has ovulated.

The first thing you will notice about this description—something most women know from their own experience—is that the menstrual cycle is complex. It's a complicated, multifarious, and repeating process that affects how women feel every day of the month, not simply the days when we are bleeding. This is important for many reasons, but chief among them is that if a woman chooses to chemically alter her hormonal cycles, she is making the decision to change the way her body works on a daily basis.

Many girls are happy to get their first period, but feelings about the process change within a year or two. The novelty wanes when women realize they are stuck with monthly bleeding for the next four-odd decades. This transition from feeling pretty good to less positive about menstruation doesn't happen just on the basis of how our bodies change. From the very moment we learn that we will menstruate, different cultural voices are vying for our attentions, subtly shaping the way we see the experience. Without a doubt, the work of second-wave feminism has improved the social conversation around menstrual issues, but even educated women with access to good health information have a surprising lack of knowledge about how their body functions and an unwillingness to talk openly about their cycles. This silence begins with menstruation and extends into decisions about birth control and sexuality. Let's examine the roots of our complicated relationship with menstruation.

The Messy History of Menstrual Politics

For probably as long as women have been menstruating, people have been puzzling over why it happens and what it means. As Thomas Buckley and Alma Gottlieb explain, "This apparently ordinary biological event has been subject to extraordinary symbolic elaboration in a wide variety of cultures."[1] In Western society, the ancient Greeks applied their best minds to the task of unraveling the mysteries of the female body. They had some serious limitations: first and foremost, they didn't have access to actual human organs, since the dissection of corpses wasn't permitted.[2] Through their observation of animal organs and also the behavior of living women, the Greeks theorized that the uterus was a multicompartmental appendage with tentacles.

Even at this early point, the question of whether menstruation was healthy or destructive, either to women themselves or to the world around them, was a point of contention. Hippocrates, the legendary doctor whose work is still acknowledged through the oath recited by modern medical practitioners, believed in a system of health based around the four "humors," chemicals in the body that he imagined must be in balance to prevent illness. To this way of thinking, menstruation was a boon because, among other benefits, it got rid of bad humors and brought the body back to equilibrium. Aristotle, born shortly after Hippocrates's death, didn't believe bleeding was such a good thing. He believed that if you wanted to find the biggest difference between men and women, you needed to look to their hearts. It was from here, the great thinker reasoned, that blood fermented and bodily energy emanated.[3] Aristotle (and many after him) believed that semen and menstrual blood were equivalent fluids with one key difference: semen left the body with great energy, while menstrual blood flowed more passively. This happened, they argued, because women's souls have less energy than men's, and therefore menstrual blood was physical evidence of women's intellectual and spiritual inferiority. In other words, monthly bleeding was physical proof that men should be in charge.

By the era of the Roman Empire, many things had come a long way. Perceptions about periods had not. Pliny the Elder, a first-century geographer and naturalist, included his observations about menstruation in his classic thirty-seven volume work *Natural History*, in which he "describes menstrual blood as a deadly poison, which contaminates and decomposes urine, destroys the fertility of seeds, kills insects, withers crops, kills flower, rots fruit and blunts knives."[4] The idea that bleeding women could damage food sources has a certain cross-cultural currency, occurring in other incarnations throughout history and even to the present day.

Following the teachings of Hippocrates, the second-century Roman physician Galen believed that menstruation had a therapeutic effect. He reasoned that if bleeding could alleviate discomfort for women, perhaps it could do the same thing for men. In this way of seeing the world, women had a built-in mechanism for getting rid of "bad blood," but men needed some help from the lancet. Galen's work became the basis for centuries of bleeding to cure everything from the flu to bad moods. This approach was both negative and positive in the way it imagined menstruation: the blood itself was unhealthy to the body, but on the other hand, it was fortunate that it found a way out.

The ideas forged by classical civilization about men and women's bodies served as a base for medieval knowledge. The early fourteenth-century tract *The Secrets of Women* (*Secreta Mulierum*) perpetuated many folk beliefs, such as the likelihood that menstruating women could ruin mirrors, and built new metaphors to explain women's supposed dirtiness at "that time of month": "The uterus in women is like a toilet that stands in the middle of town and to which people go to defecate, just like all residues of the blood from all over the woman's body go to the uterus and are cleaned there."[5] Other problematic images of bleeding equated it with "disease," "cancer," and "venomous snakes."[6] Bettina Bildhauer argues that images of pollution, pathology, and uncontrollability were coupled with notions of secrecy to reinforce a certain set of gender relationships: simply put, menstruation was used as a primary means of keeping women in their place. The theme of locating gender difference, which emerged in both classical and medieval ideas about bleeding, continued through the centuries and is still with us today. It began with ideas about blood, and eventually shifted to notions about the uterus and later ovaries. Today it is alive and well in beliefs about hormones, mood, and health.

In the seventeenth and eighteenth centuries, ideas about bleeding were changing. Michael Stolberg explains that by 1600, the "'pathological' view of menstruation was a minority position amongst learned physicians."[7] Doctors and women continued to believe that the female body was full of toxins and poisons best eliminated by periods, but a competing approach, the "plethora" model, was gaining popularity. According to this viewpoint, it wasn't that women had too many bad substances in their bodies—it was that they had too many good ones. An excess of healthy blood had no less need for evacuation than a glut of toxic blood. The "iatrochemical" model rerationalized and essentially repackaged older ideas about bodily impurities and bleeding, again likening female genitals to "a gutter."[8] If earlier centuries had identified the problem of female bodies as residing in their fluids—poisonous blood—by the eighteenth century, doctors were beginning to believe that the real root of the trouble lay in female organs, namely, the uterus.

This cultural relocation of female weakness to the uterus famously continued through the nineteenth century and Victorian era. During this time, many trends emerged that continue to impact dialogue about women's health today. As Julie-Marie Strange explains, the shift in focus to the body coincided with "increasing professionalisation" of a medical community that "used its empirical claims to assert that science had proven, and could even improve, the laws of nature."[9] This represented a change from earlier practitioners who based their opinions about women's bodies on philosophical and even metaphysical considerations and served, among other things, to obfuscate the ways in which doctors were using the language of science to transmit social ideas (in this case, the mental inferiority of women and their lack of fitness for public life). One popular stream of logic went like this: the primary biological task of a female body is to carry and bear children. This requires that extra energy be directed to the reproductive system, energy that men can use for other purposes. Because of this, if a woman chooses to direct her energies to mental pursuits, she compromises her ability to perpetuate humanity and fulfill her "duties" as a female-bodied person. Doctors saw what they perceived as "mental instability" around menstruation as evidence for this: "Menstruation exposed the vulnerability of female mental health" with characteristics such as "exalted nerve tension" and bad temper.[10] (Significantly, this moment is the genesis of modern arguments about menstrual suppression. Strange writes that medical journals into the twentieth century argued "that if women behaved as nature intended, continual pregnancy and lactation would render menstruation almost obsolete."[11]) Underlying this interpretation is a belief that women's actions are based in their bodies and men's in their mental capacities.

Already this was complicated formulation: doctors argued that menstruation was a sign of failed pregnancy, but also that the lack of menses (amenorrhea) was a cause (or at least a by-product) of ill health that led to insanity.[12] British asylums in the late nineteenth century documented patients' menstrual irregularity and tied its normal resumption to mental recovery. Psychologist Anne E. Walker explains, "The normal functions of the uterus and ovaries were seen as the basis of 'normal' femininity, with abnormalities or dysfunction resulting in madness, hysteria, or physical illness."[13]

Change was again in the air as the century drew to a close. The idea that the uterus, as one physician wrote in 1870, was the base on which God built the rest of the female body,[14] was losing currency. By the beginning of the twentieth century many doctors had shifted their concern about female difference to the ovaries, a transition that would progress to hormones by the middle of the century. In an 1881 *Lancet* article Dr. James Totherick wrote, "One might heartily wish that the word hysteria were banished from our medical language, and indeed, so far as its etymological signification is concerned, from our thoughts."[15] (The ancient idea of hysteria has, of course, never completely gone away; for a modern example, one need look no further than a 2006 *New York Times* article proclaiming "Is Hysteria Real? Brain Imaging Says Yes."[16]) The important thing to notice here is that no matter what part of the female body is under scrutiny (menstruation, the uterus, the ovaries, or the hormones), there is always a part of women's natural functioning that some people will point to as the place where difference—and supposed female inferiority—comes from.

As the nineteenth century melted into the twentieth, feminist activists and an increasingly educated female population created their own response to paradigms that portrayed menstruation as mentally and physically debilitating. They rejected long-held notions such as the necessity of rest during periods. Groups such as the Medical Women's Federation rewrote menstrual language, aiming to normalize the experience, stressing activity, cleanliness, and self-control—an insistence designed to counter the idea that periods indicated women were "out of control" and needed a man to manage them. They argued that for many women, period-associated illness and disability were self-fulfilling prophecies. If young women were taught to participate in normal activities and not to see themselves as ill, they would develop good patterns that would lead to more educational and vocational opportunities. Programs of youth education were promoted, and mothers were encouraged to give their daughters "the facts" about menstruation.

As Strange points out, while this movement represented progress in many ways, it also discouraged women from telling their daughters about menstrual difficulties.[17] If they had terrible cramps, they should keep it to themselves so as not to distort their daughters' opinions about the normalcy of bleeding. This sort of selective silence and denial of menstrual realities became a distinguishing feature of how the new woman dealt with periods. As Sharra L. Vostral notes, if you could "pass" as your nonmenstruating self, then no one could tell you when you were and weren't able to fully function.[18] If you could foster the fantasy that you didn't bleed, then the fact that you did couldn't be used to mark you as different or disabled. It relied on notions about hygiene, self-control, and femininity that reinforced rather than dismantled gender roles. Like nineteenth-century feminists who opposed contraception and invested in widely held beliefs about female "moral superiority" to gain political power, women insisted that ladylike silence about periods was the only way to avoid having female power limited by them.

This push to send periods "into the closet" happened, not coincidentally, at the same time that menstrual product makers such as Kimberly-Clark (makers of Kotex) were creating and growing their industry and claiming authority to dictate cultural standards on menstrual etiquette. Marketing products that had been originally developed to bandage war wounds, pad makers successfully appropriated both the feminist language of freedom and the sexist anxieties about self-control and dirtiness of early century activists.

From the turn of the century through the 1940s, parents were a young girl's main source of education about menstruation. Journalist Karen Houppert explains that while periods weren't positively perceived—they were shrouded in a pink cloud of secrecy—there was a general cultural consensus that if maturing girls were to be protected from the dangers of their burgeoning sexuality, it would be by providing them with a good amount of information about their bodies. She writes, "Warnings . . . were used to persuade middle-class parents that they desperately needed to teach their daughters the facts of life if they were to prevent them from sexual experimentation. Today, of course, similar diatribes imply that young girls know *too* much."[19] An important point here is that conversations about menstruation were placed in opposition to discussions of sexuality. You had theoretical conversations about bleeding so that you wouldn't seek firsthand knowledge about sexual intercourse.

A 1915 manual called *Almost a Woman* describes respectable middle-class parents debating how to tell their prepubescent daughter the facts of life. The father of the family, Mr. Wayne, urges his wife to have the conversation sooner rather than later: "I beg of you not to postpone your instruction too long. I am more and more convinced that right knowledge not only safeguards purity, but really produces true modesty."[20]

If parents were responsible for transmitting information about periods, the source of this knowledge was already an "expert class." Houppert writes, "The popular interpretation of germ theory, the social hygiene movement, and the Progressive movement led to dozens of didactic pamphlets and self-help books sermonizing about why mothers should tell their daughters about menstruation and why they should tell them about it *this* way."[21]

The center of menstrual authority shifted seismically midcentury as the growing feminine product industry began to insist that they—not parents—should be the source of youth education. Tampon and pad manufacturers, who were gaining power in the early decades of the twentieth century, had decided by the 1950s to get into the sexual maturation information business in a big way. Establishing "education departments" that produced pamphlets and films, the major product makers positioned themselves to shape and dictate the narrative that young girls would receive about their bodies. There were multiple benefits for product makers in taking on this project. First, it allowed them to build brand loyalty to their products before a drop of blood had flowed onto panties. Second, in crafting a story about menstruation that insisted it was a process that called for secrecy, cleanliness, and a certain amount of shame, companies were able to generate the very concerns that would motivate women to consume and adhere to their brands. Girls, for example, were taught that menstrual management involved extreme discretion, and then pitched products that promised easy concealment.

A deep contradiction developed between the optimistic take-home message of initial menstrual education—"periods are normal and there's nothing wrong with you"—and the lived monthly experience of bleeding—"don't talk about it and don't let anyone know that it's happening." As Karen Houppert puts it, "To a young girl, if nobody talks about something like menstruation or sex in the real world, and yet she thinks about it, then she's convinced she's weird."[22] She adds that women "may be excited about getting their period before it happens, but when the reality sets in, with the one two punch of genuine inconvenience and manufactured embarrassment, they view things differently."[23]

As new ideas and industries emerged in the twentieth century, old beliefs about menstruation found new articulation in the language of science. In 1920, Bela Schick suggested that special bacterium, or "menotoxins," might lurk in otherwise seemingly innocuous discharge. If this were true, it would explain a host of controls on menstrual behavior; perhaps the blood *could* actually kill plants or poison food. While some scientists still hold a candle for this theory, as Buckley and Gottlieb point out, it was and remains "controversial at best."[24] Still, a small group of doctors and gynecologists continue to fear that menstrual blood is chemically dangerous. Dr. Nelson Soucasaux, a Brazilian gynecologist, hypothesizes that what were once referred to as "menotoxins" are, in fact, real biological compounds including prostaglandins (lipid compounds associated with muscle contraction and inflammation response) that are responsible for, among other things, PMS and menstrual discomfort.[25]

The persistence of beliefs that menstrual blood is somehow dirty or even toxic offers more ways of understanding its cultural significance. In the 1960s, anthropologist Mary Douglas published a highly influential work called *Purity and Danger*. In it she famously defined pollution as "matter out of place." In a very literal way, menstrual blood has often been perceived this way. We think of blood as something that stays inside the body unless we are injured. Instead, it leaves the containment of the body without trauma, a phenomenon with no equivalent in males.

For Sophie Laws, concerns about the dirtiness of periods are a more basic expression of a fear of difference: "The idea that people with certain characteristics are dirty is very often found as part of the attitudes of a dominant group towards a less powerful one. It is a persistent feature of racism and anti-Semitism as well as of misogyny."[26] She explains that dirt is equated with a lack of self-control, which always has the potential to threaten existing social relationships. By staying clean, women demonstrate cultural "compliance."

A powerful image of resistance to the performance of cleanliness is found in the writing of Inga Muscio. In *Cunt: A Declaration of Independence*, the author's funny, angry love letter to the female body, she paints vivid pictures of her efforts *not* to contain and manage her menstrual flow. She writes, "In the morning I walk around the house with my Blood towel wrapped around my waist. It catches the flow when I sit down. I use it to wipe the insides of my legs. Otherwise the blood splatters on my feet, floor. I step in it and get it everywhere. Sometimes I don't clean it up right away. Messy, messy. Fingerpaints in Kindergarten messy. I like to do this for a very good reason: Because I can!"[27]

Muscio's intention is, in part, to disrupt the systems of female control that are based in menstruation. One method of noncompliance is very literally to let the blood flow. Her book is eloquent in its reconfiguration of menstrual meanings and provides a concise queer response to the heteronormitivity inherent in the dominant culture surrounding periods. While most of us wouldn't be comfortable walking around in bloody clothes, it is worth taking the larger point and thinking about the ways in which even the most independent, confident women among us try to keep bleeding a secret, and how this concealment corrodes our power and self worth.

Twentieth-Century Legacies

For centuries, the absence of a doctor's presence signaled health. Today, it is very much the opposite, and we understand medical intervention in bodily processes as proactive insurance of enhanced wellness. We take statins to lower cholesterol and bisphosphonates to strengthen bones. There are antidepressants for mood and vitamins and supplements to ward off nutritional deficiencies. Since the twentieth century, all aspects of women's sexual and reproductive health have been subject to medical management, from periods to childbirth and, of course, menopause. That trend has ebbed and flowed under the criticism of social forces like the women's health movement, which critiqued gynecological practices and pharmaceutical interventions such as hormone replacement therapy and the Pill itself. Today, however, the forces urging medical and pharmaceutical intervention are as strong as ever. Women must decide if they believe, as some doctors have argued, that it is evolutionarily more "natural" *not* to menstruate, or if HT and ET with their proven risks are still better than enduring the menopause transition without drugs.

One reason that women have been ready to pop the pills or take the tests or undergo the procedures, both historically and currently, is that both the medical and pharmaceutical communities have tended to gloss bodily processes that are distinctly female as equivalent with illness. As I have shown, this is a tradition with a history as old as medical writing itself. In the nineteenth and for much of the twentieth century, women's complaints of pain and distress were often associated with mental illness; they were often counseled that it was mostly (if not entirely) in their heads. Their ovaries or hormones might be behind the mental illness, but it was mental nonetheless. The end of the twentieth and beginning of the twenty-first century have brought a near complete reversal of this approach, with doctors claiming that, in fact, every discomfort is real, indicative of sickness, and possibly ripe for drugs or surgeries. Both of these approaches betray a conspicuous lack of room for middle ground.

In the 1970s, the women's health movement worked to raise awareness of the ways in which healthy women's bodies were "medicalized," pointing out that female difference was interpreted by the still largely male medical establishment as signs of abnormality and illness. This groundbreaking perspective saved countless women from the dangers of badly tested drugs and unnecessary surgeries. The problem with it, of course, was that it didn't leave too much recourse or sympathy for women who were genuinely suffering and dealing with physical pain. To these women it seemed as if the feminist message was "buck up, pull up your socks, and get over it." Unfortunately for all women, there were drugmakers and doctors who were all too willing to provide a caring shoulder for those who felt ignored or disrespected by the antimedicalization camp. These industry forces were right to acknowledge women's discomfort and distress, but they were wrong to capitalize on it and answer it with dubious drugs and useless medical interventions.

The crux of the problem seems to be an insistence that female symptomatology is necessarily one way or another, entirely physical or purely sociological. The body and the mind are seen as separate entities. The mind is the terrain of culture, best studied by psychology and anthropology. The body is the domain of science and medicine. The problem with this way of seeing things is that it doesn't allow for the ways that culture (including medical and pharmaceutical culture) can create sickness, and indeed the ways that aspects of the body can generate attitudes and identities. It creates a world in which science and medicine can claim the authority of absolute truth.

As Margaret Lock, a Canadian anthropologist who has worked extensively on female life transitions, explains, "Until recently the individual body has been conceptualized as a universal biological base upon which culture plays its infinite variety."[28] In other words, bodies are all the same, and any difference can be understood as purely cultural. In this adversarial world, women's health activists were on one side of the debate, and the medical community on the other. The problem with this matchup, from a feminist perspective, is that if medical language insists that it is infallible and completely objective, it suggests by extension that activist arguments are based in subjective, unscientific, and emotional rationales.

Increasingly in the 1980s and 1990s, this hard and fast division was challenged. Anthropologists—often feminist—sought to highlight the fluidity between different fields of knowledge about human beings and bodies. Rejecting a traditional binary way of seeing the body, these new scholars argued for "biocultural" approaches, meaning a way of understanding physical phenomena (such as menstruation) that took into account both social and biological factors.

Lock, both a scholar and a feminist, took a leading role in this redefinition process. Deconstructing and rebuilding earlier arguments about medicalization, Lock points out that certain dichotomies—such as mind/body and nature/culture—that were previously thought to be antithetical are, in fact, integrated. She writes, "Social categories are literally inscribed on and into the body."[29] Imagined this way, illness and pain are real, but they are also heterogeneous experiences, the children of a complex conversation between physical sensations and the tools our cultures and societies provide us with to evaluate them. Pain is not determined by power relationships, but the way that we interpret pain is. The same thing is true of wellness: you may be healthy and overweight, but if you live in a culture that perceives excess pounds as signifiers of disease, you may not feel well. Given this, one of the great successes of medicalization is that it has successfully masked the role of social forces in defining illness and deciding who is sick.

Seeing Red: Cultures of Menstruation

Understanding the ways that menstruation has been represented, imagined, manipulated, and culturally deployed to maintain gender difference has been a major feminist project of the last three decades. This cross-disciplinary effort has worked to give women new ways of understanding their bodies and well-being. In the early days of second-wave feminism, this was a simpler task: people argued that periods had been negatively construed and harshly censored, mostly by men at the expense of women. Alternately, others insisted that our own "bad attitude" about periods was a cultural aberration, that women who were removed from these negative influences would naturally use bleeding as a locus of spirituality and empowerment.

The past decades have changed this argument, nuancing it and sometimes rejecting it outright. Understanding these changes and the way that we see periods today provides a gateway for asking larger questions about the choices we make about sexuality, social roles, and ultimately, birth control.

Most women are familiar with the idea that menstruation is a "taboo" subject. For us this word means forbidden or proscribed, but it actually has a more specific meaning in anthropology, having to do with supernaturally sanctioned laws. Before the language of science and medicine claimed ultimate authority to speak about how people and bodies should and shouldn't be, that kind of last word belonged to religion. With regard to periods, the term "taboo" is generally used to talk about various cultural practices that restrict or dictate female behavior during bleeding. Areas of study on this subject are too numerous to mention, running the gamut from African tribal restrictions on women entering the forest to cultures where women spend their menses in a communal hut to Jewish purity laws.

Historically, these taboos were seen as pure impositions of male power on female bodies. Men were afraid of women and their blood, so they controlled female behavior during menses. Thomas Buckley and Alma Gottlieb challenge more traditional notions of power dynamics in menstrual practice, arguing that women may have had more agency in the creation and maintenance of these rituals than previously imagined: "The possibility should not be ruled out that women themselves may have been responsible for originating the custom in many societies . . . There is also the possibility that such seclusion, when practiced, may sometimes in effect be voluntary, a cultural option to be exercised by women in their own interests rather than those of men."[30] Seen this way, women aren't victims of cultural strictures, but rather pragmatic participants in them.

If a woman lives, for example, in a culture that believes that bleeding women endanger crops, she can use this misconception to rest from work for a few days. This is a complicated sort of power: it relies on negative beliefs about female bodies, but it nonetheless confers a certain amount of agency on exactly the community it is seeking to control. An example in our society would be a teenage girl who wants to obtain birth control pills. She may be reluctant to reveal her intention to have sex to either her parents or medical practitioner, but she has other strategies at her disposal. If she chooses to access language that medicalizes her period—saying, for example, that her cramps are intolerable—she may receive the pills she desires. This is a very limited means of gaining agency; it relies on manipulating existing ideas and structures rather than trying to forge new ones.

Another very useful distinction that Buckley and Gottlieb make is to break menstrual beliefs into categories, observing that some assume that bleeding women are a danger to their communities, while others hold that they are a danger to themselves. In the first case, menstruation puts women in a position of power and in the other, a place of vulnerability. While American cultural conversations about menstruation are usually framed in terms of the former, medical approaches to periods tend to make use of the latter.

Premenstrual Syndrome is an interesting area of overlap between these two ways of understanding female power. Women experiencing PMS are problematic, according to stereotypes, because they pose dangers (or more likely inconveniences) to others: they readily express anger at partners and coworkers, feel empowered to reject work, and engage in "unfeminine" behavior. In general, they destabilize gender expectations and traditional social roles. Medical responses, while acknowledging these concerns, also play on patient fears that they may "harm" themselves if they don't pharmaceutically address their hormonal flux. Among other problems, medical accounts of PMS list depression as a major manifestation of the ailment, which can be managed with drugs ranging from antidepressants to birth control pills.

One example of this that held bigger lessons for all pharmaceutical consumers was the transformation of the antidepressant Prozac into the menstrual drug Sarafem. This story involves not only the smart rebranding of an aging and familiar pill, but the whole-cloth creation of an illness limited to the female population.

By the late 1990s, drug giant Eli Lilly was about to lose its patent on the blockbuster antidepressant Prozac. That means that the drug could be sold under its chemical name—fluoxetine—by other companies for less money. This represented a significant financial loss for the company, and to prevent this, they did some quick thinking. In 1998, Lilly hosted a roundtable of experts to discuss whether or not some women with particular symptoms during PMS actually had a disease.[31] The panel included sixteen key experts, representatives from the FDA, and people from Lilly. The panel concluded that a disease dubbed "Premenstrual Disphoric Disorder" (PMDD) did exist and that Prozac could be used to treat it. By December of 1999, Lilly had FDA approval to market their drug for this purpose.

Lilly surprised everyone when they decided to completely rebrand the drug. Turning the pill pink and purple, they gave it a pretty, feminine new name—"Sarafem"—and embarked on a campaign to educate women not only about the pill, but about the disease itself. Because they had essentially created PMDD, women didn't know they should be taking medication to treat it. Sarafem was chemically identical to Prozac, but after the latter became available generically and dropped in price, Sarafem was a lot more expensive.

What happened here makes important points about drug marketing, but also about cultural perceptions of PMS. Saying that Lilly and experts receiving money from that company "invented" PMDD does not mean that many women don't suffer from debilitating PMS. Indeed some— although not most—women do struggle with more severe and disruptive monthly symptoms. The problem is that the "disease" was designed to fit a drug that already existed. By organizing the right symptoms and giving them a name, pharmaceutical makers also designed the cultural response to their new health problem. The pains, mood swings, and other symptoms that women experience are physical realities; the ways that Lilly and their experts train women to identify, understand, and respond to the problems are subjective and cultural.

This situation is particularly dangerous because the line between normal premenstrual symptoms and those severe enough to warrant pharmaceutical treatment are blurry. It isn't like performing a test for strep throat. This lack of clarity has made it easy to suggest that healthy women would benefit from chemical management of normal monthly hormonal fluctuations.

This suggestion is not inconsistent with a culture that locates female difference (always already only a step away from disease) in PMS and menstruation. Instead of working to identify and address sexual and gender injustices, cultural conventional wisdom points the finger at women's bodies. The problem isn't a social system that privileges men over women; it is a pathological physical difference that can be treated with drugs.

Author Sophie Laws feels that the concept of taboo inaccurately describes modern Western ways of dealing with periods, preferring the idea that periods are ruled by etiquette. She points out that the rules we make—and break—today surrounding menstruation don't have to do with religion or the supernatural, but rather with social considerations. She defines etiquette as "rules of behavior governing social relations among people of distinct social statuses or classes,"[32] and explains that etiquette works to maintain established roles by wielding the threat of social punishment. In other words, it is a way of behaving that both defines and maintains power relationships.

So what are the "rules" we follow when it comes to bleedings? For one thing, we are secretive about the process. Women go to great lengths to conceal menstrual products, especially after use. As discussed earlier, this is in part an effort to appear to the world as nonmenstruators. This silence extends to menstrual advertising, which never shows images of blood, opting instead for white, clean motifs and mysterious blue liquids. It also extends to everyday conversation. Laws notes that one of the most important pieces of etiquette involves who can and can't initiate conversations about menstruation. Men are allowed to do so publicly, making jokes or other references to the process, but female speech on the subject is considered inappropriate except in the context of intimate relationships and same-sex environments. The fact that the most acceptable way to talk about periods in a co-ed setting is in the context of jokes and statements rife with gender kitsch is because these forms of speech reinforce traditional ideas about men and women; they don't, in other words, threaten established power relationships between the sexes. The fact that men are the ones with the authority to initiate that speech further drives home the message that even when it comes to this indisputably female subject, they are still in charge.

The entire relational dynamic of menstruation functions, in Laws's opinion, to "emphasize an image of women's lives as circumscribed by men's gaze."[33] In other words, the way that men and women relate to each other on this subject functions to remind women that male priorities and desires dictate many aspects of their lives. When bleeding, women are constantly aware of themselves and of the men around them, and by extension, of the terms of their relationships to these men: "Orientation to others, to one's appearance rather than one's own feelings, are of the essence."[34] How we make others feel becomes more important than how we feel. Laws is more explicit: "My view is that menstruation is used in our culture as the basis, the excuse, for a flexible and changing set of ideas and practices which reinforce men's power over women."[35]

Our cultural silence about menstruation is not only psychologically stifling, it can be dangerous, too. Karen Houppert, a former staff writer for the *Village Voice*, became publicly interested in menstruation for the first time when she went out to buy tampons. She discovered that Tambrands—one of the largest manufacturers of tampons at the time—had both raised the price of their product and reduced the number of tampons in a box by nearly a fourth.

Houppert's frustration with the menstrual hygiene industry's profits— an approximately two-billion-dollar-a-year[36] behemoth that holds women worldwide hostage to its whims—grew into greater concerns about product safety and social perspectives. In 1995, she penned a *Village Voice* article called "Embarrassed to Death: The Hidden Dangers of the Tampon Industry" in which she argued that culturally enforced silence about all things bloody was putting women at risk by allowing the menstrual product industry to operate relatively unscrutinized. Women were so eager not to engage publicly with the subject of periods that crucial safety concerns were going unaddressed.

While the content of Houppert's article was certainly controversial, the part of the piece that really got tempers flaring was the cover. "The picture," she says, "looked like any of a dozen provocative ads for skin creams, perfumes or health clubs: a woman's sexy lower torso in profile, smooth thighs and pert butt alluringly displayed. But here, peeking out from between the woman's thighs, was a tampon string." Not surprisingly, Houppert notes, "people freaked . . . They couldn't get past the cover to the article inside."[37]

The reaction to Houppert's article functioned as literal proof of its content: important issues that affect the lives of most women could not be considered because the cultural imperative that menstruation remain invisible and private was too strong.

Breaking the Silence

I believe that both the enforced silence surrounding menstruation and the twentieth-century pressure women feel to pass as nonmenstruators have huge ramifications for choices about birth control. Just as menstrual concealment produces a fantasy of bloodless womanhood, so hormonal birth control creates a cultural fiction of contraception without cost. Given the wide array of health problems and side effects associated with the treatments, these methods are in actuality free of repercussions only for men. Just as pads and tampons conceal blood, so the female body contains the real tolls exacted by hormonal contraceptives.

It is important to note that young women learn about birth control even as they are being inducted into proper menstrual behavior. Although sex and menstruation aren't necessarily related, cultural messages regarding the two are often concordant. One of the many ways that culture, menstruation, and birth control come together is over the issue of teen sexuality. It has been well documented that average age at menarche—that is, the age at which a woman gets her first period—has been dropping over the past century. This may be for a number of reasons, including improved nutrition and greater exposure to environmental hormones and toxins. In 1976, physical development expert J. M. Tanner published an influential report in which he argued that the age at menarche was dropping by four months per decade. This otherwise unsensational report collided with growing cultural concern about adolescent sexuality and contributed to a rash of near hysterical newspaper headlines in various national publications.

Of course while menarche signals the ability to conceive children, it does not imply sexual activity. All of these breathless 1970s accounts of nubile preteens assumed a metaphorical alignment between menstruation and sex. The fact that the presence of a period indicates the absence of a pregnancy didn't seem to make a dent in the argument: earlier periods meant earlier intercourse and more unwanted teen pregnancies.

Research on early adolescence again reared its head in the popular media in 1991 in a *Newsweek* article called "The End of Innocence." While much had changed in American life, the article was remarkably similar to the ones published a decade and a half before. Both single and working mothers, those popular media villains, were implicated in pubescent precocity, along with some new culprits, such as the rise of HIV/AIDS. The language of the article is telling, noting that early periods and absent parents have combined to cause a "breakdown of authority."[38] If we dig into this, we see that several connections and analogies are being drawn: the "breakdown" of the womb lining and the "breakdown" of the traditional family, premature bleeding and premature sex, and ultimately, the presence of menstrual bleeding and a threatened social order.

Emily Martin argues that words like "breakdown" are themselves indicative of how we view the processes of the female body. She points out that looking at the values of words in scientific writings betrays the not-so-objective agendas that sometimes underpin them: "unacknowledged cultural attitudes can seep into scientific writing through evaluative words."[39] Other authors concur with this, noting, "even today, menstruation is a sad story, depicted in the literature as 'disintegration,' 'decay,' 'shrinking,' 'shedding,' 'discharge,' 'dribbling,' and 'sloughing.'"[40] By opting to use words that portray this biological process in pathological terms, doctors often indirectly suggest that menstruation is disease.

Metaphors matter, too, and the female body is often described using images of failed production, a factory that has failed to perform its job. This suggests that a woman's biological purpose is the production of a child, and a period constitutes a missed opportunity. This reflects on society's definition of the purpose of a female body, a purpose that is seen very differently depending on whether that body is rich or poor, white or black, young or old. Women themselves adopt this sort of language to describe their menstrual experiences—particularly with regard to PMS—favoring images of disembodiment and passivity, saying that they don't "feel like themselves" or are "out of control."

And we want to things to be in our control. The experiences that make us feel otherwise contribute negatively to our lives and health. Perhaps without denying the very real physical and emotional pain that women—myself included—often experience, it is possible to suggest that part of the reason women feel "sick" with menstruation is a result of the deeply ingrained notion that periods are evidence of our inability to be autonomous and functional. We know that's not true: we are great at our jobs, at managing our lives, at balancing an impressive array of commitments, roles, and tasks. We also know that as women we have to work a little harder to achieve all this—we constantly have to prove ourselves. But we convince ourselves that we are in charge. Then, once a month, we are reminded that we aren't free of inequality, that our identities, accomplishments, opportunities, and ways of relating to other people are constantly mediated by social forces. We want to prove society wrong, we want to be powerful and accountable only to ourselves, we want to be spotless.

In *The Female Thing*, cultural critic Laura Kipnis's acerbic, funny treatise on feminism and femininity, the obsession with menstrual management is tied to a larger female anxiety about dirt. It's not just blood we feel responsible for cleaning—it's houses, our faces, even our relationships. Any visible blemish on ourselves, our homes, our lives seems to be begging for a good scrub. Kipnis writes, "If women didn't menstruate . . . would the cleaning imperative have taken hold a little less successfully, and be abandoned with a little more alacrity? If women didn't have vaginas, would we take fewer bubble baths, be less susceptible to the newest miracle cleaning product's marketing campaign, let up on the cleaning standards . . . and simply not do more than 50 percent of the housework?"[41] At least for the time being, she concludes, we will wrestle with these questions. "Cleaning house, cleaning up society, cleaning up sex, scrubbing away at those unsightly nose pores: housekeeping of one sort or another remains a plight."[42] When it comes to sex—an act closely aligned throughout history with dirt—the cultural messages about cleanliness are at their loudest. No wonder, then, that so many modern women are happy to take the responsibility for contraception if it means sex without the mess of latex and spermicide and mutual responsibility. How much easier it is to let the cost of managing the potential messes of unchecked intercourse run quietly through our veins. And if sex and blood are two of the biggest points of anxiety and difference for women, it is easy to see the allure of a drug that promises to control both.

Chapter Six

Spotless: Questions and Controversies with New Menstrual Suppression Drugs

Science may be working rapidly to perfect the human body, but it is certainly not in the image of woman.

—Kathleen O'Grady

It wasn't a real advertisement, but it could have been. Smartly dressed women worked and frolicked and practiced yoga as a soothing voice-over asked, "What if you could have your period just once a year?"

"Once a year?" enthused a professionally dressed brunette. "I'd like that!"

The spoof was a *Saturday Night Live* sketch, a fake commercial for a mythical menstrual suppression drug called Annuale. While some of the ad was over the top—a written warning at the end cautioned "do not take Annuale if you plan to ever become pregnant, as it may turn your baby into a fire monster"—the most striking part of the parody was how little exaggeration was required to make a point about the way that pharmaceutical companies use direct-to-consumer advertising to entice and manipulate female consumers.

The fictional pill offered continuous hormones for forty-four weeks. As most women have become aware, real pills promising fewer or eliminated periods have become a prominent feature in the contraceptive landscape over the past decade. Far from being completely outlandish, Annuale would actually constitute a middle ground between Seasonale and Seasonique, two products that cut bleeding to four cycles a year, and Lybrel, a drug that completely eliminates withdrawal bleeding.

For many women who deal monthly with pain, mood instability, and the general hassles of managing menstrual blood, the possibility of living without periods holds tremendous appeal. Women reason that if bleeding has historically been a marker of female difference, an excuse to keep women out of the schools and professions into which they desire entry, perhaps getting rid of it altogether really is the next step in the continuing battle for female equality.

As with every new and potentially profitable pill, menstrual suppression drugs entered the public consciousness armed with powerful scientific and medical rationales. The most provocative was that menstruation itself was unnatural and avoiding it through a constant regimen of pharmaceutical hormones would bring you closer to an evolutionary ideal. Our prehistoric ancestors, argued pill advocates, lived in a state of near constant gestation and lactation during their reproductive years and would have had little opportunity to bleed. Some doctors also suggested that eliminating the period would be a great way to curtail health problems ranging from premenstrual syndrome to anemia, as well as reducing the risk of certain cancers.

Many women, however, were unconvinced. They didn't really mind getting their periods each month, and felt that the experience, however inconvenient or unpleasant, connected them to other women in a fundamental way. Some felt that there was something strange and distinctly unnatural about stopping bleeds, even if they couldn't explain why they felt this way. Quickly, women's health activists and patient advocates took on the role of "loyal opposition," pointing out that arguments for menstrual suppression played on old ideas about the dirtiness of menstruation, the abnormality of healthy female bodies, and the supposed psychological and emotional burdens of monthly hormones.

Can this "new" contraceptive method really transform women's lives in a positive way? What are the unique risks and open questions associated with continuous hormone regimens, and how can we understand the cultural conversations that impact how scientific data about them is presented?

John Rock vs. Elsimar Coutinho: A Brief History of Menstrual Suppression

The storm had been brewing since before the Pill was legalized, but it was Brazilian doctor Elsimar Coutinho who tossed the first lightning bolts. In 1999, Coutinho, a longtime researcher of contraceptive methods and one of the fathers of the injectable progestin Depo-Provera, partnered with Population Council scientist Sheldon Segal to publish *Is Menstruation Obsolete?* This slender volume argues that using and developing available hormonal contraceptives for the purpose of preventing periods would offer multiple boons, including disease prevention and improved job performance.

The book set off a firestorm, polarizing medical and cultural opinion. For some, Coutinho's work was a revelation and a testament to the promise of modern gynecological science. Contemporary medical technologies could be wed to our evolutionary needs and open up new possibilities for women's lives. For others, it was sexist medical logic taken to the extreme, attacking one of the most intrinsic processes of the female body. The only marriage here, opponents insisted, was between old ideas about women's bodies and new drug company interests.

The idea of menstrual suppression—using technology to block periods—was not a new one. Indeed, doctors have possessed the tools to help patients stop monthly bleeding since the legalization of hormonal contraception fifty years ago. Each pack of birth control pills contains a certain number of active pills—generally twenty-one—and a smaller number of sugar pills—usually seven. For decades it has been common knowledge in the halls of college dormitories that if you wanted to skip your period, all you had to do was throw out the sugar pills and skip directly to the next active one.

As we have learned, the bleeding that occurs at the end of the active pills is not the same as natural menstruation. Proponents of menstrual suppression are quick to point out that withdrawal bleeding, essentially a chemically induced period, happens when the progesterone that has been flooding the body stops abruptly.[1] While it has many similarities with a natural bleed, it is fundamentally different.

So if withdrawal bleeding isn't the same as a real period, why do pill packs contain the seven sugar pills? John Rock, that dapper, pious architect of the Pill, wanted to cast his contraceptive drug in biological terms that his church could understand—he wanted to present the Pill cycle as "natural." A loyal Catholic, Rock believed he understood how to build and explain a drug that would override church objections to birth control.

Malcolm Gladwell writes, "In 1951 . . . Pope Pius XII had sanctioned the rhythm method for Catholics because he deemed it a 'natural' method of regulating procreation: it didn't kill sperm, like a spermicide, or frustrate the normal process of procreation, like a diaphragm, or mutilate the organs, like sterilization."[2] It was easy to argue that estrogen and progesterone were "natural"—the body made these hormones (forget for a moment that the ones used in the Pill were made in a laboratory). For couples using the rhythm method, progesterone produced a "safe" period; Rock reasoned that his pill worked the same way but extended that safe time to the entire month. It was an adjunct to, not a substitute for, a natural contraceptive method. The pope was initially persuaded by this logic and offered tentative approval in 1958 for Catholic women who suffered from dysmenorrhea and uterine problems. As Gladwell notes, "If Rock wanted to demonstrate that the Pill was no more than a natural variant of the rhythm method, he couldn't very well do away with the monthly menses. Rhythm required 'regularity,' and so the Pill had to produce regularity as well."[3]

So for the sake of consistency, Rock convinced Gregory Pincus, the Pill's co-parent, that despite the fact that bleeding could be completely prevented by continuous hormone use, it shouldn't be. Instead, a week of placebo pills would be included to emulate the body's natural cycle. It was an imitation of life, but a symbolically powerful one. Rock felt it would keep the drug in the good graces of the church, and besides, he reasoned, it would create greater psychological comfort for new female patients who would already be dealing with so much change. Having a period, even a chemically induced one, would provide a measure of normalcy.

Imagine John Rock's heartbreak when after so much chemical and rhetorical maneuvering a new pope ultimately rejected his brainchild: in an official 1968 letter entitled "Humanae Vitae," Paul VI officially banned oral contraceptives, deeming them "artificial."

To the minds of many advocates of menstrual suppression, the withdrawal bleed is a relic of a time when science had to bend to the cloth, when appearances trumped good sense. Paul Blumenthal, a professor of obstetrics and gynecology at Stanford University School of Medicine explains, "The fact that birth control pills were prescribed as monthly cycles for all these years is the reflection of what someone thought women would want as opposed to what was physiologically necessary."[4]

Many scientists never gave up the idea that women need not go through a week of pads and tampons if they were already taking the Pill. Elsimar Coutinho came to New York in 1959 as a guest investigator at Rockefeller University for Medical Research. It was a heady time in hormone research, and Coutinho had the chance to work with some of the men who had made the Pill possible. He also met Sheldon Segal, an endocrinologist who helped the young doctor begin framing his ideas about the potential of hormonal contraception. Coutinho returned to Brazil but not before beginning work on a new progesterone, medroxyprogesterone acetate (MPA)—Depo-Provera—which Upjohn, the pharmaceutical company, hoped would help prevent late-term miscarriages. While clinical trials proved the drug ineffective for that objective, the doctor found that his progesterone had a powerful effect on ovulation. This research led Coutinho to develop Depo-Provera as the "first long-acting injectable contraceptive,"[5] a treatment that had the unintentional side effect of reducing and even eliminating menstruation.

In 1976, a British veterinarian named R. V. Short published an influential essay, "The Evolution of Human Reproduction."[6] He argued that continual menstruation is a by-product of modern life rather than a natural evolutionary event. This perspective was based, among other factors, on the lack of menstruation in other nonhuman primates and on the much more limited menstruation of women in particular "primitive" societies. The conclusion was clear to Short: perpetual periods were not, evolutionarily speaking, the biological rule. And the problems they caused, including increased cancer risks, anemia, and premenstrual syndrome, "highlighted the importance of developing a non-steroidal contraceptive that would allow a woman to return to the reproductive state that was the norm for our primitive ancestors—amenorrhea."[7]

Short's ideas also grew out of his beliefs about population control. The 1960s and 1970s saw a growth of political concern about the potential ramifications of third world population growth. In a 1972 essay Short wrote, "Many economists have predicted that the rich nations of the world are destined to grow richer at the expense of the poor nations, who are doomed to become poorer. It seems doubtful that mankind could survive the ensuing racial and national tensions if there was to be an increasing polarization between the haves and the have-nots."[8] His solution to this impending international class war: simply reduce high birth rates in poor countries. In light of this, the argument in favor of curtailing menstruation with hormones for the benefit of preventing anemia and other nutritional problems in women in non-Western nations takes on new significance.

Medically, Short relied heavily on the work of Dr. Katharina Dalton, particularly with regard to PMS and its potential to encourage crime and antisocial behavior in women. Although women have experienced some premenstrual complaints, including variable moods, for thousands of years, it was Dalton who gave the set of symptoms a name in 1953. This British doctor worked tirelessly for decades to publicize the condition that she christened, and in addition to opening a clinic, she penned the popular handbook *Once a Month* in 1978. The book drips with overheated descriptions of hormone-crazed women wreaking havoc; Karen Houppert writes that it "reads as if hordes of angry women are ripping at our social fabric with bared teeth."[9] Although revered by some, Dalton has been broadly criticized for questionable methodologies and bad science: "The problems with Dalton's research are numerous, ranging from a lack of control groups to the use of non-representative samples to unjustified conclusions to unwarranted universalizations."[10]

However dubious the political underpinnings of Short's work and however shaky the science, his conclusions about menstruation and evolution were popular. Among the mainstream gynecological opinion makers to take up his theories were the editors of *Williams Obstetrics*, a leading gynecological textbook. Zahra Meghani notes that the book characterizes bleeding as "an inherent hormonal disorder." She adds that the "implication is that menstrual suppressant contraceptives ought to be used as 'treatment' for all females of childbearing age, barring those contemplating pregnancy."[11]

By the 1980s, drugmakers still had not capitalized on a potential market for period suppression (and even Depo-Provera would not be approved in the United States for another decade). In part, this was because research suggested that women did not want to get rid of periods. A 1983 World Health Organization study that looked at female populations in ten nations found that despite common menstrual complaints and negative cultural perceptions of bleeding, women perceived the event as natural and had no desire to suppress it.

Elsimar Coutinho believed this was because women harbored misperceptions of the event—they still believed, as classical thinkers did, that it freed the body from toxins. Others felt it served as a signifier of femininity and youth. To the doctor's mind, periods served few positive purposes and caused many problems. It was a desire to correct "mistaken" beliefs that led to the publication of Coutinho's influential book *Is Menstruation Obsolete?*

Written in Blood: The Case against Bleeding

In *Is Menstruation Obsolete?* Coutinho and Segal start from Short's evolutionary argument against periods and expand it with additional medical and cultural justifications.

The most controversial and powerful claim remains, of course, that menstruation is somehow fundamentally unnatural. Prehistoric women, the book argues, would have had few, if any, menstrual periods. This was for two reasons. First, those ancient females would have been perpetually pregnant and lactating (which provides some natural prevention of periods). Second, when they weren't busy birthing and breastfeeding, our ancestors were on the move. They were walking and gathering and eating a lot less food than us, all factors that could have contributed to a level of body fat low enough to prevent menstruation. Today, our stagnant, infertile, modern lives have made our bodies behave in ways that nature and evolution never intended. Segal writes, "It has also not escaped scientific attention over the years that modern woman, endowed with essentially the same gene pool as her Stone Age ancestors, has a totally different reproductive pattern."[12]

While certainly it is true that women had more babies before the advent of reliable, readily available birth control, it is always valuable to be skeptical of scientific claims based on imagined but unprovable histories. Canadian health activist Kathleen O'Grady writes, "There are questions concerning the accuracy of Coutinho's perpetually pregnant ancient woman. We have little evidence to pronounce conclusively that women rarely menstruated in the past. Rather we have ample evidence to suppose that women were regularly practicing birth control methods (and hence menstruating) in countless cultures."[13]

The prehistoric woman is a favorite character in any scientific or political rationale that seeks to establish something "natural" about women's bodies. This happens, at least in part, because of her relative evolutionary proximity to the animal world and her lack of surviving cultural artifacts. There are, of course, already logical flaws in this theory: first, it assumes that animals lack culture; and second, it assumes that just because evidence of culture as exemplified by surviving artifacts does not exist now, it never did. In fact, it is the lack of hard evidence about ancient peoples that makes them particularly useful for promoting social agendas about how bodies should be and what they should do. We can easily imagine these distant ancestors across the hazy imprecision of time; they must certainly have been closer to some imagined origin where humans lived totally as nature intended.

What evidence we do have supports the notion that prehistoric women lived with culture differently, but just as surely, as we do. In her essay *Childbirth in Prehistory: An Introduction*, archeologist Elisabeth Beausang refutes Coutinho's claim that childless women were without exception infertile; to this group she adds women who were "socially excluded from the possibility" and "women who for some reason choose not to give birth." She writes, "The fact that the biological variables can and are manipulated and modified by cultural practices and circumstances has to be acknowledged as a possibility even for prehistoric times."[14] In other words, while they lacked our technologies for pregnancy prevention, they still had the ability to make choices to have or not have sex at certain times, and perhaps to not have sex at all. Women had fewer choices, but they did not completely lack agency.

Perhaps this is the crux of the issue: whenever ancient woman is imagined, she is seen as powerless, completely subject to the harsh controls of the natural world and of the men in her community. It is from this "ideal" that doctors and cultural critics build an idea of what women (and men) should want and how they can make choices about their bodies. Referring back to the arguments of Margaret Lock, we can see that a popular belief in a strict nature/culture binary is easily exploited and coupled with authoritative language to create the impression that certain things are "natural," and therefore good, as opposed to "unnatural" products of a corrupt, unhealthy postindustrial society.

Coutinho and Segal actually confuse the nature/culture binary even as they use it to justify their claims. In the book's first chapter they write, "For the hundreds and thousands of years of the prehistoric epoch, with life based on hunting and gathering, the role of women was perceived as producing a child, preferably a man-child."[15] Even as they argue that early women—read "women in their natural state"—don't menstruate, they betray the preferences of certain cultures for the baby to be a boy.

Zahra Meghani writes that a feminist analysis "reveals that these theorists' recourse to ideas of evolutionary-suitedness is strategic." She makes this point humorously, pointing out that that bipedalism—walking upright—"is not categorized as a pathological evolutionary aberration although it is both unique to humans and causes some percentage of the population to experience various physical ailments, such as fallen arches and back pain, impairing their ability to function well in society."[16] And yet there are no cries in the medical community to return to moving on all fours.

Menopause provides another example of the way that women's histories are reimagined to promote certain cultural perspectives. Even today, the notion that women before the twentieth century didn't live long enough to cease menstruating persists. In the 1990s, when drug companies had significant interests in pushing hormone treatment for all peri- and postmenopausal women, it was common to hear that menopause wasn't natural and was a "disease" of modern life that required pills to cure it. Statistical analysis by, among others, Margaret Lock has shown that these claims were based on oversimplification, and in fact, a visit to former centuries would have revealed many gray female heads.

While "natural" does not necessarily mean "correct" or "positive," it is frequently interpreted this way. Menstrual suppression is often explained in terms of female empowerment, but a hard look at the evolutionary logic behind it betrays a reactionary argument about women and biological destiny. In looking at nonhuman primates, Coutinho and Segal write, "Regardless of the social structures in which they live, it is rare to find a menstruating nonhuman primate free-living in the wild."[17] What are we supposed to assume about life in a "natural" condition from this statement? First, that females do not live alone. Second, that the male primates in their community are in charge. Third, that they do not bleed and are most likely pregnant. Even though we are talking about apes and not humans, the message is clear.

The Perils of Periods: PMS, Anemia, and Other Menstrual Hazards

Whether or not women *should* get periods, why might they want to avoid them? At the top of the list of reasons is that old scourge of womankind, PMS. On this subject, suppression advocates get nearly hysterical in describing the debilitation women experience. Most of the really dramatic work cited goes back in one way or another to Katharina Dalton. The laundry list of hazards includes common complaints like mood swings, headaches, and menstrual cramps, and moves on to increased rates of suicide, "inattention to cooking recipes, failed examinations, tardiness at classes or meetings, low marks at school, involvement in car accidents, mishaps at home or work, even committing crimes or felonies,"[18] and "marital conflicts, mistreatment of children, aggressiveness and work directed indiscriminately toward subordinates and superiors alike, excessive food intake, and alcohol abuse."[19]

What woman *wouldn't* want to prevent such problems? Thank goodness we now have estrogen and progestin pills to keep us from the fate of becoming bad-cooking, child-abusing, husband-hating, boss-disrespecting, fat, alcoholic, suicidal criminals.

Most women have some experience with PMS, and those experiences, however unpleasant, should tell us that this sort of portrait is not only hyperbolic, but absurd and insulting. What becomes clear here is that there exists a deep anxiety over women's roles. While women have been experiencing premenstrual pains, to greater and lesser extents, for as long as they have been bleeding,[20] the subject has received inordinate attention in the last hundred years as our culture has tried to cope with women's dramatically changing roles. Our preoccupation with PMS is related to a new focus on the importance of women's hormones over women's organs in defining biological difference. It constitutes an extension of historical claims about women's instability and lack of self-control from the limited period of bleeding to the constant flux of the menstrual cycle.

If the period becomes the moment of crisis where all the uncertainties about who women should be are laid bare, it is clear, looking at this list of symptoms, what we are worried about. When hormonally compromised, this thinking insists, women express distinctly unfeminine behavior, like unharnessed anger, desire, appetites, and a general lack of self-control and grace. If this list of PMS symptoms is to be believed, women are equally unable to perform traditionally male roles. They are noncompliant to authority in job settings, inefficient and clumsy at work, and unable to perform in academic contexts.

The real problem seems to be the same one we have been struggling to reconcile since the second-wave feminist movement—that is, the sense that women "want it all." Periods—and more specifically, cultural ideas about premenstrual syndrome—provide a forum for expressing the opinion that if you try to be everything, you will be nothing. Modern women can try to pass as men for most of the month, filling traditionally male roles, but at some point their hormones defeat them. And at that moment they can't even be good women anymore.

An infuriating message, to be sure. It is on this point, I would argue, that Coutinho and his cohorts are mistakenly but genuinely trying to provide compassionate options for women. These doctors feel that if the signs of menstruation (and although it goes unspoken, presumptions about female weakness) are removed, then no one in a woman's community—not even the woman herself—can argue that she is unable to capably fill whatever role she would like.

This might seem like a pragmatic solution. But it proposes that instead of addressing the social inequities and generations of negative misperceptions of female bodies, women should instead accept that the flaw is within them. It is a biological solution to a problem that has social, political, and physical dimensions. This does not make room for female empowerment, but rather replaces one type of control (social and political) with another (pharmaceutical).

This is not to deny the reality of PMS as a source of suffering for many women. In an excellent history of PMS since the Renaissance, Michael Stolberg debunks the notion that it is a twentieth-century illness and is therefore purely or even largely a construction of a sexist medical establishment. Stolberg writes that contrary to many claims, "premenstrual suffering was frequently described as a very common complaint by physicians and women alike," adding, significantly, "this is far from denying the role of cultural and social influences. Repeatedly, over the centuries, the interpretation and even the very perception and experience of the nature and timing of premenstrual suffering were profoundly reconfigured and transformed."[21]

As with menopausal symptoms, such as hot flashes and night sweats, PMS difficulties can range from nonexistent to debilitating. For most women, their period brings nothing more than inconveniences, but a smaller group will find their lives complicated, damaged, or disturbed by them. Diane, a woman in her midtwenties who works for a woman's health organization, shared her story with me. Growing up in rural Idaho, she suffered each month with almost unbearable pain. Because her family was deeply religious, birth control pills were not an option. When she was finally offered hormonal contraceptives as a solution to period pain, Diane was already in her twenties. "It totally changed my life," she says. "I don't like the idea of being constantly medicated, but right now, this makes my pain manageable."

For this tiny but significant group, menstrual suppression drugs may provide one option for alleviating suffering, particularly if they are already taking hormonal birth control. In small short-term studies, menstrual suppressants have been modestly more successful in alleviating period-related symptoms than traditional oral contraceptives.[22] One of the difficulties, however, of drawing definitive conclusions about treatment is that PMS is a constellation of symptoms rather than a clear, distinct malady. You can't test for it like a blood disease or cure it with antibiotics like an infection. That fact makes separating physical and social factors next to impossible, and it becomes hard to know which patients would benefit.

Another problem that distinguishes PMS is that prescribing hormones to treat it would necessarily be a long-term prescription. When the revelations of the Women's Health Initiative made clear the irresponsibility of prescribing HT in the long-term, it was—and is—still possible to prescribe the drugs in the short term for the treatment of menopausal difficulties such as hot flashes and vaginal dryness. However, since we lack long-term safety data for menstrual suppressants, the wisdom of prescribing them for the treatment of PMS, even in extreme cases, remains an open question. It is certainly not responsible to suggest the drug for PMS management in most women who are not otherwise seeking hormonal birth control.

What of other period problems? In particular, Coutinho is concerned with preventing two serious chronic problems, endometriosis and anemia.

Endometriosis happens when the tissue that lines the uterus grows outside the organ or on the ovaries, pelvic area, or bladder. Endometrial tissue, whether it grows where it's supposed to or in a place it shouldn't, responds to the hormonal messages the brain sends out. It builds up in response to hormones over the course of the month and breaks down. Unfortunately, when this breakdown doesn't happen inside the uterus, blood and tissue have nowhere to go and become trapped in the body. This can cause scar tissue and cysts. It is frequently very painful and can lead to fertility problems.

Menstrual suppression drugs may be a good option for treating pain associated with this condition because they block the chemical messages from the brain that would cause errant cells to build up and bleed.

It is worth mentioning that this is different than claiming that continual menstruation *causes* endometriosis, as Coutinho and Segal argue. While it is true that continuous menstruation aggravates the condition, it is still a leap to claim that it is responsible for the rise in the incidence of the disease that doctors have observed in the past century. It may turn out that this is the case, but until we have more information, it is irresponsible to market menstrual suppression drugs preventatively.

Anemia is a disease in which the body doesn't have enough red blood cells. Consequently, as blood flows through the body, it struggles to carry enough oxygen to the heart. It is treated and prevented by taking an iron supplement and also by making an effort to eat foods that are naturally rich in the mineral. For women who suffer from anemia, menstruation can cause further problems because the associated blood loss depletes iron stores.

In the United States, anemia is a tricky issue because while more women suffer from it than men, many women get too much iron. Period defender and author Dr. Susan Rako writes, "While we've heard a lot about 'iron-deficiency anemia,' and we know that we need enough iron in our diets to keep ourselves healthy, we know considerably less about the risks of excessive amounts of stored iron. Few of us have any idea how iron-rich our diets may be."[23] Rako, author of *The Blessings of the Curse*, the only book to take on menstrual suppression, believes that menstruation provides a natural way for women to rid their bodies of excess nutrition that can potentially contribute to serious health problems such as heart disease.

Anemia is a more serious threat for women in developing nations, where, as Zahra Meghani points out, its major cause is "inadequate sanitation facilities, resulting in high incidence of hookworm disease."[24] She adds that "it is unclear how suppressing monthly menstruation is any part of a sound solution and quite clear how awesome a potential market the Third World can be for menstrual suppressant contraceptives."[25]

The Advent of Menstrual Suppression Drugs

The wording of the FDA letter was harsh and unequivocal: Duramed Pharmaceuticals, at the time a division of Barr Laboratories, would have to make serious changes to their advertising campaign for the new drug Seasonale or face serious consequences.

Seasonale, the first pill to be specifically marketed for the purpose of menstrual suppression, was approved for use in the United States on September 5, 2003. The pill had been on the market for a little over a year when the letter went out in December 2004. It had gotten off to a slow start, but hopes for the drug were very high, with sales projections that warmed the hearts of company executives.

The FDA's complaint was that Duramed was minimizing the risks of their new drug, specifically downplaying the significant intermenstrual bleeding and spotting patients experienced when taking this pill. It was, undeniably, a serious marketing problem. How did you convince patients to buy a drug for the prevention of bleeding that had the major side effect of causing . . . well . . . bleeding?

In the early 1980s international opinion suggested that women weren't interested in eliminating periods, but this had started to change by the 1990s, perhaps due in part to books like *Is Menstruation Obsolete?* and the subsequent media coverage of its ideas. A multicountry survey published in 2003 found that there was "gradual acceptance of amenorrhea associated with contraception."[26] Women were opening up to the idea of stopping their periods. Results from a questionnaire survey of countries in Asia, Africa, and Europe found that only black African women seemed to like their periods and that other women "would opt to bleed only once every three months, or not at all."[27] Study authors concluded that "providers tended to overestimate the importance of regular menstruation to their clients."

This was all very good news for Duramed, who was in the process of winning an FDA green light for their birth control pill that would do just that—limit menstruation to every third month or a total of four periods a year.

An American study published in 2004 found that out of 1,470 women questioned, 59 percent expressed interest in either partial or complete suppression of menses. One-third would be willing to never bleed at all.[28]

Approval for the drug was based on a study population of 682 women who were randomized to Seasonale and a traditional oral contraceptive (Nordette) for one year. At the end of that time they found the drug's efficacy and toleration to be similar to traditional birth control pills. There were indeed fewer periods but still a large number of bleeding and spotting days due to breakthrough bleeding. This problem decreased with usage, but was responsible for some patients discontinuing use before the year was over.[29]

In taking issue with Duramed's marketing of the drug, the FDA pointed out that the pill's labeling cautioned patients to weigh the desire not to bleed menstrually against the likelihood of bleeding intermenstrually and noted, "More Seasonale subjects, compared to subjects on the 28-day cycle regimen, discontinued prematurely for unacceptable bleeding."[30] How many women were having unplanned bleeding? According to the FDA, "During the first Seasonale treatment cycle, about 1 in 3 women may have 20 or more days of unplanned bleeding or spotting."[31] In other words, patients had a similar number of bleeding days as women taking traditional oral contraceptives. However, those on Seasonale didn't know when those days would occur.

While bleeding decreased with time, the FDA pointed out that the use of the word "initially" when describing the breakthrough incidents was inaccurate, because even after a year of use, 42 percent of users were still reporting bleeding or spotting.

Finally, the FDA took issue with the advertisement's suggestion that limiting periods had "no adverse effects" and that there was medical agreement on this fact. They pointed out that in reality the drug was associated with "numerous risks" and that "the TV ad misleadingly suggests that Seasonale is safer than has been demonstrated by substantial evidence or substantial clinical experience."[32]

Four years later, it was Wyeth's turn to debut their new drug Lybrel. While Seasonale cut bleeding to four weeks a year, Lybrel sought to eliminate it completely. This time, the study population included 2,134 women between the ages of eighteen and forty-nine with regular menstrual cycles. The trial lasted for nineteen months,[33] during which time patients were asked to record in diaries whether or not they took the drug and any instances of bleeding that occurred. Only 921 of these women were still taking the pills a year later—that's less than 50 percent of the original study population. Of the women who stopped taking the drug, 396 discontinued because of uterine bleeding.[34] Other statistically significant side effects included increases in blood pressure and weight gain (although this was small, averaging less than two pounds).

After a year, 58.7 percent of women reported no bleeding or spotting, which means that 41.3 percent were still spotting after a year of use—that's two out of every five subjects. And 79 percent of women reported no bleeding (blood flowing heavily enough to require sanitary protection), which means that 21 percent of women—one in five—were still experiencing bleeding that required menstrual protection. Bleeding and spotting did decrease with use: 93.9 percent experienced spotting with the first pill pack, while only 21 percent did by the thirteenth—but many women continued to experience problems. Again, far from offering women mastery over their menstrual cycles, the pills made bleeding even less predictable.

The FDA hesitated with approval in June 2006, citing, among other things, the need for additional analyses of their clinical data, especially data concerning pregnancy rates, bleeding patterns, and discontinuation rates among study participants (with such a large dropout rate, this shouldn't have come as a surprise for Wyeth). Wyeth received an "approvable" letter, meaning that an eventual full FDA approval was likely, but not assured.[35]

The issues must have been resolved by May 2007, because the FDA officially gave Wyeth the nod to start marketing. The approval letter cautioned, "Health care professionals and patients are advised that when considering the use of Lybrel, the convenience of having no scheduled menstruation should be weighed against the inconvenience of unscheduled bleeding or spotting."[36]

Just the Facts Ma'am: The Basics of Menstrual Suppression Drugs

There are currently several different hormonal methods that a woman can use to stop her periods (although as I have shown, this is an imprecise process at best). Depo-Provera and the hormonal IUD Mirena use only the hormone progestin to accomplish this end. In both cases the suspension of periods was an unanticipated side effect and originally seen as the price of using a more effective contraceptive, not a selling point of the drugs.[37] The vaginal ring (NuvaRing), a clear flexible device that releases estrogen and progestin when placed in the vagina, has been tested for extended use,[38] as have alternative distribution devices like the estrogen patch—although far less study is generally available on these devices, let alone on the specifics of use for eliminating or curtailing menstruation.

Seasonale offers estrogen and progesterone for eleven weeks and sugar pills for one week (when withdrawal bleeding happens), and Seasonique, a more recent product from the same manufacturer, replaces the week of sugar pills with pills containing low doses of estrogen. Lybrel offers continuous estrogen and progesterone.

Another option is the use of birth control pills that reduce the number of inactive pills and therefore the days of bleeding. This class constitutes a sort of middle ground between traditional OCs and newer menstrual suppression drugs. Some brand names include Yaz, Loestrin, and Alesse.

Traditional oral contraceptives, when used continuously by skipping inactive pills, provide the same results as using Lybrel. Some doctors believe this is a better option for women who choose to eliminate periods because it avoids the expense of buying a new drug and opens up the possibility of using cheaper generic prescriptions. Washington state–based gynecologist Leslie Miller advises, "I don't think women need another brand name contraceptive like Lybrel."[39] Bi- and tricyclic birth control pills should not be used for this purpose because the shift in hormones is too rapid without the inactive week, and irregular and spotty cycles are usually the result. If you are considering this regimen, talk to your doctor about whether it is the right option for you.

Menstrual suppression drugs work through the same mechanisms as older OCs—they prevent the brain from sending messages to the reproductive system to develop egg follicles. They also stem the growth of the uterine lining, so that if fertilization does occur, implantation is less likely, and they cause cervical fluids to remain inhospitable to sperm.

New menstrual suppression drugs carry approximately the same health risks as older OCs. The *American Family Physician* advises patients that they found "no difference in safety or effectiveness between cyclic and continuous or extended-cycle combined contraceptives" and that "patients' satisfaction and adherence is similar for all types."[40] Taking the drugs in the short term doesn't seem to harm the uterus[41] or fertility. In a trial to test the ability of women to return to menstruation and ovulation after use of menstrual suppression, a researcher found that "99 percent of 187 participants experienced either a return to menses or become pregnant within 90 days after stopping the study drug."[42] Keep in mind that these participants took Lybrel for an average of one year—not a long time—and that 187 is a small study population.

Of course, new drugs always open up long-term safety questions that only time and further scientific study can answer. The question is what difference, if any, continuous exposure to hormones makes when compared with interrupted exposure over time. Remember that the longest trial of new menstrual suppression methods has lasted only two years. While this may seem like a long time, in the scope of comprehensive understanding of drugs, it is relatively short. Many side effects take decades—and populations of thousands taking a given prescription—to emerge. The Society for Menstrual Research cautions, "Long-term studies that address potential risks beyond the uterus, such as breast, bone, and cardiovascular health are still needed. Furthermore, there is an urgent need for studies that address impacts on adolescent development, since young women and girls are a target audience for cycle-stopping contraceptives."[43]

Indeed, the question of how menstrual suppression drugs might affect very young girls differently is an important one. Recall the case of Depo-Provera, the first menstrual suppressant. Often given to young girls because they are less reliable with daily pills and the injection need only be given every three months, the drug has been shown to cause a loss in bone density, leading to the placement of the FDA's mandatory black box warning on patient package inserts.[44]

Similarly, menstrual suppression drugs are frequently marketed to women who suffer either painful or erratic periods. Young women in the first year or two of menstruation are far more likely to experience both of these problems, and it makes them a particularly lucrative population for drugmakers. Just as many women suffer greater discomfort for a few years at menopause (on average, 2.5) as cycles are winding down, so do girls adjusting to their hormonal and menstrual fluxes need time to let their body transition. For this reason, many gynecologists advise that girls not be given the drugs until they have had a chance to menstruate naturally for at least a year. It is hard to argue that a woman who has never experienced nonmedical periods has had adequate personal experience to make comprehensive, informed decisions about the value of such events.

There are serious practical concerns with menstrual suppression drugs. Something so basic that many don't consider is that women use menstruation—and withdrawal bleeding—as a tool for determining whether they are pregnant. If a woman becomes pregnant and continues taking hormone drugs, serious complications may occur. Diethylstilbestrol (DES) was an estrogen drug given to women in the 1960s and 1970s to prevent miscarriages. It did not ultimately accomplish this task; however, it did cause sexual and reproductive problems for mothers, babies, and even the offspring of children born using DES. One of the important lessons of DES was the danger of exposing fetuses to estrogen drugs, particularly after the first months of gestation. It seems possible that a mother taking menstrual suppressants could have a similar outcome.

Delayed discovery of a pregnancy raises other issues for a woman who does not wish to carry it to term. Since accessing second trimester abortions in the United States is very difficult, prompt discovery of unwanted pregnancies is paramount for many women. Even where they are legal, terminations get more expensive with time, and a delay can make a procedure cost prohibitive.

For these reasons, the FDA recommends taking a pregnancy test each month when using drugs that eliminate or curtail bleeding, just to be on the safe side.[45]

There are other benefits to menstruation. Susan Rako points out that in focusing on ovulation and bleeding, doctors ignore related dynamic, ongoing hormonal processes. She insists there is a "popular ignorance of the particular health benefits that accrue to women as a result of normal hormonal fluctuations and the monthly bleed . . . Women's reproductive hormones play a part in the normal functioning of every organ system in the body."[46] Indeed many of the complexities of female hormone cycles are still ill understood and pronouncing them useless is both premature and dangerous.

An example of the hazards of such thinking can be seen in changing ideas about the safety of performing oophorectomies in women. For generations, doctors insisted that once reproduction was over, organs such as the uterus and ovaries served no function except tempting the possibility of female cancers. For this reason, hyster- and oophorectomies became some of the most common surgical procedures in American life. To this day, one in three American women will have had her uterus surgically removed by the time she dies. It has since come to light that the ovaries do much more than make eggs and, by extension, babies. The ovaries continue to produce important female hormones even after menopause. Their removal, particularly before the menopause transition, increases a woman's chances of dying from many illnesses. William Parker, a California-based gynecologist and medical school professor, found that in a group of 10,000 women, for every 47 who are saved from ovarian cancer by the surgery, an additional 838 will die from coronary heart disease when compared with women who kept their ovaries.[47] A reductionary understanding of parts of the body and their processes can lead to avoidable tragedies. Women have historically been subject to an undue amount of these.

In the media blitz that surrounded the approval of both Seasonale and Lybrel, the Society for Menstrual Cycle Research provided a tempering voice. After a 2007 meeting, the Society released a paper calling for more research on long-term effects of the drugs. In addition to pointing out the importance of examining psychological factors as well as biological ones, they stress that these drugs "suppress the complex hormonal interplay of the menstrual cycle. The impacts of this cycle on women's health are not completely understood."[48] They conclude that "authentic choice is only possible when accurate and comprehensive information is widely available."[49]

A "Natural" Choice

For many women, the fluctuations of the menstrual cycle provide unique opportunities for understanding their lives, their societies, and their emotions. This brings us back to the problem of negative cultural messages and how women can manage and understand their bodies in a world that wants to control, pathologize, and interpret them.

The various marketing campaigns for both Lybrel and Seasonale present a great example of how difficult this can be. They universally assume that women don't like to menstruate. Tracy Clark-Flory writes, "To view the Lybrel Web site, you might think that women everywhere have been waiting desperately for the chance to postpone their periods . . . It turns out that not all women want to cure the curse. Wyeth's own research says so."[50]

Having assumed that no woman would want to miss out on the opportunity to suspend bleeding, drugmakers proceed to play on conflicting ideas of technology and nature, youth and affluence, illness and lifestyle, and of course, female liberation and traditional women's roles.

I scan for examples of menstrual suppressants in the media and find *Sex and the City* author Candace Bushnell pushing Seasonale as though it were a pair of Manolo Blahniks. And an advertising campaign for Loestrin 24 follows the adventures of a fictional character named Cammie—as hip, urban, and well off as the characters in Ms. Bushnell's book—as she negotiates life in New York City. Cammie is in her midtwenties with a boho apartment in Alphabet City loaded with fashionable clothes and a rocker boyfriend who fronts an indie band. For Cammie, a period that lasts only three days is a state-of-the-art-accessory—like an iPod or a designer handbag. In both these commercials, period control is sold as a marker of affluence and style, a natural accoutrement to modern life.

Such focus on modernity, technology, and choice functions in direct contradiction to arguments about the so-called naturalness of menstrual suppression. It's not about what all women have been doing for generations; it's about what modern women can and should do right now. Drugmakers' stress on lifestyle factors betrays their hopes that menstrual suppression will be adopted not to treat abnormal or problematic menstruation, but rather as just another lifestyle option for healthy women, like attending a yoga class or eating grass-fed meat.

In selecting "chick lit" imagery, pill makers have chosen a nuanced archetype that is at once independent and current and also fundamentally tied to traditional notions of female desire. Jaclyn Geller, among others, has pointed out that the characters in the television version of *Sex and the City* initially resist, but ultimately succumb, to social conventions regarding love, sexuality, and the social world.[51] Carrie Bradshaw is both content in the nontraditional family structure her friends provide and desperately searching for the perfect man.

Likewise, period suppression drugs seek to convince women in the language of independence and self-sufficiency that they should cede control of their bodily functions to a drug company. Yaz, another period shortener, blasts punk music that effuses, "We're not gonna take it!" Again, the rhetoric of cultural resistance is employed with the goal of ensuring pharmaceutical compliance. Much like early twentieth-century menstrual product makers, pill pushers have realized how effective co-opting the language of feminism can be.

A Seasonique advertisement depicts two identical but differently dressed women who identify themselves as "emotional" and "logical." Emotional wants to take menstrual suppressants, but she is scared—it just doesn't seem right somehow. Logical assures her that it is safe and, in fact, the rational and smart thing to do. This advertisement works on many levels, not the least of which is that it plays on women's internalized fears of being perceived as irrational and driven by their feelings—something considered more true before and during menstruation. The advertisement encourages women to identify with the confident, scientific, self-controlled voice of logical over the insecure, timid persona of emotional. Even as this commercial plays on images of modern, take-charge women, it exploits deep and historic stereotypes of women in general and menstruating women in particular.

As the Society for Menstrual Research points out, "Historically, nasty surprises with hormonal therapies for women (e.g., heart disease and hormone therapy for menopausal women, the link between oral contraceptives and blood clots, DES and various health problems) have taken many years to surface."[52] Until we have more extensive long-term data on the repercussions of suppressing periods and exposing the body more continuously to synthetic hormones, use of the drugs for lifestyle purposes should be limited. Susan Rako doesn't mince words: "Manipulating women's hormonal chemistry for the purpose of menstrual suppression threatens to be the largest uncontrolled experiment in the history of medical science."[53]

That said, menstrual suppression drugs provide another choice for women, and that is a good thing. If a patient takes the drugs and finds that she feels good on them, that they improve her quality of life or improve her health in one way or another, she should feel confident taking them as long as she does so as an informed consumer who understands all the risks and unknowns. As one (male) commentator reasons, "Pills can liberate you from old burdens. They can also impose new ones. I'm glad women are free to take Lybrel. I hope, in the future, they'll also feel free not to."[54]

Like Candy: The Politics of the Morning-After Pill and Bringing Hormonal Contraception Over the Counter

Medicine is always a political process.
—L. L. Wynn and James Trussell

Susan Wood is not prone to grand gestures. A serious woman with strik-ing white hair and deadpan delivery, she had been working at the FDA's Office of Women's Health (OWH) for several years when she decided, in late summer of 2005, to walk out on her job. She had been closely mon-itoring the FDA's debate about the approvability of Plan B—the so-called morning-after pill—for over-the-counter status. Wood was furious over what she saw as the FDA's willful disregard for scientific evidence show-ing Plan B to be safe, and its apparent decision to treat the drug as a special case not subject to the usual evaluative methods. Why was this contraceptive drug being treated differently than other pills sold to both sexes? Why was it being held to a higher standard?

The controversy over Plan B has stretched over many years and illumi-nates critical controversies and patterns in women's health care. It has touched on fundamental issues of patient access; the right of doctors, hos-pitals, and pharmacists to refuse medicines on moral grounds; and the ability of women who aren't medical professionals to assess the appropri-ateness of contraceptive methods for themselves without gatekeepers. As L. L. Wynn and James Trussell of Princeton University's Office of Population Research write, "New medical technologies are good to think with. Their very novelty makes them prime subjects for debate over the meaning of medicine and science in a social and political order. Examining these debates can reveal cultural categories, social conflicts, and the relationship between individual bodies and the body politic."[1] Old cultural enemies clashed over this new drug, and pharmaceutical control became, as it has been in the past, a potent metaphor for talking about female reproductive control.

What can women learn from the long journey of Plan B, and what issues remain with this drug? Should the Pill follow in the footsteps of its sister drug and become available without a doctor's prescription? What must female patients understand about the social, political, and governmental forces—such as the FDA—that make key decisions about which methods will be available and under what terms?

The FDA Gets Political Over Plan B

The FDA has been playing a significant role in American women's health for many decades.[2] In the past fifty years, several women's health tragedies have changed the way the organization does business. One of these involved a woman at the FDA named Frances Kelsey, who in her first month of work for the organization in 1960 withheld approval of Thalidomide, a morning sickness drug for expectant mothers that was available and popular in Europe. Kelsey didn't think the evidence was there, and after Thalidomide was shown to cause serious deformities in infants whose mothers had used it during gestation, her newer, stricter standards were put in place to make sure that patients were protected.

The FDA approval process involves a flawed but rigorous set of standards. In order for a drug to be approved, its maker must demonstrate that their product is both safe (it won't cause any terrible side effects) and efficacious (it works for the purpose for which it is being approved). A pill may meet one of these criteria but fail on another one. For example, the medicine Vioxx helps ease joint pain, but it has been found to cause cardiovascular problems. Other pills are safe but ineffective.

Pharmaceutical makers must demonstrate these qualities in a series of trials called phases 1, 2, and 3 before a pill is approved for public use. Prior to initiating this series of tests, animal trials must first demonstrate basic safety. Once that is accomplished, phase 1 trials begin with a small number of human subjects, generally between twenty and fifty. During this time, drugmakers and scientists can experiment with dosage and check for any obvious safety problems. A phase 2 trial expands the testing to a couple hundred patients. By the time a phase 3 trial occurs, testing the medication on potentially thousands of people, it is well on its way to becoming available. But since it often takes decades and tens of thousands of patients taking a drug in a real-world setting before side effects and even general usefulness are determined, most drugs' true safety and efficacy remain open questions even years after the FDA gives them the green light.

In 1998, the first dedicated emergency contraception (meaning the pill was made for the sole purpose of preventing pregnancy after sex), Preven, was approved for use in the United States. A year later Plan B hit the American prescription drug market.[3] The drug is a progestin-only (levonorgestrel) preparation that, when taken within a certain window of time after having unprotected sex, offers defense against pregnancy by stopping ovulation, potentially (though not definitely) impairing sperm mobility and preventing implantation of a fertilized egg.

Women have been using "morning-after" options since the 1960s. In 1974, a Canadian gynecologist named Albert Yuzpe published instructions for just such an option that remained the primary means of emergency contraception for decades.[4] The Yupze regimen advised patients who wanted postcoital protection against pregnancy to take larger doses of already available birth control pills. Sure, it might cause nausea, vomiting, and even dizziness, strange bleeding, and headaches, but it was better than having an unplanned pregnancy or an abortion. Plan B simply streamlined this process by providing a prepackaged two-dose option for women whose contraceptive had failed them or who had not used protection.

In 2003, the Women's Capital Corporation (later acquired by Barr Pharmaceuticals, Inc.) sought over-the-counter approval for their pill. The initial process went smoothly, and the advisory committee voted overwhelmingly—twenty-three to four—in favor of letting women decide for themselves if Plan B was a good option for them. This vote happened after a day-long hearing in which medical experts and individuals were given an opportunity to testify. Both liberal and conservative groups had their say, and over sixty medical organizations, including the American Medical Association and the American Association of Pediatrics, spoke in favor of OTC approval.

Despite overwhelming support from the medical community, not everyone thought that changing Plan B's status was a good idea. Using arguments that were often at first based on medical literature but that grew increasingly emotional and ideological, groups such as Concerned Women for America and the American Life League argued that increased access to emergency contraception (EC) would endanger young women. Among other social maladies, Plan B would promote promiscuity and risky sexual practices, it would remove a girl's ability to say no to lusty male suitors, and it would perhaps provide a way for pedophiles and perpetrators of incest to hide their crimes. Wynn and Trussell have pointed out that these arguments relied on sexual paradigms in which women lack powerful and autonomous sexual desire and instead serve as the gatekeepers for supposedly less controllable male urges.

In retrospect, the looming questions that still haunt EC—for example, the exact mechanism through which the pill prevents pregnancy—were already circulating in the room. Pro-life activists equated Plan B with abortion. Others worried that removing doctors from the path to pills would cause a fundamental disruption of the doctor-patient relationship.

Also evident from the start was the role of George W. Bush's administration in influencing FDA decision making. Of the four committee members who voted against OTC approval, three were Bush appointees with noted conservative and pro-life positions. Two, W. David Hager[5] and Joseph Stanford, were doctors who refused prescriptions for conventional oral contraceptives to all unmarried patients. Another committee member, Susan Crockett, was on the board of the American Association of Pro-Life Obstetricians and Gynecologists.[6] (Further evidence of the Bush administration's desire to inform medical policy through whatever means necessary came to light with the departure of former US Surgeon General Richard Carmona, who went public with the ways he was censored by the president, including being forbidden to discuss contraception.[7]) These committee members' objections were inconsistent with the conclusions of medical experts: while political groups disagreed about whether the drug should travel over the counter, doctors and scientists were overwhelmingly in agreement that the pill should be available. When it came to safety and individual efficacy, there was no reason not to let women make up their own minds about Plan B. When the hearing concluded, OTC approval seemed likely to happen in short order.

Plan B then traveled up to the FDA's Office of New Drugs, which also agreed that the drug should be given OTC status. Soon, though, problems began mysteriously cropping up. The FDA began asking for data that wasn't required of other drugs, such as actual-use studies and information on patient label comprehension. While it is certainly admirable to ask in advance if patients will be able to understand drug instructions, these questions hadn't been posed with regard to other medications. The FDA was making up new rules to delay the approval of OTC status for Plan B.

In particular, the FDA dwelled on the health of women under age seventeen who might take the drug.[8] The crux of the issue, again, was not medical concern, but rather anxiety about adolescent sexuality and who would make decisions about it. The answer, as far as the government was concerned, was clearly not teenage girls.

In May 2004, the FDA sent Barr a nonapprovable letter suggesting that there was no quick fix for emergency contraception (when the FDA issues an approvable letter it means that while there is more work to do—perhaps further study or providing the FDA with more data—there are clear and easy steps to take to ensure the drug will pass muster). Immediately, many interested parties in the women's health and medical worlds cried foul and began publicizing the oddities of the FDA's decision. A 2005 report from the Government Accountability Office (GAO) found that "the decision was . . . highly unusual and . . . was made with atypical involvement from top agency officials and may well have been made months before it was formally announced."[9] Undaunted, Barr resubmitted their application in the summer of that year.

And then things went quiet. The FDA made no formal claims on the subject; they simply stopped moving on the issue of emergency contraception. Nothing happened as months rolled by. Susan Wood wasn't the only one who was frustrated. Senators Hillary Rodham Clinton of New York and Patty Murray of Washington withheld approval of new FDA commissioner Lester M. Crawford in protest (he had served as acting commissioner throughout the debate). A condition of his acceptance was assurance that the status of the pill would be resolved by September 1 of that year (2005).[10] Once Crawford was put in power, he immediately set about blocking Plan B.

It was a hot Friday afternoon in August 2005 when the controversy, which had been building for years, came to a head. Crawford finally announced the FDA's decision: Plan B's OTC status would not be approved at that time. The process would be opened for public commentary and the final decision would be indefinitely delayed. Wood, Clinton, Murray, and countless women and activists knew what this meant. It was effectively another no for emergency contraception.

Wood decided enough was enough. "The point of my resignation was to help clarify the problem—that the FDA was totally out of whack," said Wood four years later.[11] Plainly, there was much to be clarified, about the role of a conservative religious administration in making secular and sexual health policy, the tendency of organizations like the FDA to treat women's health and products as special cases, and of course, the desire of established authorities, both governmental and medical, to maintain more direct control over women's contraceptive choices.

Within three months, Crawford was gone, a victim of personal controversies more than public missteps (he was accused of having an inappropriate relationship with a staff member as well as of financial improprieties). When he left, women who had been burned in the Plan B brawl and betrayed by Crawford didn't mince words. Clinton noted, "With the resignation of Dr. Crawford, the FDA has a real opportunity to restore its battered reputation and nominate a leader with vision and drive to ensure that the FDA upholds its gold standard of drug regulation."[12]

It would be another year before Plan B was finally approved for OTC status on July 31, 2006, with the significant caveat that it would be available only to women eighteen and older. Approval had taken three years and three different FDA commissioners, and it revealed how FDA leadership, tied to political ideologies, was capable of distorting and hijacking the drug approval process.[13] As a new FDA commissioner, Margaret A. Hamburg, takes the helm, the challenge of fixing an institution with a vast range of systemic problems, serious financial challenges, and a badly damaged public image remain.[14] After becoming the head of the massive organization in the spring of 2009, Hamburg noted that top priorities for the FDA include creating more transparency so that the public can understand how decisions about drugs are made. "The FDA has been seen as a cold regulatory agency and also something of a black box," Hamburg explained. "We have a chance to open it up and make sure the American people have the safe, high-quality foods they need, the safe and high-quality drugs and medical equipment they need."[15]

A Failure to Communicate: Key Issues in the Plan B Debate

One persistent concern about allowing over-the-counter access to any drug, and particularly women's health drugs, is that it leads to a break-down in the doctor/patient relationship. Women ultimately need to see providers, for many good reasons beyond preventing drug side effects. But in the case of Plan B, one of the main problems with going through a doctor is timeliness: the sooner EC is used, the more effective it is. If taken within twenty-four hours, it may reduce the risk of pregnancy to .4 percent, while if a patient waits until forty-eight to seventy-two hours after intercourse, this risk goes up to 2.7 percent.[16] Because EC is by definition used in unexpected or unanticipated situations, making a doctor's appointment can pose a serious barrier to getting the drug quickly enough for it to be most helpful.

A second major issue is economics. If a patient has to pay for a doctor's visit, the price of emergency contraception rises from around $50 to closer to $200. This would make the drug more expensive than consistently taking the Pill. It would pose serious access issues for young patients, particularly teenagers, who don't necessarily have ready access to that amount of money.

Opponents of OTC access for EC are quick to romanticize the doctor/patient relationship as essential to female well-being. How, they ask, can women—particularly young women—be expected to make this sort of decision on their own without expert guidance?

This perspective ignores many of the realities of the modern dynamic between practitioners and patients. Female patients rarely have time for a conversation with their doctor in a health care environment that pushes doctors to fit in as many patients as possible and to delegate most care to nurses and aides. When female patients do see doctors, they are hardly peers engaging in a conversation. The doctor controls the right to dispense desired drugs and has the right to refuse certain care options. Female patients often (wrongly) construe personal questions about their intimate lives as judgment. They may be embarrassed about choices they view as irresponsible. And to top it off, patients must pay for the privilege of having this so-called conversation. This is not to suggest that the vast majority of doctors don't act out of concern and compassion for their patients. But it is necessary to acknowledge the fact that the doctor/patient relationship isn't an equal one.

Considering these power dynamics, the remarkable thing about the EC debate is that it has redrawn some traditional positions. The majority of medical organizations and experts endorse over-the-counter status, despite the fact that this has meant a reduction in physician power. Why would doctors—who are so often excessively territorial and protective of their role as pharmaceutical gatekeepers—be willing to give up control of Plan B? One reason, surely, is that the majority of medical and professional evidence suggests that that giving OTC status to Plan B was the correct course. Many doctors are no doubt driven by a desire to provide patients with the most efficient care.

Plan B provides doctors with an occasion for activism on both sides of the political spectrum. A fascinating example of this involved Boston doctor Rebekah E. Gee and the corporate behemoth Wal-Mart. Gee prescribed emergency contraception to a patient in 2005. That young woman, a mother of three, tried to fill the prescription (as she did with all her medicines) at the Wal-Mart pharmacy. Gee notes, "Through her experience, I became aware of Wal-Mart's refusal to stock Plan B."[17] Long a bastion of so-called red state values, the retail giant declined to provide the drug on moral grounds. Rather than stand idly by, Gee and colleagues partnered with a Boston law firm and reproductive rights groups to file a lawsuit demanding that Wal-Mart provide emergency contraception, according to a Massachusetts law demanding that pharmacies stock all "commonly prescribed medications." The suit was successful, and after Gee and her associates threatened to pursue the issue state by state, Wal-Mart decided to carry the drug nationally. For her efforts, Gee received threatening e-mails and letters, including some that accused her of being like Hitler and trying to "'depopulate' the human race."[18] Gee takes this in stride, noting, "Our government has been burying its head in the sand, pretending that sex does not happen. This agenda sets women back decades, threatening their right to achieve equality in society."[19]

Emergency contraception is big business, and with that comes big power; sales jumped from around 10 million in 2004 to 40 million in 2006, and then doubled again to nearly 80 million in 2007.[20] These numbers have continued to grow as the drug has gone OTC in over forty nations. This opens up the fascinating possibility that drugmakers, who have so often reinforced traditional power relationships in the interests of promoting their products—often acting against the best interests of women—can also serve to create fault lines that challenge the medical establishment. This has the unintentional effect of providing opportunities for enhanced autonomy among female patients.

As we know, medical autonomy for women has always been hard to come by. Wynn and Trussell point out that in the drama of emergency contraception, female patients are always cast as the victims, a pattern consistent with portrayals of other drugs that supposedly make having sex easier. Just like the Pill before it, Plan B is accused of making it easier for men to force women to have dangerous sex. Despite the fact that many registered sex offenders have been documented filling Viagra prescriptions on the public dime under Medicaid, Plan B is the drug that has come under fire for "facilitating the sexual exploitation of women."[21]

This focus on female bodies can be attributed in part to their potency as a metaphor for the *social* body. When female bodies become uncontrollable—when sex and reproductive issues are placed in female hands—it threatens existing social orders. Traditional power holders, like political and religious leaders and some members of the medical community, use this thinking to convince people that it is necessary to mediate and stabilize the threat of female sexuality. If we control women's choices about their bodies, we can temper confusing and uncomfortable social shifts.

Such anxieties about sexuality are particularly felt with young women and girls, in this case leading to the initial restriction of OTC availability to women eighteen and older. But it's obvious that restricting EC access isn't doing much to stabilize our society. The United States has a teen pregnancy rate that is considerably higher than other industrialized nations.[22] Emergency contraception could be particularly useful for younger women[23] who have less predictable sexual patterns and less access to traditional birth control methods.

The Plan B issue has always been characterized by disagreements about whether or not EC could be considered a form of abortion. Perhaps most obviously at issue is the basic definition of pregnancy. Most major public health groups define pregnancy[24] as starting after the implantation of a fertilized egg in the womb. At this point the body comes to understand that it is carrying an embryo, and the dividing cells continue maturing. But some members of the pro-life community have moved in recent years to locate the beginning of a pregnancy (if not the beginning of life) before this, at the moment where sperm meets egg and fertilization occurs. This is a new gloss on an old argument: instead of debating whether life begins at conception, pro-life forces are attempting to redefine the meaning of conception. Those who claim that emergency contraception is abortion have been forced to conjure up old-fashioned images of silent film–style villains and damsels in distress, because the usual tools of pro-life groups—specifically, images of developing fetuses—are impossible to deploy in the Plan B context.

It is estimated that half of fertilized eggs are never implanted and leave the body before any biological changes indicative of pregnancy occur. Many things can cause this to happen, including breastfeeding. Indeed, this is one way that lactation acts contraceptively. According to this way of thinking, breastfeeding women should avoid sex entirely because they might fertilize an egg that would be prevented from implanting and in that way inhibit the growth of life.

EC proponents have sought to avoid this messy debate by repeatedly stressing that the method works by inhibiting ovulation, not by preventing implantation. While certainly EC does the former, it may do the latter as well: no one is sure. The fact that science lacks a basic functional understanding of EC opens it up to the accusation that it works as an abortifacient. In fact, the same questions that exist about EC also endure with more traditional oral contraceptives.

Plan B is a strange drug that doesn't fall neatly into established categories. Even though EC works like birth control pills, the fact that you use it *after* sex makes it seem more like an abortifacient; when opponents of the pill speak about it, the fact that it isn't one doesn't matter. For reasons that are more conceptual and ideological than scientific, postcoital contraception unsettles and confuses people. We are used to the idea that contraception must involve forethought, and that a failure to plan will (and in the minds of some should) have consequences. Because it is taken after sex, Plan B seems to be "breaking the rules." In doing so it has created a murky fluidity among legal but contested medical options, like abortion, and more generally accepted forms of health care, like birth control pills.

This is a middle ground that has been effectively exploited by those who seek strict social controls on female reproduction. Efforts to restrict women's options that started with abortion and have moved on to EC can easily advance to the Pill or the IUD. Ambiguities that exist about the ability of EC to prevent implantation also exist with more traditional hormonal contraceptives. By making a psychological association between EC and abortifacients because they both happen after sex, and using this to argue that anti-implantation mechanisms constitute abortion, religious and cultural forces opposed to birth control are able use EC as a gateway for implying that contraceptives generally are a form of abortion and should be restricted or eliminated.

Facing the Zygotes: Language, Conscientious Objection, and Contraceptive Politics

Definitions matter in this negotiation. When word began to spread in the summer of 2008 that the Bush administration was planning to institute a "conscience rule" that would support the rights of health care workers to deny giving care that they found morally objectionable, women's health activists were quick to point out that one of the major issues at stake was when pregnancy began. Ostensibly, the bill was about abortion; it would ensure that religious persons were never forced to participate actively or passively in the termination of pregnancies. A deeper look suggested that broader issues were at stake, particularly an effort to redefine when pregnancy starts and blur the lines between birth control pills and abortion. Lawyers for the National Women's Law Center noted, "This gives an open invitation to any doctor, nurse, receptionist, insurance plan or even hospital to refuse to provide information about birth control on the grounds that they believe contraception amounts to abortion."[25]

The rule was officially announced in December 2008, about a month before Bush left office, and it went into effect on Barack Obama's inauguration day. The rule missed being enacted by its original November 1 deadline but happened anyway under a "White House directive" for "extraordinary circumstances."[26] Writing in the *New York Times*, journalist Robert Pear noted, "Administration officials were unable to say immediately why an exception might be justified in this case."[27] The rule said that "providers—including hospitals, clinics, universities, pharmacies and doctor's offices—can be charged with discrimination if an employee is pressured to participate in care that is 'contrary to their religious beliefs or moral convictions.'"[28] It had the potential to affect low-income communities in particularly adverse ways, since it applied specifically to publicly funded institutions and communities where people had fewer resources to choose from if the health care they needed wasn't being provided. Mary Jane Gallagher, president of the National Family Planning and Reproductive Health Association, noted, "We worry that under the proposal, contraceptive services would become less available to low-income and uninsured women."[29] The Obama administration immediately announced plans to roll back the rule, but the process could take months to finalize.

How many doctors object to providing certain kinds of care? A study published in 2007 in the *New England Journal of Medicine* suggests that the number is substantial: 52 percent of surveyed doctors objected to abortion as a response to botched birth control, and 42 percent felt that parents should be involved in deciding whether to prescribe teenagers contraceptives.[30] The article's authors estimate that as many as 14 million Americans may be going to doctors who don't believe they have an ethical obligation to provide a patient with all their medical options if they find some of those possibilities objectionable, and 100 million Americans have doctors who don't think they should be required to provide referrals for pills, procedures, or surgeries to which they object. These statistics offer a snapshot of how far-reaching the Bush-style conscience rule could be. On a practical level it is clear that patients need to be proactive in educating themselves about their medical conditions and calling doctor's offices in advance of appointments to insure that their chosen practitioner provides all the services—or referrals—they might need.

For young, uninsured, and low-income women, this poses particular challenges. Women who struggle to afford a single doctor's visit find that refusal of services at one office may mean an inability to receive desired care. Indeed, while advocates of sexual education often rightly point a finger at abstinence-only programs (which received $1.3 billion of federal money under Bush[31]) when looking at teen pregnancy statistics, it is worth asking how free and open access to birth control services might impact these numbers. As one doctor notes, refusal of services "represents the latest struggle with regard to religion in America," noting that doctors who insist on conscientious objection want "an unfettered right to personal autonomy while holding monopolistic control over a public good."[32]

Several pharmacies also claim the right not to dispense Plan B or conventional contraceptives. So-called pro-life drugstores, such as the one that opened in Chantilly, Virginia, in 2008 and became the subject of a *Washington Post* article, are springing up around the country in states that allow druggists to refuse to provide products to which they object.[33] The group Pharmacists for Life provides a national list of pharmacies that don't stock contraceptive products. While some bioethicists feel that this sort of movement accurately represents the diversity of American opinions about these drugs, others worry that, particularly in rural areas, the new policies might create large geographic regions where birth control services are simply unavailable. At the very least, women's health advocates argue, pharmacies that refuse to stock contraceptives should disclose this fact in some overt way, perhaps by noting their policies in store windows or by posting them on their Web site.

Few would argue that opponents of abortion should be forced to perform or assist in the procedure. Also at issue, though, is the right to refuse to provide patients with complete information about their medical options as well as the right to refuse to provide referrals. While the first issue is understandable, already legally protected under the Civil Rights Act of 1964, and largely uncontested, the second and third are more controversial.

One of the least compassionate aspects of the Bush administration's conscience clause was the singling out of policies aimed at ensuring that hospitals, even religiously affiliated ones, offer EC to rape victims. Research prior to OTC status indicates that when it came to providing resources for rape victims, emergency rooms and hospitals were falling down on the job. A 2002 report found that only 21 percent of rape victims received emergency contraception between 1992 and 1999.[34] While these numbers have steadily improved over the last decade, they still remain strikingly low.[35]

Many states have taken steps to mandate that the drug be offered to women who come to emergency rooms after sexual assaults. Because the efficacy of EC declines rapidly with delayed administration, hospital refusal to provide the drug could be particularly devastating for rape victims. In some cases conservative lawmakers, such as Connecticut governor Jodi Rell, have contributed to legal compromises to ensure that women who need the drug receive it.[36] The Connecticut rule dispensed with earlier requirements that women take both an ovulation and a pregnancy test before the drug could be administered, and state bishops decided not to fight the change. In Pennsylvania a similar bill stirred controversy and resistance from Catholic groups and other religious organizations who believed that EC amounted to abortion and opposed it even for rape victims. Amy Beisel of the Pennsylvania Catholic Conference explained, "If we believe that life begins at conception, then we are talking about treating two patients."[37] Representative Dan Frankel countered, "This is not an issue about abortion . . . this is about protecting women who have been victimized."[38] These state skirmishes were hard-won, and the new rule threatened to undo the fragile peace that had begun to grow on former battlegrounds. Lawyer and historian Dorothy Roberts singles out the tendency to "pit a mother's welfare against that of her unborn child" as a particular feature of a society that tries to withhold reproductive autonomy from female populations.[39] Here we see this strategy of control taken to the next level: the psychological and physical well-being of women at their most vulnerable—after a rape—is pitted against the *idea* of an unborn child.

By late February 2009, the Obama administration moved to discard the Bush conscience rule. By that point seven states and two family planning groups had filed lawsuits to contest the policy.[40] One official noted that problems with "the Bush provider-refusal regulation" included the fact that it was worded so vaguely that "some have argued it could limit counseling, family planning, even blood transfusions and end-of-life care."[41] The decision followed other reproductive health actions taken in Obama's first thirty days where women's rights figured prominently. In addition to removing the conscience rule, Obama laid the groundwork for dispensing with the so-called global gag rule, a Reagan-era policy that refused American funds to international family planning groups that offered or even just referred women for abortions.[42]

Lest women feel too optimistic about the new administration's efforts to increase their reproductive rights, let it be known that the Obama administration capitulated with record speed when Republican lawmakers singled out contraceptive spending as an example of pork in the giant economic package. Commentator Ellen Goodman noted, "Searching through the economic stimulus plan for a villain, the balky Republican leadership jumped on a provision to allow states to expand family planning under Medicaid."[43] In defending his fledgling health care plan in the early fall of 2009, Obama said unequivocally that he did not plan to use public dollars to fund abortions, despite the fact that they are legal medical procedures. Women's health provisions have again been singled out, treated differently, used as political currency, and made into an example. It is a reminder that post-Bush optimism needs to be tempered by the realities of reproductive struggles that will no doubt continue to endure.

A victory for emergency contraceptive advocates that was not tied to the new administration happened in March 2009, when the US District Court for the Eastern District of New York ordered the FDA to offer Plan B without prescription to seventeen-year-olds within thirty days, and gave the organization a mandate to reconsider the original decision for women of all ages. Judge Edward R. Korman noted that the FDA had "acted in bad faith and in response to political pressure."[44] It was a vindication for Susan Wood and the other health advocates who had fought to publicize the strange case of Plan B. For young women who are still barred from access, it is important to know that several states offer programs where patients can obtain the drug directly from pharmacists, usually for a small consultation fee. These programs were put in place in response to the initial rejection of OTC Plan B to make access easier for women who didn't have the time or financial resources for doctor's visits.[45]

Politics Aside: Safety and Efficacy of Emergency Contraception

Once we detach these little pills from the big rhetoric that surrounds them, what information do patients need in order to use them safely and wisely?

The single biggest misconception about emergency contraception is that it is equivalent to medication abortion. Many young women who could benefit from the drug are reluctant to use it because of this very common error. Emergency contraception will not induce abortion if a patient is already pregnant. Mifepristone and misoprostol, the drugs taken to cause an abortion, work in ways that are totally different from EC. Mifepristone is an antiprogestin that prevents progesterone from protecting a woman's pregnancy and letting her body know that further ovulation isn't necessary. As a result, the uterine lining begins to shed—as it does in a monthly period. The second drug, misoprostol, induces uterine contractions that cause bleeding and the expulsion of the embryo.

Plan B has the opposite effect on a woman's hormones. It provides the body with a massive dose of progestin (levonorgestrel), helping to prevent ovulation by convincing the body that it is already pregnant. Despite being used after sex, EC is (as its name implies) contraception, meaning it *prevents* pregnancy—not abortion, which ends pregnancy.

There are several forms of postcoital birth control. The most famous, of course, is Plan B. For many reasons it is the simplest form of emergency contraception, consisting of only two small white levonorgestrel pills that may be taken together or twelve hours apart. In the summer of 2009, the FDA approved Plan B One-Step, a single 1500 µg dose of levonorgestrel.[46] In addition, at least twenty-three approved brands of birth control pills can be used for emergency contraception,[47] including combination (estrogen and progestin) and progestin-only pills; progestin-only pills are found to have fewer side effects and to be more effective. Patients who choose to use regular birth control pills must take the suggested dose in two installments spaced twelve hours apart. If you are considering this, be sure to speak with your doctor or consult a health care professional (clinics like Planned Parenthood can offer comprehensive information). Because you may experience severe nausea and vomiting, you might want to take an antinausea aid such as Dramamine or Bonine to settle your stomach.

In general, Plan B and hormonal emergency contraception have good safety profiles, and there are no long-term side effects. But because they offer a large dose of powerful chemicals, there are usually short-term side effects. These are generally painful but not dangerous, usually akin to bad menstrual symptoms. Common problems include cramping and abdominal pain, dizziness and headache, breast tenderness, spotting or bleeding, and tiredness. As with traditional oral contraceptives, EC can interact with certain drugs, particularly those that are metabolized through the liver such as St. John's Wort, potentially decreasing its effectiveness.

Because EC disrupts the menstrual cycle, it is likely that those who take it will experience cycle irregularity. Your period may come earlier or later than you expect, or your flow might be different from your usual menses. Repeated use of the drug over a short period of time may cause a more serious disruption of periods and even menstrual chaos. Since the extent of this damage isn't known, it is advisable to use emergency contraception only as a backup method, not as a primary form of birth control. One extremely rare but serious possible problem is ectopic pregnancy.[48]

Another highly effective type of birth control that can be employed after sex is the insertion of a Copper-T IUD. The IUD can be inserted up to five days after intercourse[49] and is 99 percent effective at preventing pregnancy. The decision to have an IUD put in is a serious one and is far more complicated to reverse than taking a pill. IUDs generally remain in the uterus for years (three to ten) and are not a short-term solution to any problem. Still, this method may be more foolproof in terms of pregnancy prevention than chemical alternatives.

Many health experts recommend that women keep emergency contraception on hand as a precautionary measure. This advice comes in response to studies showing that women are more likely to use the pill if they already have it. Michael T. Mennuti of the American College of Obstetricians and Gynecologists (ACOG) explains, "We hope to make EC a forethought, not an afterthought."[50] The shelf life of Plan B is forty-eight months,[51] long enough to make the fifty dollar investment worthwhile.

Access remains an issue for many patients. Estimates vary about how many pharmacies carry the drug. A study of Los Angeles–area stores found that 69 percent had the drug on their shelves, 19 percent referred callers to other providers, and the remaining stores refused to provide information or hung up the phone.[52] A survey in New York City is more encouraging:[53] between 2002 and 2006 the percentage of stores stocking Plan B rose from 55 percent to 87 percent, and by the spring of 2007 the number was up to 94 percent, an accomplishment that Council Speaker Christine Quinn called a "major victory in the fight to protect the reproductive rights of all women."[54] In general, access to EC is better in cities than in small towns,[55] and the number of stores that stock the products has improved since OTC status was granted.[56]

In all of the ideological scrambling over emergency contraception, one of the FDA's most basic criteria—how well emergency contraception works—has been pushed to the corners of the conversation. Indeed, while EC boasts hearty safety statistics, serious questions remain about how well it actually prevents pregnancy. For activists who support greater access and education around Plan B and other EC methods, the hope surrounding the drug is multifaceted. First and foremost, they hope that it will help reduce teen pregnancy rates and unwanted and unplanned pregnancies in the larger female population. In the United States it is estimated that 3.5 million unplanned pregnancies occur each year,[57] 30 percent of them in teenagers.[58] Before the battle over OTC status, some scientists and population experts estimated that that this number could be reduced by half if emergency contraception was broadly used.[59] With several years of use, studies were unable to demonstrate a significant reduction in unwanted pregnancies between women with increased access to the drug and those who needed to go through doctors. The question remains: do unwanted pregnancies remain high because EC doesn't work as well as medical experts believe, or is it because even patients who can procure the drug don't use it?

While certainly some women remain unaware that a postcoital option exists, they are increasingly the minority. One trial found that "some 64 percent of reproductive-age women surveyed in 2004 said that there was something women could do to prevent pregnancy following sex, and 75 percent of those women mentioned emergency contraception."[60] Studies show that awareness of the drug has exploded, due in part to heavy media coverage of controversies surrounding its status. So why are so few young women taking advantage of backup contraception?

When I talked to a group of college women at a small school in the Northeast, they were informed about the availability of Plan B as an option and very clear about the willingness of their school health services to provide it. One girl explained to me that she has taken Plan B a couple times despite using both condoms and the pill: "I take Microgestin and my boyfriend uses condoms every time. But once or twice the condoms have broken, or I've forgotten to take my pills. So, yeah, then we've used the morning-after pill." Perhaps low use is simply a process of education, and with a few more years of increased availability, more women will opt to turn to EC in unanticipated situations.

Much seems to hang on how patients interpret the word "emergency."[61] While there isn't currently a limit on how often the drug is used, EC is intended to be employed only when other strategies have failed. A frequent argument against the easy availability of emergency contraception—one of the few to be voiced by those on both sides of the political spectrum— is that it might encourage people to rely on less effective methods of birth control or even engage in high-risk behaviors like unprotected sex with the belief that the potential consequences of these lapses can be accounted for after the fact. A deep concern on the part of conservative opponents seems to be that knowledge of Plan B will lead men to pressure female partners into condomless sex. Some cite studies that show a return to unsafe sex practices following the development of powerful drugs to treat AIDS in the 1990s.[62] Most studies suggest that these fears are unfounded, and that the availability of these drugs doesn't lead to riskier behavior.[63] However, at least one study has indeed found that EC knowledge can lead some to take more chances. In my conversations, a theme that emerged again and again was that the women who were informed about EC were more likely to be using other contraceptive methods and were among the most educated and motivated when it came to protecting their health.[64] Far from taking a devil-may-care approach to contraception, these women were doing everything they could think of to prevent pregnancy *and* sexually transmitted diseases.

Efficacy still dogs the drug, and even large meta-analyses fail to find a reduction in pregnancy even when EC is readily available.[65] One source of concern is that access studies, which fail to demonstrate a reduction in unplanned pregnancies, do show that women with greater access to EC are more likely to take it.[66] So if more women are using the drug, why aren't pregnancy numbers down? Two different but deeply related efficacy issues are up for discussion here: the first is the ability of the pill to prevent pregnancy in an individual woman, and the second, its ability to reduce pregnancy on a population level.

Official efficacy rates suggest that EC reduces the risk of pregnancy substantially. One estimate figures that if one hundred women engage in sex without protection in the second or third week of their cycle, eight will become pregnant. Another study finds that with combined Emergency Contraception Pills (ECPs: pills that have both estrogen and progestin), only two will become pregnant (a 75 percent reduction) and with progestin-only pills, only one woman will conceive (an 89 percent reduction).[67] Other figures are not so optimistic, figuring efficacy as low as 49 percent.[68] Writing in the journal *Contraception*, Elizabeth G. Raymond, Jennifer Liku, and Eleanor Bilma Schwarz note that estimates placing efficacy in the 80 and 90 percent range are "probably false,"[69] and figure the real reduction is closer to 50 percent, noting that "a robust estimate of the efficacy of emergency contraception is not currently available."

Why is it so hard to tell how well EC works? These authors note the difficulty of mounting a trial to assess this, citing, among other problems, ethical concerns with creating controls. In other words, scientists can't ask a group of women who have engaged in unprotected sex not to take the drug or give them a placebo, so getting good comparative data is tricky.

What seems undisputed is that for individual women, taking emergency contraception provides some real, if variable, protection against pregnancy. Though use is still relatively low—one British report estimates that only one in ten women wishing to avoid pregnancy turn to emergency contraception when they are at risk[70]—it is safe to say that EC is a valuable resource that women should be able to access at will.

From Emergency to Everyday Use: Should the Pill Go Over the Counter?

The fortunate lack of a safety disaster in the Plan B experience has renewed old controversies about whether traditional birth control pills should follow emergency contraception over the counter. Some countries, including Spain and Russia, already offer the Pill without prescription.[71] Other nations, including the United Kingdom, have been cautiously piloting programs to test the safety and feasibility of such a move.[72] By late 2008, two London districts had received permission to offer OTC birth control pills.[73] The program will work through something called patient direction, in which a doctor can authorize a pharmacy to provide pills without prescriptions to a certain group of patients. Women will still need to have their blood pressure checked and their medical information reviewed to ensure that they don't have compelling contraindications.

Momentum for making the change away from prescriptions built in 2008 when the prestigious medical journal the *Lancet* recommended that offering the Pill directly to consumers would cut ovarian cancer risks. In the dramatic article scientists estimated that in the fifty years the Pill had been available it may have prevented as many as one hundred thousand deaths.[74] The authors concluded, "This latest study raises the question again of whether oral contraceptives should be made more widely available to women to protect them from ovarian cancer. We believe that the case is now convincing. Women deserve the choice to obtain oral contraceptives over-the-counter."[75] Learning a lesson from the history of emergency contraception, advocates of nonprescription pills realized they needed a health imperative to spark acceptance of this controversial, if not new, idea. Much like the relegalization of contraception in the United States from the 1920s to the 1960s, as well as the initial legalization of the Pill, the case for access has been couched in terms of disease prevention rather than female sexual empowerment.

Other experts are quick to point out that neither the evidence nor the issues are so clear cut. Rosanna Capolingua, the president of the Australian Medical Association, says efforts to remove prescription requirements from the Pill will not advance women's health: "We've known about the link between ovarian cancer and the Pill for some time, but it [the Pill] inherently has other risks and so that's why it's important that it's prescribed by a doctor who can assess a woman's particular circumstances."[76]

In other words, prolonged hormonal contraception is more complicated than EC. It requires more understanding and knowledge of an individual's health issues and can have more serious outcomes if used incorrectly. More conditions make the Pill a bad idea, and there are a greater number of problems that need to be constantly monitored by a doctor.

And so the role of doctors as administrators of women's health again comes to the fore. Access to hormonal contraception has long been a powerful incentive for women to maintain regular relationships with health care practitioners. Many public health care experts fear that removing the requirement that the Pill be prescribed would eliminate many women's most powerful motivation for having yearly Pap smears, HPV tests, and other evaluations that can be powerful indicators of wellness or infection. Indeed, whatever ovarian cancer prevention might be achieved through increasing access could easily be eliminated by increased cervical cancer if women fail to have their yearly exams.

When I spoke to Amy Allina of the National Women's Health Network, a grassroots women's health group in Washington, DC, that takes no money from drug companies or device makers (and that therefore tends to be able to criticize potentially dangerous drugs more frankly), she told me that while the network's position on over-the-counter OCs "has evolved slightly" over the years, what hasn't changed is the feeling that the benefits of increased access to the Pill should outweigh the risks of women taking the drug without expert medical advice, if such a change is to happen.[77] It is likely that when women take the Pill without consulting with a doctor or nurse, women who shouldn't consider hormonal options—particularly those with increased cardiovascular risks or undiagnosed diabetes—will take the drug.

The problem, Allina explains, is that it turns out that doctors don't have a great track record with filtering out women who shouldn't be on the Pill. So even if they *do* consult with a doctor, women who should not be prescribed the Pill often are. In fact, studies suggest that when women are handed a list of health considerations and given the opportunity to self-educate, they do a better job than doctors at spotting potential health red lights (the only place where this doesn't seem to be true is with undiagnosed hypertension). Unfortunately, the ability of women to self-educate and administer medicines is largely left out of the conversation.

So is the problem that women who want hormonal contraceptives can't get them? Dr. Sarah Jarvis of the Royal College of General Practitioners in the United Kingdom argues that the problem for most women is not access to pills, but rather adherence to daily regimens: "Compliance is low with oral contraceptives. In one study of women using oral contraception, 47 percent missed one or more pills per cycle, and 22 percent missed two or more."[78] In other words, the problem isn't that women can't get pills—it's that they can't seem to take them correctly. But a survey in the United States suggested a contrary position: 41 percent of those surveyed who were not currently using oral contraceptives said they would start if they were able to get the drug without going through a doctor.[79]

While many women may like the idea of bypassing medical professionals on their path to reproductive independence, economic issues may preclude this reality for a large number of people. Granting oral contraceptives OTC status would mean that they would no longer be covered by insurance. This would pose a serious problem for low-income women and at least an inconvenience for others. And it would be difficult to send one pill over the counter without allowing others to follow. The reason for this is that so many oral contraceptives are "me too" drugs—pills that are similar enough to existing drugs that they have used existing safety data to gain FDA approval. If one company received permission to market their pill over the counter, any other pill that used the same safety data for green-lighting would have to go over the counter as well.

Because of this, those wrestling with the OTC issue suggest that perhaps progestin-only pills (POPs) should go over the counter and combined pills (those with estrogen and progestin) remain with prescription status. This way, those who rely on insurance to pay for pills could get them, and those who wanted to buy them in a drugstore without a prescription could also be accommodated. This isn't a perfect plan. Because POPs are newer, we have a lot less information about their efficacy and their unique concerns. Sending POPs over the counter creates a risk of "classing" the pill and creating a situation where women who would need to rely on POPs would be stuck with a product about which we have less knowledge.

For now, women's health advocates are gathering information and trying to think through the potential positives and pitfalls of changing the way that women get birth control. "It's all so complicated," Allina told me. "How this plays out in the reality of women's lives is really the question. Is it more of a barrier to access to sit in a clinic for two hours and pay for a doctor's visit? Or is it more of a barrier to pay a higher price for the drug? It's a tough question."[80]

The issue of gaining insurance coverage for contraceptives has been a feminist battleground for decades. Women are no strangers to navigating political minefields on the way to picking up their birth control pills. Today it is estimated that only 15 percent of indemnity insurance plans and 39 percent of HMO plans cover all FDA-approved contraceptive methods. Only twenty-seven states require insurers who cover prescription drugs to pay for contraceptive drugs and devices,[81] and many of these have conscience clauses and opt-out policies for employers and insurers. This means that women spend 68 percent more money out-of-pocket on health care than their male counterparts.[82] Still, the proportion of insurers who cover contraceptives has skyrocketed in the past decade and is three times higher than just ten years ago.[83]

For low-income women, there is good news and bad news. The good news is that family planning coverage is mandatory in the Medicaid program. Title X programs, which provide services for women at varying income levels but largely focus on people below the poverty line, fill an important gap in coverage for women who don't qualify for Medicaid. This program also provides family planning services, but (and here's the bad news) the program is chronically underfunded. Since 1980, this resource, which provides contraception to 4.2 million women, has seen its funding slashed by 61 percent.[84]

Ironically, the contraceptive equity movement really gained steam when insurers who refused birth control coverage began paying for erectile dysfunction drugs. Women from both sides of the political spectrum saw the injustice of covering drugs that may lead to unplanned pregnancies while refusing to pay for prescriptions to prevent them. While this comparison has proved powerful, Gretchen Borchelt, senior counsel for health and reproductive rights at the National Women's Law Center, notes, "Certainly we want to think more broadly than just Viagra."[85]

When Margaret Sanger and the early mothers of modern contraception allied their movement with the medical profession, they made a bargain: contraception would be a health issue, not a sexual one. In exchange for legality and respectability, women would cede some level of autonomy and authority. The unwillingness of insurers to cover sexual health products breaks this time-honored arrangement. Either contraception is medicine or it is not. If it is not, then women shouldn't have to go through gatekeepers to get it. If it is, then it should be covered like any other prescription pill.

Chapter Eight

Running in Cycles: Fertility Awareness and Natural Birth Control

I'm dreaming now: of adolescents knowing how their reproductive systems work before they become sexually active and before they choose a birth control method; of women and men being as aware of our fertility as we are about our sexuality.

—Katie Singer

Something was in the air as I took the podium to talk to a group of graduate students in Washington, DC, in February 2009. I hesitated as I began to speak, sharing the history of hormonal contraception and moving on to the current issues surrounding birth control today. When I opened up the conversation for questions, hands flew up. I expected some to be annoyed about my cautious attitude toward the Pill or perhaps curious about new drugs like menstrual suppressants. Instead, the women wanted to know about fertility awareness.

"Given the lack of innovation in pharmaceutical contraception and the dangers of existing methods," asked a quiet, chicly dressed redhead, "what is the future of birth control? Is it fertility awareness?" Mumbles of agreement spread around the sunny conference room.

It wasn't the first time I had faced this question. In the past year or so, friends had begun to inquire in hushed tones about the possibility of natural birth control. We had all been raised in the church of the Pill, and such talk was blasphemous. The reasons to fear natural methods were well known: they were unreliable, risky, and the near-exclusive practice of quite another church. And yet as my friends edged closer to thirty and problems with other types of birth control persisted, they began to chip away at the gospel of pharmaceutical infallibility. They came to me because I was a well-known heretic.

What are the facts and fictions surrounding natural birth control methods, particularly fertility awareness? Is it indeed a viable method of managing fertility, simply a useful system for acquiring knowledge of one's body that should have little to do with contraception, or an unreliable crackpot method suitable only for religious fanatics and pharmaceutical alarmists? How do religious and social relationships affect the acceptance and availability of knowledge about this type of fertility control, and are those historical alliances shifting?

History, Naturally

A surprising fact about the Fertility Awareness Method (FAM), either as a method of birth control or a tool for improved gynecological health, is that it is a modern method that stands alongside the Pill as a twentieth-century innovation. Although women have been manipulating their fertility for as long as they have been menstruating, good knowledge about the ovary and how it functions has emerged slowly over the past two thousand years. While interest in the uterus was more profound until the end of the nineteenth century, these olive-shaped and sized organs have attracted ample speculation and misinterpretation over the course of recorded human history, and only in recent years have we come to fully understand what they do and how they do it.

It is impossible to know who was the first individual, driven by curiosity, eccentricity, or perhaps something darker, to open the abdominal cavity of a female animal or human and notice these tiny matching organs sitting like ears on the sides of the uterus. Aristotle observed that castrating animals seemed to have an effect on their sex drives but didn't extend the possible implications of this information to humans. His influential theory of human conception, which continued to inform doctors for well over a thousand years, was the "seed and soil" model: the female body provided rich "soil" in which the male "seed" could thrive. In this system, the ovary was essentially irrelevant. Other doctors and philosophers quickly began to consider that perhaps the ovary had a direct role in reproduction, and second-century Roman physician Galen believed that it made a kind of sperm. But interest in the ovary stalled—or at least slowed precipitously—for about a thousand years.

Then in the sixteenth century, Fallopious (1523–1562) explored the existence and function of the tubes that bear his name and compared the ovaries with the male testicles. It was around this time that the two oval female glands acquired their name. Despite changes, many doctors continued to believe that follicles and ovulatory material were a product of, rather than a partner in, conception.

Regnier de Graaf (1641–1673), a Dutch physician and anatomist, believed that the ovary was important and had been misunderstood and underestimated by those who came before him. De Graaf rejected older notions that ovaries were appendages and dismissed false analogies between male and female reproductive systems. He wrote in 1672 that he believed the whole organ was a giant egg, just like the kind laid by birds. De Graaf based this conclusion, in part, on experiments conducted with the recovered ovaries of corpses, which he boiled and tasted.[1] He insisted that the taste was similar in texture and flavor to avian products. In all of this questionable experimentation, de Graaf noticed something important: he became one of the first to accurately describe the corpora lutea (what ovarian follicles become after ovulation has occurred).

By the end of the seventeenth century, three distinct schools of thought had emerged concerning what ovaries actually did and their role in making babies: the first held firmly to the Aristotelian view that men were the active agents in conception and women were simply loyal farmers who nurtured their crops. The second believed that the ovary itself was the site of conception. A third, approaching something closer to (although still distant from) the truth, believed that the ovaries were female testes that produced some sort of reproductive product (although it would still be many years before the clear differences between these male and female organs would be spelled out).

In the eighteenth and the early nineteenth centuries, doctors continued to worry about the exact anatomy of the ovary. Many ideas, some ahead of their time, were in the air, including the notion that the actions of the organs controlled menstruation. These ideas were noted, although largely ignored, by a medical world that still believed that menstruation had a purgative quality and therefore functioned to relieve the body of toxins, not in response to hormonal fluctuations.

As with so many discoveries about women's bodies (and bodies in general), more substantial knowledge about the ovary began to emerge in the nineteenth century, in part in response to an increase in the desire of doctors to perform surgeries on them. In the 1840s Félix A. Pouchet, a French naturalist, debunked the belief that the ovary functioned in response to sexual intercourse. Pouchet was used to working with animals, and like so many before and after him, drew mistaken analogies between human and nonhuman bodily processes. He believed that menstruation was equivalent to heat in nonhumans and proposed therefore that ovulation must happen during menses.[2] His belief that bleeding signaled the start, rather than the end, of the menstrual cycle would haunt the practice of natural birth control well in to the twentieth century. Other thinkers, such as Adam Raciborski, thought that Pouchet was wrong. In 1843 Raciborski published his observations about recently married women. He noticed that those married after the twelfth day of their menstrual cycle were less likely to become pregnant than those married in the first half of the month.[3] Still, the damage was done, and the notion that midcycle sex was safest for pregnancy prevention was popularized.

These decades of uncertainty and the contraceptive systems that emerged based on faulty science created a deeply held distrust on the part of women and their partners of the use of bodily indicators alone to predict fertility. To this day, many educated people believe that natural methods rely exclusively on such outdated and mistaken ideas about the female body.

By the 1870s doctors had discovered ovulation, and this realization triggered a shift in focus away from the uterus as the center of female health. It also set scientists on a path that ended with the discovery and isolation of sex hormones and the eventual development of contraceptive methods based on them. By 1905, another Dutchman, Theodor Hendrik van de Velde, showed that women ovulated only once during an individual menstrual cycle. Then in the 1920s two doctors independently made a breakthrough:[4] Hermann Knaus of Austria and Kyusaku Ogino of Japan both found that in women with normal menstrual cycles, ovulation occurs approximately fourteen days before the onset of menstrual bleeding.[5]

Before women knew how their ovaries worked in relation to their menstrual cycles, they couldn't avoid or engage in sex strategically to control fertility. It just wasn't possible. Once better information became available, exactly how best to use this information remained—and to some extent remains—an open question.

In this sense, methods of contraception based on fertility awareness are twentieth-century innovations. They are developments contemporary with the Pill, and historically postdate older methods like condoms, cervical caps, and IUDs.

Becoming Aware: Different Methods of Natural Fertility Control

One of the most confusing things about understanding natural contraception is realizing that there are several different methods and combinations of methods that have been used over the past seventy-five years.[6] They are different in ideology, approach, terminology, and efficacy. Understanding these distinctions is the first step in evaluating whether and to what extent fertility awareness can play a role in your own contraceptive choices.

When I call these methods "natural," I mean only that they involve no chemical, surgical, or device intervention to prevent pregnancy (although of course many people use them in combination with other methods, particularly barriers). I am specifically not making any sort of moral or ideological judgment about what people should or shouldn't do to manage their fertility. As a person who has used pills, barriers, and occasionally fertility awareness, I believe that there will be a different answer to the question of how or whether to prevent pregnancy for every adult engaging in heterosexual sex. And as I hope my discussion of the mythical cavewoman in previous chapters has made clear, I have no interest in theorizing about what is natural or unnatural when it comes to sex.

There are four major types of natural contraception: calendar (which uses a woman's menstrual cycle to guess when she will ovulate and therefore avoid sex for several days around that time), those based around fertility signs like cervical fluids and cervical position, those that analyze changes in basal body temperature, and approaches that use devices such as saliva tests or fertility monitors to estimate when ovulation has occurred. Other approaches combine various aspects of these different methodologies. Calendar-based methods (such as the rhythm method) and systems that use abridged monitoring of fertility signs don't work nearly as well as comprehensive regimens that look at temperature, cervical fluid, and other physical indicators that ovulation is going to happen. This latter system is usually called the fertility awareness method, or FAM. Experts who teach FAM lament the association of what they consider a reliable way to control fertility with much less predictable methods based largely on guesswork.

It is frequently noted that FAM and the rhythm method are two different things. When people say this, they mean that calendar-based systems and those that rely on monitoring signs of fertility are discrete. I have found that terminology around different methods is very confusing. Some calendar-based systems, such as the Standard Days method, are referred to as subtypes of fertility awareness in some studies, but this isn't accurate. The important thing to ask when analyzing a method of natural birth control is whether it depends on looking at a calendar, looking at what is going on in your body, or both.

Calendar-Based Methods

Q: What do you call people who use the rhythm method?
A: Parents
—Old Catholic school joke

The first category of natural birth control, under which the rhythm method falls, includes those systems that are calendar based. These methods rely on estimating when ovulation occurs based on either an average menstrual cycle or calculations made by observing an individual's previous menstrual cycles. Couples practicing this type of birth control simply avoid sex during the days when it is believed that ovulation is occurring.

Calendar-based natural family planning systems are known to be significantly less effective than observational approaches, and the reasons for this should be obvious: if they are based on an average menstrual cycle— such as the classic twenty-eight-day model—they operate on the assumption that one woman's body will work like another's. If a method uses a women's past cycles to guess when she is fertile, it assumes that she won't experience any cycle variability over time. All women know that menstrual cycles are inconsistent, both among women and over the course of an individual woman's life. Some women are different month to month. One woman may have regular twenty-nine-day cycles, but her friend may experience a thirty-two-day cycle and then a twenty-five-day cycle. Even if a system is based on a woman's own menstrual history, it is not necessarily accurate, because a number of factors (illness, stress, and travel, to name only a few) can cause even the most regular among us to have an atypical month.

Advocates of calendar-based systems argue that they are simpler to learn and less difficult to practice than other methods. This sort of assumption is based on the belief that women are too lazy to take their temperature every day, as well as other ideas about the abilities of uneducated women to fulfill and understand the tasks involved in using a technique that involves observation of fertility signs.

The problem with this sort of approach—and its implicit assumptions—can be seen in a 1999 study involving teaching fertility awareness to Mayan women. In designing the study, researchers working with the Population Council wrote:

> More than half of Mayan women have never attended school. Given such low educational levels, the ease with which a method can be learned could affect both adoption of the method and its effectiveness. A blanket calendar method with simple rules of abstinence that are applicable to all couples would appear to offer advantages in its simplicity over other natural methods that require observations of cervical mucus or basal body temperature.[7]

Researchers admitted, however, that the workability of their plan would depend on the women they were instructing having, on the whole, regular menstrual cycles. They were basically saying that something was better than nothing.

What they found, of course, was that even women who claimed to have regular cycles often had striking inconsistencies when compared with other women and individually from month to month. Researchers concluded that because their cycles "may not be very regular," a calendar method—in this case the Necklace system—might put women at "an unacceptable risk of pregnancy."[8]

Again, the problem here is the assumption that there is such a thing as a regular menstrual cycle. Indeed, the only thing that seems regular is variability. The misconception among women and health care professionals that most women bleed every twenty-eight to thirty-one days is responsible not only for countless unplanned pregnancies, but also for the unnecessary medicating, often with oral contraceptives, of women for menstrual irregularities.

Still, new systems based on this relatively old way of performing natural family planning continue to be developed. The Necklace method, which involves using beads to count supposedly fertile and unfertile days, is a variant on the Standard Days method, which relies on creating a fixed system of days during which couples abstain (or use alternate contraception).

The Standard Days/Necklace method was developed and tested in the 1990s by researchers at the Institute for Reproductive Health (IRH) of Georgetown University (a Catholic university). Standard Days[9] was developed, in part, in response to a belief that it would be too difficult to educate populations—particularly international populations—about more precise but complicated natural contraceptive techniques.[10] Victoria Jennings, one of the researchers who tested Standard Days, notes, "These methods are just too complicated . . . It takes two weeks to train a provider on these methods at minimum, and eight sessions with a client to learn how to use these methods."[11]

In studies published in the journal *Contraception* in 2002 and 2004, Standard Days was studied in populations of women in Bolivia, Peru, and the Philippines. Women were given a CycleBeads necklace and followed for thirteen cycles. Study authors announced proudly that only 43 of their 478 participants became pregnant (around 12 percent), an efficacy "comparable to that of male condoms" and "significantly better than that of other barrier methods (female condom, diaphragm, cervical cap, or spermicides)."[12] It is important to note that only women with regular menstrual cycles—between twenty-six and thirty-two days—were included in the study.[13]

This was all quite exciting, and Georgetown wasted no time in marketing CycleBeads to the general public. The necklace is composed of thirty-two plastic beads: nineteen coffee-colored beads, split by twelve glow-in-the-dark white beads, and one tomato red bead. At the center of the string sits a black cylinder with a shiftable black ring. On the first day of a woman's period, she moves the black ring to the red bead. Each day she moves it ahead one bead, first over the initial set of brown beads, then onto the white ones, and eventually back to brown. When a woman hits the white beads, she considers herself fertile and either abstains for twelve days or uses alternative contraception (this choice is a touchy issue for natural family planners, who are still, on the whole, religiously motivated and opposed to barrier contraception). By July 2004, the IRH estimated that thirty thousand women had started using the method.[14]

I asked Toni Weschler, author of the most influential FAM guidebook around—*Taking Charge of Your Fertility*—about CycleBeads. Weschler is warm and patient, but she didn't hesitate to offer her opinion:

> As far as menstrual beads, don't get me started! *Awful.* For one thing, they are no different than the rhythm method, since they don't account for potential variation in the day of ovulation! And they are only effective for women with consistent twenty-six to thirty-two-day cycles. They tell all these women that they are fertile between days 8 through 19, regardless of what their unique cycle might be any given month. Which begs the question, why should they even use the silly beads at all. Why not just make a blanket statement that if you have cycles between days 26 and 32 days, consider yourself fertile between days 8 and 19, and don't waste your time with the beads? Also, in any given month, the woman could ovulate much earlier or later than normal, and bingo—an unplanned pregnancy![15]

Feminist women's health centers offer an alternative calendar method based on a woman's individual cycle history. To practice this method, a woman records her cycles for eight to twelve months, noting their length and the number of days of bleeding in each. After this time, a woman can subtract eighteen from the length of her shortest cycle, noting this as the first fertile day. She can then subtract eleven from the length of her longest cycle, noting this as her last fertile day. So if the shortest period is twenty-seven days (27 − 18 = 9) and the longest period is thirty-one days (31 − 11 =

20), a woman can estimate that her first fertile day is the ninth day of her cycle (with the first day of bleeding serving as day one) and her last fertile day is the twentieth day. She would then need either to abstain from sex or use alternative contraception for twelve days.[16] Because women's cycles change throughout their lives, this number should be recalculated each month, adding the most recent cycle's information. As noted above, however, the fact that even a woman with very regular periods experiences periodic variations casts serious doubt on this sort of system.

Monitoring Fertility Signs

In the 1930s, when John Smulders, a Dutch physician, and other doctors were settling on a formula for the rhythm method, Father Wilhelm Hillebrand, a Catholic priest, was working on a system to curtail pregnancy by monitoring basal body temperature (a woman's waking temperature after at least six hours of sleep). As fertility expert Katie Singer notes, "Before ovulation, your body is cooler. After ovulation, your temperature will warm up and stay warm."[17] This rise in body heat happens because of progesterone, the hormone released by the ovarian follicle once an egg has burst forth and the follicle has retreated to corpus luteum status. By monitoring and recording daily temperatures, women can tell with some accuracy if ovulation has taken place.

In the early 1950s, Dr. John Billings, an Australian doctor and father of nine, pioneered a method of fertility control based on watching changes in cervical fluid (sometimes called cervical mucus), substances produced by the cervix that can aid or impede the ability of sperm to survive. The cervical fluids respond to hormones during the menstrual cycle, and in the days before ovulation, become sticky and stretchy, like an egg white. Once ovulation has passed, the cervical fluids become creamy, pasty, or they dry up completely. Significantly, while Billings first advocated both temperature and fluid methods, he eventually decided this combined system was too complicated and decided instead to encourage only fluid monitoring.

Today, a modern day version of the fluid-only approach is the TwoDay method[18] of fertility control. Another product of Georgetown's IRH, this technique councils women to ask themselves two questions each day. The first is "Did I note any secretions today?" and the second is "Did I note any secretions yesterday?"[19] Researchers studying the method explain, "If she noticed no cervical secretions of any type today or yesterday, her probability of getting pregnant from intercourse today is very low."[20] To test this system, trial authors observed 450 women in Guatemala, Peru, and the Philippines. Of the 52.7 percent of women who completed the trial, forty-seven got pregnant. This method makes many assumptions, among them that women can differentiate cervical secretions from other kinds of vaginal discharge (such as fluids having to do with sexual arousal) without other types of information. One senses, reading the literature, that Georgetown isn't entirely happy with this method; even in a study supporting TwoDay's efficacy, they promote Standard Days. Still, they note, the advantage of the TwoDay method is that women with longer and shorter than normal cycles can use it as well.

By the 1970s, Catholic groups had started to teach methods that combined temperature recording with observation of cervical fluid and cervical position (which changes, like fluid, in response to hormones throughout the menstrual cycle). These approaches, called "symptothermal" methods, became the basis for FAM, the type of natural birth control that has been shown to be by far the most efficacious.

In the decades before the 1970s, most resources regarding natural contraception came from and were administered by the Catholic Church. Katie Singer explains that this often caused problems because it limited access to classes and information to those whose relationships and sexual practices fell within Church-approved models.

By the time Singer was learning about the method years later, things hadn't changed very much. She describes her introduction to fertility awareness, which came after years of struggling with contraception she didn't like and persistent yeast infections: "I began learning fertility awareness primarily by taking classes and reading literature put out by Catholic organizations. Many statements in the literature didn't suit me. Despite my discomfort, I started to observe and record my fertility signals."[21] In 1997, after developing an enthusiasm for the method, Singer tried to take a class with a local expert in New Mexico, where she lived. The woman told her politely that she could give Singer an application for the class, but couldn't accept her because she was unmarried and had "genital contact."[22] Singer went on to write a lovely, comprehensive book on FAM called *The Garden of Fertility* and to counsel women both on the method and on other important aspects of health—such as nutrition—that can profoundly impact menstruation and conception.

Perhaps because of the association of natural birth control with religious values and—to those on the outside of these institutions—prejudices, it has been difficult to build alliances between educators who are experienced in teaching natural family planning and women's health organizations and clinics. As a result, many educated women are unaware that these options exist.

Toni Weschler began teaching fertility awareness in the early 1980s. Weschler embraced a symptothermal system that synthesized taking basal body temperatures and watching changes in cervical fluids and position. In 1995 she published *Taking Charge of Your Fertility*,[23] a truly radical book that instructed women in how to use fertility awareness methods to prevent or encourage pregnancy, and also simply to improve awareness of reproductive health, all from a secular, feminist perspective. Weschler's point is that the FAM is the only method of family planning that is useful at all points in a woman's reproductive life, from menarche to menopause, and if she chooses, for contraceptive and reproductive purposes. While *Taking Charge of Your Fertility* explains how to use FAM to prevent pregnancy and also to monitor gynecological well-being, Weschler tells me that the book attracts many more women who are looking to get pregnant. She theorizes that the book's title may be part of this trend. It is telling that women pursue detailed, complex information about their bodies and menstrual cycles only in the context of trying to have a baby, when such knowledge would be useful in so many other contexts.

Another option for predicting fertility is to use devices such as fertility monitors and saliva tests to predict when ovulation is about to happen. Ovulation predictor kits test for the presence of luteinizing hormone (LH). Bursts of this hormone are usually followed by ovulation within twelve to thirty-six hours. Fertility monitors can be inconsistent, but they represent a technology that is still developing and changing, offering the promise of improved predictive powers in the future. A 2004 test of one such monitor, the Clearplan Easy, found that it has the potential to help women narrow the window of time during which they can consider themselves fertile. However, fertility devices can still only predict ovulation around two days in advance. Since sperm can live for five days, this means a woman using a fertility test can easily become pregnant from sex that happened days before ovulation. Because of this, these technologies are best used in combination with other methods, such as the observation of cervical fluids.[24] As Weschler notes, "These monitoring tests can be superb in adding yet another piece of evidence to corroborate the other fertility signs that women observe, and I personally believe that the more signs you chart, the more effective the method will be."[25]

Rules of the Road: A Basic Outline of FAM

The method popularized by Weschler is exactly the more complicated set of practices that worried the researchers at Georgetown and women's health educators all over the world. And yet, Weschler insists, it is simple and can be practiced in just minutes a day. What is outlined below is a basic description of the method—it is not intended to teach its use. Anyone interested in learning or practicing fertility awareness should talk to a doctor or health care professional, get a book specifically on the subject, or take a class on the method.

The first step is to get a chart where you can record various information throughout the month, including start date, cycle day, waking temperature, vaginal sensation, position of cervix, cervical fluid, whether you have sexual intercourse, and any other information that might be relevant in understanding the cycle—for example, recording food cravings or mood swings might help to diagnose and treat premenstrual syndrome. These charts can be found in books and photocopied or downloaded online. Fertility charting has, like everything else, gone digital in recent years. Jane, a thirty-something midwesterner tells me that she uses an online service that stores her charts and allows her to update from her phone.

On the first day of your cycle, begin taking your temperature with either a digital thermometer or a basal body glass thermometer upon first waking. This means leaving the thermometer by your bed and sticking it in your mouth before you get up, go to the bathroom, brush your teeth, have breakfast, or move in any significant way. Some people believe that taking the temperature vaginally is more accurate, and if you are having trouble with taking it orally, you can try this, but make sure to be consistent—don't switch between oral and vaginal readings in a certain month. To be accurate, you should have gotten at least three hours of sleep. It's best to take the temperature at approximately the same time each day, as each hour of variation can cause slight inclines in temperature and can skew your results. Record your temperature on your chart, connecting the circles each day to form a line that goes up and down as the month progresses and shows how your body changes day to day.

The day your temperature rises noticeably—at least two-tenths of a degree higher than it has been for six days—use a ruler to draw a straight line across the entire chart at one-tenth of a degree above the highest temperature for the previous six days. Once your temperature has stayed above this "coverline" for three consecutive days, you can assume that ovulation has occurred and that you are no longer fertile for the month. If your temperature goes up but doesn't stay above the coverline for three days, you must start counting again when it returns to a level above the line.

Remember this can be complicated by many things, from daylight savings to changing time zones to having a lot of alcohol the night before to having a fever. It is normal to have outlying temperatures that aren't the result of ovulation, and you must be very careful when deciding that ovulation has indeed occurred.

After taking your temperature each morning, you should check your cervical fluid. This can begin as soon as you finish your period. Weschler advises, "Focus on vaginal sensations throughout the day (i.e., Does the outside of the vagina feel dry, sticky, or wet? Does it feel like you are sitting in a puddle of eggwhite?)"[26] When using the bathroom throughout the day, check fluid by using clean fingers to separate the vaginal lips and use either tissue or fingers to gather a small bit of secretion between the thumb and pointer finger. Feel the fluid on your fingers before looking at it and notice if the texture is dry, creamy, pasty, or sticky. Observe the fluid and slowly draw your fingers apart. When women are preparing for ovulation, fluid will often stretch between fingers to distances of an inch or two and be clear in color like an egg white. Record observations about cervical secretions on your chart, being sure not to confuse other fluids—

such as semen, spermicide, or wetness resulting from sexual arousal—with cervical mucus. Because these substances can confuse charting, be sure not to chart if you have just had sex or used another form of contraception that involves spermicide (such as a diaphragm). Also be aware that many prescription drugs, including antihistamines and antibiotics, can affect cervical fluid. Try to check this fertility sign at least three times a day. With practice, women can identify their "peak" day: the last day of high-quality cervical fluid before ovulation happens, and, as the name suggests, the best day for having sex if pregnancy is desired.

Cervical position can be determined by squatting and inserting just-washed fingers into the vagina and feeling the entrance to the uterus. The cervix, a tiny pink nub, serves as the boundary between the womb and the vagina. At the beginning of the cycle, the cervix is low and hard. As days pass and hormones begin to flow, it slowly rises and begins to open and soften, preparing to welcome sperm as ovulation becomes imminent. (Women who have delivered children vaginally will always have a slightly open cervix). Once ovulation is over, it returns to its original low, closed position.

Keeping track of these three signs will help a woman determine when she is fertile. During fertile days, sex should either be avoided or a barrier method of contraception used. Remember, hormonal contraception like the Pill is incompatible with natural methods because women taking estrogen and progestin for birth control don't have true menstrual cycles and don't usually ovulate. Use of condoms, female condoms, diaphragms, and cervical caps is compatible with fertility awareness as long as you are able to correctly observe cervical fluids.

There are many things that can happen biologically that complicate or compromise FAM, including breastfeeding, perimenopause, chronic illness, thyroid problems, polycystic ovaries, and profoundly irregular cycles. Much like calendar-based methods, these contraceptive techniques work better for women with more regular menstrual cycles. Unlike calendar methods, FAM and symptothermal methods can account for more natural variation between cycles. If you fall into any category that makes using FAM more complicated, be sure to seek special counseling and assistance before attempting to use the method, and be aware that you may have risks that other women don't have to deal with.

Clinical evaluations of symptothermal fertility control suggest that they are highly effective. When used correctly, they approach hormonal con-traceptives in their ability to prevent pregnancy. Of course this varies much more than other methods with imperfect use: when mistakes are made, it is an unforgiving method. A 2007 German study found that in a group of nine hundred women, fewer than two out of every hundred became accidentally pregnant, a failure rate of between .4 and .6 percent.[27] Unlike many scientists studying FAM, who worry that subjects will find the method too complicated, lead researcher Petra Frank-Hermann isn't concerned about the ability of women to follow FAM guidelines: "The women or couples who want to learn the method have to buy a book, or attend an NFP [natural family planning] course, or get some teaching by a qualified NFP teacher. Learning STM [symptothermal method] is usu-ally no problem. There are precise rules that work. However, in contrast to the oral contraceptive pill or other family planning methods, STM needs more engagement and time to learn it."[28] I believe that this confi-dence in the abilities, motivation, and intelligence of adult women is warranted. If we want to take serious steps toward reproductive health, this sort of respect on the part of researchers and health educators is fun-damental.

Making It Work: Questions and Controversies with Natural Birth Control

The major issue for most women when making a decision about birth control is efficacy: does it work, and how well does it work?

Sometimes it can be difficult to assess the efficacy of natural birth con-trol because the multiplicity of methods and the complex process make it hard to study. Perfect use failure rates range from less than 1 to 9 per-cent,[29] and actual use rates are often unavailable or inconsistent, but are much higher, undoubtedly in double digits. Many trials have serious methodological problems, including high dropout rates, which make con-clusive data hard to come by.[30]

Determining if something works, however, means more than pulling apart ideal and actual use rates in a study. It means weighing risks and ben-efits in a real-world context. While fertility awareness has many upsides—lack of chemical intervention in the body, practically no financial cost, and improved awareness of overall reproductive health, to name just a few—it also has significant considerations. First, it is a method best practiced by committed couples. While this aspect is in some ways a result of how the technique has been framed by the religious communities who have nurtured and developed it, it is important to note that FAM doesn't provide protection from STDs and is a method that relies heavily on good partner communication. Second, it is a method best practiced by those for whom an unwanted pregnancy would not be devastating, either because they are able to have a child or have no moral objection to abortion.

When women opt to practice natural birth control, particularly FAM, they take responsibility for their reproductive choices in a way that is unique and radical. There is no pharmaceutical "big brother" sitting over your shoulder making sure that you don't mess up. If you use this technique and get pregnant, you have no one to blame but yourself. But I see that as a good thing in many ways. Much of the conversation about birth control insists that if women have the means to control fertility, they will have more choices. Most of these means, however, fail to trust women with the basic abilities and motivations to act in a manner that reflects their desires and expresses autonomy.

Women want to be in control. For this reason, when they encounter natural birth control for the first time, they are often seized with the passion of a convert. This can be good and bad. It provides the energy to be diligent in learning and performing the method, but it can imbue women with a false sense of knowledge about their body. Some become convinced after a month or two of use that they "know" when they are ovulating. Others lose zeal with time and continue practicing some aspects of the method but not others. Toni Weschler addresses these tendencies, noting, "One word of warning about taking shortcuts: once you decide not to chart every day, it can be very tempting to slack off and either chart even less than recommended, or stop altogether, convincing yourself that you just *know* when you're fertile."[31] Weschler says that this sort of overconfidence is one of the top reasons that women have unplanned pregnancies using the method. If you want to use this type of birth control, be warned that there are no shortcuts.

A young graduate student from a northeastern American college shared her story with me, illustrating the perils of this thinking:

I first went on a pill—I have no idea which one—when I was a senior in college. I had some menstrual irregularities and a doctor (he attempted to describe the menstruation process to me by using a lawn-mowing analogy—why he thought I didn't understand it at age twenty-two, I have no idea) prescribed something to get me back on track. Whatever it was, it was horrible. I became a complete emotional basket case. I was on it for only a month, and it made me clingy, weepy, and just plain strange. Anyway, the experience has made me a little wary of birth control pills ever since.

Before I got married (last August), my husband (then, fiancé) and I had to decide what we would use once we got married. Since he is generally prone to avoiding medications of any kind, and due to my previous experience, we decided to go with something more "natural." A friend of mine recommended FAM. I started learning about it, and I loved this method—it's fun, for those who enjoy understanding the biology—and since my husband's a scientist, he likes to learn a little about it too.

Here's a big caveat, however: I cannot exactly be a poster child for this method. I, admittedly, have been almost exclusively using the temperature shift as a guide for fertility. Also, the method basically says, if you want to be "safe," abstain from sex whenever you might be fertile, and use a condom at all other times if you are trying not to get pregnant. We didn't really do that—instead we would use condoms when I suspected I was fertile, and nothing when I thought I was "safe." That said, we got pregnant.

The mother-to-be adds thoughtfully, "The moral of my story is that if you really want to avoid getting pregnant, or at least have more control of your fertility, you should follow whatever method you use to the T. If you're on a pill, take it every day at the right time. If you're using more natural methods—do everything suggested."

It should go without saying (but I will say it!) that any method of natural birth control should involve watching and observing your cycles for a significant amount of time before you begin to rely on it for contraceptive purposes. This time should be measured in months—plural, multiple, many—if not years.

With this method, practice makes perfect. The more you chart and come to understand your body, the less likely you will be to make a mistake. Given this fact, many women wonder why training in fertility awareness from a noncontraceptive perspective (that is, to fully understand menstrual cycles and maintain good gynecological health) isn't offered to younger women.

One of those people is Toni Weschler, who received hundreds of letters from women over the years asking why they didn't receive this useful information when they were just starting to bleed instead of the same old talk about how to conceal and silence periods. Her response was a book that adapted FAM for the younger set, leaving out specific information on how to use the technique for birth control. *Cycle Savvy*[32] details the basics of menstruation and ovulation (and how to observe and track them) for girls ages fourteen and older. This sort of knowledge can aid, among other things, in helping to diagnose period problems without resorting to potentially dangerous early drug interventions. It can also help catch really serious problems, such as ovarian and reproductive cancers, before they become fatal. On a more basic level, it can take the fear out of normal but frightening events like spotting, sharp abdominal pains around menstruation, and of course, mysterious discharge. *Cycle Savvy* is a truly revolutionary book in the way it reimagines menstrual education: it assumes that young women should be given the tools to understand what is happening in their bodies, not just told that it is normal and handed a tampon. Or told they are not normal and put on the Pill.

Even in its redacted form, Weschler's book caused controversy. Some women had tried various methods of FAM and had unexpected pregnancies. They didn't want their daughters to suffer the same fate. Other, more usual suspects, simply didn't want young women having too much information about either their bodies or sex. Janice Crouse, a senior fellow at the conservative Concerned Women for America's Beverly LaHaye Institute, explains, "I think it is inappropriate. Instead, I think that we need high ideals for our teenagers, to teach them the value of self-control because those are the disciplines that you need for your whole life. Providing this type of information says that teenagers are hostages to their hormones."[33]

While there are many problems with this sort of thinking, the most obvious is that it relies on older models of "feminine" virtues, in which women are instructed in silence and self-control: like it or not, this thinking insists, biology is destiny. The second problem that it misconstrues the basic message of fertility awareness. In fact, it's precisely when we fail to understand how hormones work that we become hostage to them. Not knowing why something in the body happens the way it does and living in fear of it is an awful sort of mental captivity. As journalist Catherine Price notes, "I've never bought the argument that if you give teenagers more information they're going to run out and have more sex. I'd instead suggest that any girl who's going to devote time to taking her temperature and checking out the daily position of her cervix is not the girl we need to be worrying about. We need to be worrying about keeping the 'mysteries' of the female body so mysterious that young women end up accidentally pregnant."[34] Researcher Beth Roth backs up this opinion, noting, "An adolescent girl's lack of understanding of her menstrual cycle and inability to identify the fertile and infertile phases of her cycle directly contributes to contraceptive risk-taking behavior."[35]

Concerns about a woman's ability to understand and use fertility awareness are not limited to young women. Many adult women struggle to convince their partners that they are capable of successfully implementing the method. When I asked Katie Singer about broaching this sometimes difficult topic, she pointed out that men are fertile every day, but women only a handful of days each month. And yet most methods require women to bear the day-to-day burden of birth control. All the experts I consulted feel that FAM is a cooperative method and that male partners should be involved; in fact, they argue, it is the only method that requires both men and women participate.

The same sorts of conversations about personal responsibility, autonomy, and capability that are being had over dinner tables and in bedrooms are also happening publicly in clinical and educational settings around the world. As I sat through a presentation of contraceptive options from a young representative of Planned Parenthood last year, I marked the absence of any mention or acknowledgment of natural methods. This absence was especially pronounced as the conversation included discussion of methods not currently marketed in the United States (Norplant) and methods with very low efficacy rates (contraceptive film). Why, I wondered, are fertility awareness techniques, whether you believe they work or not, so controversial that we can't even discuss them? When women are forced to seek out information about FAM through backward channels and pass it along like contraband, is it any wonder that those who choose to practice it often stumble?

Part of the problem, of course, is distrust between Catholic groups and secular (often feminist) women's health educators. While these alliances have been improving, they still leave much to be desired. Some of this problem is ideological: feminist educators have grown out of a tradition accustomed to fighting for broader contraceptive access, while conservative and Catholic powers were trying to foreclose options. Feminists look to expand access to methods to larger and more diverse groups of women, while Catholic groups often seek to tightly control who can receive contraceptive information and how they can get it. Marcos Arévalo of Georgetown writes, "Even the option of developing a referral system between family planning programs and NFP [natural family planning] NGOs is not possible in many settings because the ideological differences between the two severely limit the success of such a system."[36] Other problems are practical: it takes significantly longer to correctly train staff in how to teach FAM and longer still to convey the method to patients and clients. This difficulty is further compounded by the lack of resources for women who want to learn FAM. It is much easier to write a prescription for oral contraceptives.

The result of this is that communities of women who would greatly benefit from knowledge about FAM—particularly low-income women who struggle to afford expensive hormonal methods—cannot receive training or instruction. Indeed, for secular women, only those with enough money to pay for classes starting at a hundred dollars and up can get education in the few progressive fertility awareness centers that exist.

For many communities of women internationally, fertility awareness methods provide an option that is acceptable and easily accommodated to more traditional lifestyles. Nevertheless, many nonreligious organizations have favored educating physicians internationally in pharmaceutical alternatives, even though these methods are often not readily used or accessed by many communities of women.

Many women who don't choose FAM as a method of birth control would still benefit from learning how to chart and becoming familiar with their personal menstrual patterns. For one, observing your cycles will help you notice gynecological problems that range from the annoying to the life threatening: a greatly abridged list of these includes vaginal infections, abnormal bleeding, cervical and ovarian cysts, polycystic ovarian syndrome (PCOS), endometriosis, breast lumps, PMS, and even gynecological cancers. It gives us the tools to start learning about our complex hormonal cycles and comforts us with the knowledge that our private patterns are normal. In light of these many benefits, it seems unjust that most women are never schooled in these basics. And there is so much to know: there are multiple lifestyle changes that can help to normalize erratic periods, cut down on PMS, and basically alleviate period pain without drugs, including improving nutrition, avoiding environmental pollutants, and simply getting a good night's sleep in a completely darkened room. Singer explains some of these and notes that simple changes can help to integrate many aspects of our increasingly fractured modern lives: "I've come to see how consumption of organic butter, my thyroid, hazardous waste in our oceans, my menstrual cramps, and my relationship with my partner are all connected."[37] If, as Singer says, most women aren't even in preschool when it comes to their periods, perhaps doing a little charting is a good place to begin addressing this dearth of education. But most women will never get the chance. They will go on the Pill or another hormonal contraceptive and not look back until (for some of them) they are ready to have children. They will never wonder what their menstrual cycles could have taught them or if in getting rid of monthly cycles they lose something important.

Fertility awareness is still young. The challenge now is to integrate it with other available methods in discussions of contraceptive options. It offers women so many benefits beyond birth control. While many important questions about ease and efficacy linger, to let this valuable tool languish in the shadows as it has for so many years does not benefit women. To hold the past against a still-developing method limits knowledge and choices. Giving women the best information possible and letting them make their own decisions is truly the only way to achieve gender equality in medical care.

Chapter Nine

One Less? Facts and Fictions about HPV Vaccinations

The debate surrounding the HPV vaccine might be characterized by two slogans:
"Just do it" versus "What's the hurry?"
—Alan K. Cassels[1]

The news exploded in the world media during the summer of 2006: the world's first anticancer vaccine had arrived. Gardasil, a shot that fights four forms of human papilloma virus (HPV), had been cleared by the FDA for use by American girls. Other countries raced to follow suit. If you were a woman, a doctor, or a parent at that time, you probably had an opinion about it. Most new vaccines are controversial, but Gardasil started a firestorm.

For many who had eagerly anticipated its debut, Gardasil was a wonder shot. For the first time, public health officials started to imagine a world where cervical cancer was all but eradicated. Women clamored to get their daughters vaccinated and potentially protect them from the suffering, and even untimely death, that cervical cancer could bring.

Amid all the elation there were dissenting voices. Almost from the beginning, parent groups, grassroots health advocacy organizations, and cautious doctors warned that the HPV vaccine was new and might not be either as effective or as safe as its makers dreamed. The discomfort stemmed from two issues: the speed with which Gardasil was embraced by health establishments and the strategies employed to ensure public compliance. Within months, Merck, the drug firm that created the shot, began an aggressive lobbying campaign to convince congresspeople and lawmakers to create mandatory school vaccination programs that would require middle-school girls to have the three-course series of shots as a condition of public school entry. Politicians, eager to win points with female voters as well as powerful lobbyists, sprang into action.

And then the young girls started to faint. Some experienced pain after the vaccine was administered. Some even endured paralysis within weeks of getting the shot. Doctors—including Gardasil's architect, Dr. Ian Frazer—were quick to suggest that the problem was simply nerves, hysterical schoolgirls inventing illness where there was none. Parents, however, were more concerned. Were they putting their daughters at risk or saving them from a dreaded fate? Women began to wonder why the drug was being tested—and in some cases forced—upon only female bodies. Why weren't nations rushing to push the shot on boys as well?

What is the truth about this novel option in women's health care, and how can we separate the medical realities from the important social contexts and histories that surround and threaten to overwhelm them? How can we move toward an understanding of HPV vaccination that both appreciates its awesome potential and is realistic about its unanswered questions and limitations? In a book about contraception, it may seem strange to focus on a health measure that has nothing to do with preventing pregnancy. However, HPV vaccination is an important new option in the world of sexual health, and the story of this shot holds lessons for women in other health contexts.

The Smear vs. the Stab: Cervical Cancer Prevention from Papanicolaou to Frazer

If the new HPV vaccines entered the world with a bang, the most successful anticancer intervention to precede it—the Pap smear—entered with a whimper. George Papanicolaou, a Greek doctor and reproductive scientist, noticed something unusual while examining exfoliated vaginal cells in an attempt to map reproductive cycles. The doctor realized that abnormal cellular growth—the sort that led to cancer—could be identified. Perhaps, he reasoned, cervical cancer could be predicted based on these changes.

Papanicolaou took his discovery to a prestigious eugenics conference in 1928. In retrospect, he was doomed from the start. Among other problems, his paper was riddled with errors; for example, instead of the word "cancerous," he wrote "conscious."[2] Conference attendees were lukewarm on his bold new theory, and Papanicolaou would have to wait another thirteen years—until 1941—for the full impact of his work to be understood. In his classic paper published in the *American Journal of Obstetrics and Gynecology*,[3] Papanicolaou again suggested that observing cervical cells for changes and abnormalities could be a way to forecast the emergence of cancer.

If 1941 brought enthusiasm for this idea, it also brought controversy. Pathologists didn't like the test because it was time consuming and imprecise. Gynecologists, however, were enthused, and by 1945, the procedure was being advised by the American Cancer Society. Still, adoption of the smear into routine practice was slow. Many doctors resisted offering "Paps," and many patients didn't want them anyway. A 1961 *New York Times* article revealed that two fifths of American women had never heard of the test, and even more felt it was unnecessary.[4]

Today, of course, the Pap smear is an American institution. It is estimated that 86 percent of women between eighteen and sixty-four[5] have put their feet in the stirrups at least once and let a doctor scrape a few cells from their cervix. For most women, it is a yearly ritual akin to—although certainly not as joyful as—a birthday. The result has been astounding and has transformed cervical cancer in the developed world from a scourge to a relatively uncommon event.

Certainly women still die of cervical cancer: in 2005 in the United States, 11,999 women were diagnosed with the illness and 3,924 died from it.[6] The death rate is approximately 1,100 in the United Kingdom, and around 400[7] women succumb each year in Canada.[8] Compare these tragic but modest numbers with the international death rate from cervical cancer—more than 237,000 each year, making up 9 percent of female cancer deaths[9]—and you begin to get a sense of how different the illness is for women depending where in the world they live. In America, of the several thousand women who die each year, 60 percent have either never had a Pap test or haven't had one within five years of their diagnosis.[10]

In the developing world it is a very different picture, and cervical cancer is still a leading cause of cancer death. Because annual exams require constant and repeated access to health care services, reaping their benefits remains a significant challenge for women in poor nations.

Recent years have brought new screening techniques, including genetic testing for HPV and liquid Pap tests. These screening methods are still in development, but they may eventually prove practical and cost-effective alternatives to annual Pap smear screenings for many women.[11] Still, annual screening remains one of the most successful cancer interventions of all time. As bioethicist Sigrid Fry-Revere notes, "The American Cancer Society sees its fight against cervical cancer as a success story even without Gardasil. When the disease is detected early through Pap testing, the survival rate is more than 90 percent."[12]

When a woman has a Pap smear, her doctor scrapes a small amount of tissue from around the cervix. In a traditional smear, the cells are examined by a skilled technician and checked for changes or abnormalities. For most women, having a Pap smear is the best option right now for cervical cancer screening. Newer liquid-based Pap smears add samples to liquid and use machinery to separate cervical cells from blood mucus and debris before examining them. Liquid smears may be better at finding certain types of cancer, and they offer the option of having a simultaneous test for HPV with the same sample. But liquid tests are also more expensive, and the difference in cost from a traditional Pap smear may not be covered by insurance. They also produce more false positives, especially if a woman is very young or taking oral contraceptives.

An HPV test, which also involves analyzing a cervical swab, examines DNA to check for thirteen types of the HPV virus. While in some ways the HPV test is more sensitive, the Pap test is more specific.[13] Because of this, if a woman's insurance covers both, the tests can be partnered so that one test catches what that the other misses. The American Cancer Society notes that the HPV test isn't usually recommended for women under thirty because HPV in this community is so common[14] and in most cases resolves on its own without intervention. But for older women or young women with unclear Pap smear results, it is a valuable tool whose unique advantages are coming to be understood.

The Pap smear may yet have room for improvement, but the test is already so precise that the National Institutes of Health have eased their test frequency recommendation from every year to every three years if a woman has had three consecutive normal smears. Still, many women continue to have them annually, and there is nothing wrong, safety-wise, with that.

The Approval and Selling of Gardasil

Flash back to 1991: Scottish-born biochemist Ian Frazer was conducting research at an Australian hospital in Brisbane. He and colleague Jian Zhou realized they had found a way to create a vaccine for HPV.[15] The original project was designed to take five years; it took a little longer but still progressed with great momentum. Indeed, the HPV vaccination would both benefit and suffer from the lightning speed with which it entered international medical consciousness. In the end, Frazer and Zhou's work would become the basis of two HPV vaccines: Gardasil and Cervarix.

Perhaps it all went so fast because the story of HPV vaccination is that of a race between rival drugmakers to corner the market on a potentially radical new technology. The contest was between two fierce competitors: on one side was Merck, with a quadrivalent vaccine—a shot that resisted four strains of HPV. On the other side was the British pharmaceutical giant GlaxoSmithKline (GSK), whose shot, Cervarix, offered protection against only two strains of HPV but promised stronger protection against them. GSK had been working on their shot for a longer period of time, but Merck beat them to the market. After reviewing four clinical trials,[16] the FDA voted to give Gardasil the green light on June 8, 2006.[17] Health Canada followed on July 18, 2006.[18]

It would be another nine months before GSK submitted their application to the FDA. When they did, GSK insisted that clinical trials would prove their product superior.[19] Two years later, Cervarix finally received approval in the United States in October 2009 and is now recommended by the Centers for Disease Control and Prevention (CDC) for use in American women, as well as in the European Union[20] and the United Kingdom (where this British product is offered to young girls at no cost through the National Health Service). GSK has a lot of ground to make up, and perceptions that their shot simply does less by protecting against fewer strands of HPV and not offering protection against genital warts is a serious obstacle to overcome. Still, the CDC's Advisory Committee on Immunization Practices declined to recommend Gardasil over Cervarix.

The FDA's 2006 approval of Gardasil was for girls between the ages of nine and twenty-six. This meant that older women would have to pay out of pocket for the shot with no hope of insurance reimbursement. In the same month that the FDA approved the vaccine, a CDC advisory panel voted unanimously to recommend the vaccination for all girls aged eleven and twelve.[21] Panel members explained their decision, noting, "Despite the seemingly high cost . . . all of the cost-benefit analyses the committee reviewed showed that the vaccine was a cost-effective intervention."[22] Such confidence in the affordability of HPV vaccination was surprising given that Gardasil had just become the most expensive vaccination in history with a price tag of $360 for all three suggested doses.

While the CDC panel recommended Gardasil, it never suggested that the shot be mandatory. Even if they had wanted to require it, they couldn't have; the ability to compel a vaccination belongs to individual states, and there is no national immunization law in the United States.[23] Curtis Allen, a CDC spokesman, noted that it was never CDC's intention to force Gardasil on women; rather, the goal was to spread the good word about its potential benefits. Indeed, he insisted, mandatory programs usually take years to build: "In the past, mandates have generally been enacted several years after a vaccine is introduced and recommended."[24]

Despite this, many states and lawmakers interpreted the FDA and CDC's fast embrace as a call to action. In September 2006, a rapid ninety days after approval, Michigan became the first state to propose requiring Gardasil as a prerequisite for school admission, and Texas governor Rick Perry issued an executive order calling for mandatory school vaccinations. In short succession, twenty-three state legislatures created bills to require that Gardasil be administered to their girls.

As quickly as these schemes were rolled out, they were rejected, overturned, and rolled back in. Texas passed a bill blocking Perry's order[25] after it was revealed that he and other state legislators collected $44,000 in contributions from Merck-hired lobbyists.[26] Other states, particularly in more religious parts of the South, rejected plans on grounds that they might seem to condone teenage sexuality. Others buckled under mounting public pressure from parent and patient advocacy groups.

Most of the proposed programs were opt-out alternatives—in other words, parents could block their children's vaccinations on religious or ethical grounds, but the assumption was that unless otherwise notified, schools would expect girls to be vaccinated. In the end, only Virginia's mandatory plan held—with a very liberal parental objection clause. The rewards for Virginia's compliance demonstrate the way that pharmaceutical makers can use financial incentive to influence public policy: only months after Virginia governor Tim Kaine signed the Gardasil legislation, Merck pledged to pour $193 million in additional funds into its Elkton, Virginia, plant where the vaccine is manufactured.[27]

New Hampshire pursued an alternate opt-in approach with great success. Instead of requiring young girls to be vaccinated, the state made Gardasil optional and free for anyone between the ages of eleven and eighteen.[28] The results were overwhelming: within months, doctors were unable to fill all the requests for vaccination. It wasn't a perfect system; for one thing, the program consumed a large percentage of the state's immunization budget, taking funds away from other shots. Another problem was that insurers refused to pay for shots in girls who fell within the free age group, creating further stress on the already overtaxed system. Still, the New Hampshire case proved instructive for other states, including South Dakota and Wyoming, which created similar programs.

The Canadian government allocated $300 million for Gardasil, and provinces rushed to design programs. Ontario was the first, with a massive opt-in program designed to make the shot available to eighty-four thousand eighth-grade girls.[29] Women's health activists balked at the speed with which these strategies were enacted and pointed the finger at drug company maneuvering. Anne Rochon Ford, coordinator of the group Women and Health Protection, noted, "It is staggering how quickly and secretly this has all happened and that points to some pretty active footwork behind the scenes."[30] At the same time, Britain raced to create a program that would work in their National Health Services. While a program for twelve- and thirteen-year-olds (with catch-up plans) wouldn't be put into place until the end of 2007 and implemented the following year,[31] many parents began paying out of pocket for daughters' shots. Australia, creator of and one of the first nations to embrace Gardasil, offered the shot free to women between thirteen and twenty-six until June 2009.[32]

Perhaps because it wanted to establish its product as the industry leader, earn government contracts, and build brand recognition before Cervarix had a chance to catch up, Merck launched a shock-and-awe campaign to have Gardasil accepted as the best standard of care. The aggressive marketing effort employed several strategies. First, it worked with women's groups like the bipartisan Women in Government to pressure female lawmakers to push the vaccination.[33] Second, it launched a powerful direct-to-consumer advertising campaign that targeted both young girls and their parents. Ubiquitous images of strong, energetic women engaging in a range of activities and triumphantly proclaiming "I'm gonna be one less! [victim of cervical cancer]" graced television screens, and advertisements played on the Web site YouTube.com and in movie theaters before summer blockbuster films.[34] Third, Merck began a program of physician education, hiring doctors to give lectures to their peers for substantial sums of money (as much as $4,500 per talk).[35]

It wasn't just that Merck wanted to trounce GSK before the latter brought its product to market. Merck also wanted to fix some of its own lingering financial and public image problems, not the least of which was its huge legal debt and market loss incurred after the blockbuster second-generation nonsteroidal anti-inflammatory drug (NSAID) Vioxx was pulled for contributing to cardiac problems and death in users. Only a year after its approval, Gardasil was going a long way to helping Merck erase this painful history with one billion dollars in profits.[36] As a writer for Bloomberg News noted, "The recall of the Vioxx painkiller . . . cut 31 percent for the shares in three months," adding, "Profit may rise in 2007 for the first time in three years."[37]

It wasn't long, though, before it became clear that the pharmaceutical giant and their allies were striking a sour note with the public. For one thing, any questions raised in the media about Gardasil, any suggestion that the shot was less than an unqualified miracle were met with ridicule. Abby Lippman, a professor of public health, was the lead author of lucid, stinging piece in the *Canadian Medical Association Journal* (*CMAJ*) that posed serious questions about HPV vaccinations even as it acknowledged the tremendous health barriers the new technology crossed. The response was fast: Lippman "was vilified in Salem-witch-trial manner for failing to toe the party line"[38] with scathing letters to the editor from doctors and public health authorities as well as articles and commentary in other news outlets that painted the activist as a crazy health alarmist. As one Canadian journalist noted, "Whether you agree with the point of view or not, she did what scientists should do: ask questions."[39]

An even more direct example of drugmakers seeking to suppress contrary opinions happened in Australia, where a university professor was reprimanded and ordered to apologize to CSL, the Australian firm that created Gardasil and licensed it to Merck, for making negative comments about the vaccine. Professor Andrew Gunn, a senior lecturer at the University of Queensland, had expressed his views on national radio, noting that Gardasil's problems included "its marketing as a solution to cancer of the cervix when at best it's expected to prevent about two-thirds of cases; the incorrect and dangerous perception that it might make Pap smears unnecessary; and the difficult question of the best age to give a vaccine whose effect might yet prove to wear off before many recipients even start having sex."[40] Each of these caveats is legitimate and far from radical. It will be decades before efficacy rates are available for cervical cancer prevention. During this time women may desert other screening methods if they believe they are safe without them. Finally, the duration of the vaccine remains an open question. These concerns had been voiced by doctors and health experts in major publications including the *Journal of the American Medical Association* and *CMAJ*. But the University of Queensland, which had a financial and research relationship with CSL, ordered the professor to issue a mea culpa.

Clarifying the Objectives of HPV Vaccination

Part of the problem in the beginning was that while Gardasil was a vaccine, Merck marketed it like a drug. Didier Hoch, president of Merck's joint venture with French drugmaker Sanofi-Aventis, noted, "In most countries, Gardasil is becoming accessible at the speed of a pharmaceutical drug, which is a first for a vaccine."[41] While drugs tend, for better and often for worse, to burst onto national scenes, demanding attention and rapid acceptance, vaccines usually follow a slower course, often taking five to ten years to gain universal acceptance. They also tend to utilize public health channels, like vaccination programs, for administration rather than promoting themselves directly to potential consumers. The *New York Times* stated, "The lightning-fast transition from newly minted vaccine to must-have injection in the United States and Europe represents a triumph of what the manufacturers call education and their critics call marketing," adding, "In two years, cervical cancer has gone from obscure killer confined mostly to poor nations to the West's disease of the moment."[42]

This hybridization confused the public. Generally, vaccines are seen as a "greater good" measure, where individual choice and need are sublimated for the betterment of the community. This is because typically, the infections prevented by shots are transmitted through casual contact and are not effectively treated with other methods. Vaccines are used broadly in the population to gain so-called herd immunity. In other words, if enough people in the population become resistant to a disease, in time there will be no one to catch it from. When it comes to potentially fatal diseases such as smallpox, the needs of the community as whole trump individual concerns.

But as we know, HPV isn't transmitted by casual contact. As Abby Lippman and her colleagues put it, "Is the aim of the vaccination program the eradication of high-risk HPV types from the population? Or is it to reduce the number of deaths from cervical cancer? These different goals require different strategies."[43]

Ian Frazer clearly takes the earlier perspective, equating the shot with Jonas Salk's polio vaccine.[44] Echoing Frazer's "big picture" approach, many media outlets often convey the message that Gardasil is about obliteration: one Australian paper explains that "the new cervical cancer vaccine is expected to almost eradicate human papilloma virus (HPV) infections in Australian women by 2050 if the high rate of immunization amongst girls continues."[45]

While this would indeed be a noble goal, it is unlikely for many reasons. Even if herd immunity were possible—and this is a controversial point—Gardasil is only effective against four strains of HPV: 16, 18, 6, and 11. The first two are indeed serious infections, accounting for up to 70 percent of cervical cancers. However, there are at least forty known strains that can cause cancer, and neither Gardasil nor Cervarix provide such complete protection against dangerous HPV strains that there is no longer a need for further and continuous screening.[46] In this context, HPV vaccinations fall somewhere between Salk's polio vaccine and a yearly flu shot.

Many prominent health officials are quick to affirm that the vaccines won't broadly eliminate the disease. Catherine DeAngelis, editor of the *Journal of the American Medical Association*, notes, "The HPV vaccine does not create herd immunity, although it would probably reduce the prevalence of HPV infections." She adds, "The primary justification for HPV vaccination is to protect women from long-term risks, rather than to prevent immediate harm to others."[47]

For Lippman, this confusion of issues isn't accidental; it is a deliberate effort on the part of drugmakers to burn the candle at both ends, to take advantage of public desire to do something good for womankind while also exploiting drug marketing techniques that speak to individual preventative health desires. In her estimation, it is an effort to "confuse the issue of epidemics with details of the ways in which women with cervical cancer suffer." In other words, cervical cancer is terrible, but the pain of women who battle it shouldn't be exploited to promote false notions of Gardasil's efficacy. As another activist notes, "There's nothing wrong with drug makers publicizing their products, but the lure of lucrative government contracts can prompt them to play fast and loose . . . Merck has greatly exaggerated both the threat of the disease and the ability of [Gardisil] to prevent it."[48]

Syringes and Surrogate Endpoints: Gardasil and the Race to Stop Cervical Cancer

Efficacy questions have plagued both HPV vaccines since their introductions. These include serious uncertainties about how effectively the shots prevent both HPV and cancer, and how long their protections endure.

Clinical trials have measured success with surrogate endpoints. That means the trials compare the HPV rates of women who have received Gardasil shots to those of a control group of women who didn't receive the vaccine. Because cervical cancer is so predictable—that is, because we know how to identify dangerous cells well before they progress to cancer—it would be unethical to let women who develop certain abnormalities progress without treatment.[49] Instead, scientists use a "surrogate," an indication that cancer may be coming, to assess if the shot has made an impact. In this case, they measure lesions that develop from irregular cells.

This is complicated because it is estimated that 40 percent of these lesions disappear on their own.[50] It is likely that many of the "cancers" seen in trials would have resolved—and created natural immunity—without need of intervention. Because of this it will take at least a decade, and perhaps several decades, to determine whether the shot actually prevents cancer.[51] Surrogate endpoints can provide only an idea of real-world effectiveness.

The announcement that HPV was a hair's breadth from being cured came as a surprise to many who were either unaware that the illness existed or unconcerned about contracting it. I first learned of HPV in high school when I heard a religious commentator on television comparing it with HIV, declaring with certainty that if teenagers knew of this scourge, they would never have premarital sex. The most frightening part of the preacher's message: he warned that HPV couldn't be stopped with condoms like other STIs.

In fact, HPV is still dramatically underdiscussed in conversations about sexual health, particularly with young people. Pregnancy, AIDS, and even other common STIs like gonorrhea, chlamydia, and herpes get more attention, despite the fact that HPV is the most common sexually transmitted infection.

The dearth of education likely has at least two major causes. The first is that HPV is usually symptomless (although some strains can cause genital warts). Cancer takes years (sometimes decades) to develop and is a rare outcome. The second major reason that parents aren't trying to frighten teenagers about HPV is that around 90 percent of infections resolve on their own within one to two years.[52] Like most viruses, once it has been fought off, the body is immune to whichever strain it previously suffered from.[53] While more than 90 percent of HPV will never even progress toward cancer, let alone actually become malignant, more than 99 percent of cervical cancers are believed to be caused by HPV.[54]

There are, unfortunately, many strains of the virus. Estimates range from 150 to 1,000. Of these, around 40 are known to cause cancer,[55] and types 16 and 18—the two strains fought by both Gardasil and Cervarix—are responsible for up to 70 percent of cancers.[56] So while the HPV vaccinations target only a very small number of possible virus strains, they do target the forms of the virus thought to be most dangerous. Because neither vaccine accounts for all cancer-causing strains, it is essential that women continue having regular Pap smears or comparable viral screening throughout their lives, regardless of vaccination status.

The virus acts by entering cervical cells and shedding its DNA. The infected cells begin producing viral proteins and spreading the infection. Such growth, if it continues for years, can become cancerous. The vaccine works like most vaccines: it introduces proteins that mimic the viral ones—not enough to cause illness, but enough to trigger the body to produce antibodies preemptively. If the body comes in contact with the virus later, it is prepared to fight it off.

It is estimated that 50 percent of sexually active people will contract HPV at some point in their lives, 6.2 million in America each year.[57] A study published in the *Journal of the American Medical Association* in 2007 found that HPV rates increase in a given population between ages fourteen and twenty-four, after which point they slowly but steadily decline through age fifty-nine.[58] The study calculated several statistics important to the Gardasil discussion. First, it found that around 26.8 percent of women in the United States are infected with the virus at any single moment, with the highest percentage at between ages twenty and twenty-four (44.8 percent). This percentage was closer than expected to the rate of infected women found in studies of vaccine efficacy among sexually active women. In other words, it suggests that vaccination has limited benefits for women who are already having sex. Second, study authors noticed that while overall infection rates were high, very few women suffered from types 16, 18, 10, and 6—the strains targeted by the vaccines. In fact, only 3.4 percent of infected women had any of the four, and of the high-risk strains 16 and 18, rates of infection were 1.5 percent and .8 percent, respectively.[59] A 2007 trial found that the vaccine didn't help women who had already been infected recover more quickly, nor did it help treat prior infections.[60]

Another unanswered question with potentially huge ramifications is the issue of how long immunity lasts. Some vaccines provide lifelong protection, while others require periodic updates, or "boosters," to maintain effectiveness. As Abby Lippman and colleagues asked in a controversial *CMAJ* article, "Will boosters be needed to maintain this limited coverage, and if so, when?"[61] Most estimates assume that coverage will last at least five years, although some data suggests it may be closer to three or four. If boosters are needed, the consequences for large-scale vaccination will be significant. First, it may upset the optimistic cost effectiveness projections, making giving the shots to all teens too expensive.[62] Second, and perhaps worse from a health perspective, it may render young people temporarily immune during the time they are most able to fight the infection only to make them vulnerable at older ages when they are less able to heal and more likely to progress to cancer.

As one writer notes, "Cancer data show that the average cervical cancer patient is forty-seven and most likely contracted HPV, which incubates for up to fifteen years before becoming cancer, in her thirties."[63] Since studies show that HPV rates are highest in the midtwenties, this data suggests that women become less able to fight off infection as the years pass. They are more likely to face HPV in their twenties, but more likely to see it morph into something truly dangerous later in life.

Merck, who insists that its shot will last, has possibly been playing fast and loose with the science on this subject. Diana Zuckerman of the National Research Center for Women and Families explains that while no product called a booster is currently available, Merck did give an additional dose of the shot to girls before measuring their antibodies at the five year mark.[64] If this is true, it means that the drugmaker basically gave women an additional dose and then claimed that the original three were still working several years on. Zuckerman notes that the shot has only been shown to last for two years and explains that Merck "isn't talking publicly about a need for a booster shot . . . perhaps because the vaccine is expensive and most people wouldn't be willing to pay $400+ for a vaccine that lasts less than 5 years."[65]

Even if vaccinations last indefinitely, which seems unlikely, receiving them may make young women less likely to get Pap smears and utilize screening methods essential to thorough cancer detection and prevention. As long as annual exams remain tied to oral contraceptive access, however, it seems likely that many women in developed nations will continue to have them, at least in their twenties and thirties. Just as worrying is the possibility that vaccination will lead to a drop in condom use, particularly in high school and college populations. While earlier studies have suggested little to no benefit from condoms in the prevention of HPV,[66] more recent work has in fact found a great benefit from using a good, old-fashioned rubber. An article published in the *New England Journal of Medicine* found that "among newly sexually active women, consistent condom use by their partners appears to reduce the risk of cervical and vulvovaginal HPV infection."[67] How much protection did condoms users get? One study found that women whose partners used condoms reduced their HPV risk by 70 percent, and even those whose partners used condoms only half the time had a 50 percent reduction when compared with noncondom users. Other lifestyle interventions that cut HPV risk include eating better and smoking less.

Another concern, according to the *New England Journal of Medicine*, is that suppressing certain dangerous strains—namely HPV 16 and 18— might allow other varieties of the infection to emerge and change and be more dangerous than anticipated,[68] altering the natural history of the virus.[69] If HPV types not prevented by the shot start accounting for a larger percentage of cancers, it could render the vaccine less relevant from a public health perspective.

While slightly older women are more likely to get cervical cancer, young women still suffer from it. One thing that makes cervical cancer headline grabbing, despite its comparative rareness in developed nations, is the young age of women afflicted by it. While cervical cancer accounts for a smaller number of total cancer deaths, it makes up a larger number of fatalities in women under forty. As a result, there is a greater feeling of senselessness with each loss of beautiful, vibrant girls and women cut down in their prime. Doctors promoting the shot emotionally recall patients who never had a chance to realize their life's promises. One Canadian doctor described a young talented pianist, who "after years of dedicated study, was scheduled to give her first piano recital in Toronto."[70] Alas, this young woman ignored irregular discharge until it became unusual bleeding. By that point it was too late, and she died within months.

HPV vaccines have been approved in some countries for use in women between twenty-seven and forty-five as well as in their younger sisters. The FDA rejected Merck's bid to extend their approval in the United States.[71] This was due in part to a lack of evidence that older populations, the vast majority of whom are sexually active, will see any health benefit from the shot.[72] In Australia, where use in older women was approved for Cervarix, the controversy was no less pronounced: Dr. Gerard Wain wrote in the *Medical Journal of Australia* that "to suggest that the vaccine will offer patients some theoretical potential benefit if they are prepared to pay for it does not reflect sound evidence-based, equitable, health-care provision."[73] In other words, if you are already having sex, it is possible that the shot will bring no benefit and certain that Pap smears and other screening tools remain your best strategy for cancer prevention. Gardasil for grown-ups isn't dangerous but is more akin to a four-leaf clover than a magic bullet. Women over twenty-six in America can still get Gardasil, but as an off-label prescription, they have to pay out of pocket for it.[74]

Those who opt to seek out Gardasil on their own may find it difficult to locate doctors offering the injection. Because of the high price, many have been reluctant to offer Gardasil, equating having the product with "handling expensive crystal with no margin for error."[75]

Even for those whose insurance companies cover Gardasil, it may be difficult to seek compensation. Most insurers pay part of the cost for women who fall within the FDA-recommended age group, while some cover only administrative costs.[76] Insurance company inconsistency about reimbursement makes some doctors less likely to carry the vaccine. Slow uptake of the vaccine, coupled with the poor economy has caused Merck to cut its sales estimates by $500 million. To compensate, the company is pursuing other ways of expanding sales, "such as reimbursing doctors who give the vaccine to uninsured patients."[77]

Parents, Schools, and the Battle over HPV Vaccination

Alarms sounded around the globe when, in the spring of 2007, a group of Australian schoolgirls experienced mysterious adverse reactions, including fainting and paralysis, after being injected.[78] Ian Frazer, the Australian inventor of Gardasil, unwisely portrayed these incidents as psychosomatic or hysterical. Australian women's health activists responded by chastising this assessment: "We shouldn't dismiss the bad experience of these girls just because we really want the vaccine to work. Women's health is more important."[79]

In America, a conservative group called Judicial Watch used the Freedom of Information Act to gain access to adverse event reports, which they then revealed to the public with sensationalist gusto. The 1,637-page report (which covered 136 serious side effects and a small number of deaths) was described by the organization's president, Tom Fitton, as "a catalog of horrors."[80]

Parents' initial optimism about Gardasil shifted to wary caution. Ontario's enormous opt-in program, which offered the vaccine to girls for free within an approved age group, began to fail. An early survey of parent attitudes toward the shot had found high approval, with 75.3 percent claiming they intended to give their daughter Gardasil.[81] By November 2007, it was clear that perspectives had changed, and vaccination rates in Ontario were under 50 percent.[82] Journalist André Picard observed that part of this parental resistance might be due to governmental "hard sells": "The hallmark of public health communications has, for far too long, been proselytizing, 'If we say everyone should have the vaccine, everyone should have the vaccine, trust us.'"[83] This sort of paternalistic approach might have worked fifty years ago, Picard notes, but in the age of the Internet, health consumers are educated enough to want to see the evidence.

In 2008, there was more bad news: two girls in Europe—one in Germany and another in Austria—died unexpectedly after receiving Gardasil. As with previous deaths in the United States, the European losses were associated with, but not tied to, use of the vaccine.[84] The European Medicines Agency felt compelled to review the vaccine's safety and announced that while it found that adverse events occurred, the two deaths could not be definitively shown to be the result of Gardasil and that the benefits of getting the shot outweighed the risks.[85] Still, it threw gas on the fire. Parents began asking questions very loudly that ranged from reasonable to outlandish: Would Gardasil lose effectiveness with the years? Could it cause reproductive problems or infertility?[86] They worried about birth defects and chemicals like aluminum in the vaccine causing degenerative diseases.

By 2008, Judicial Watch again raised the issue of more than eight thousand adverse events and seventeen deaths.[87] While the FDA reports "cleared" the vaccine from responsibility in most of the fatalities, today the question remains: does Gardasil cause more—or more serious—side effects than other common vaccines? Some sources say yes. An article published in *CMAJ* on September 1, 2008, noted that anaphylaxis (allergic reaction) is five to twenty times higher with the HPV vaccine than other vaccines,[88] but added that overall adverse event rates "were very low."[89]

Others interpreted the *CMAJ* data differently, arguing that "although there may be underreporting, the rate . . . is consistent with the rate of anaphylaxis following several other vaccinations."[90]

Whatever the reality of shot-related side effects turns out to be, the FDA saw fit to expand warnings on the vaccine's packaging in June 2008 to include "joint and muscle pain, fatigue, physical weakness and general malaise."[91] Two months later, the *Medical Journal of Australia* reported that some patients had experienced pancreatitis after getting the shot.[92] In the winter of 2008 the total number of adverse events in America was over nine thousand and included twenty-seven deaths. A pharmaceutical industry publication noted that 20 percent of all vaccine adverse events in 2008 were related to Gardasil, despite the fact that it isn't required like many childhood vaccines.[93]

We must ask the same question about Gardasil that we ask about all vaccines: is the illness serious enough to warrant the risks and side effects? It is important to put in perspective that most adverse events were not serious, and some of the more serious complications—like Guillain-Barré syndrome, a rare condition where the immune system mistakenly attacks the nerves, potentially causing paralysis[94]—have been seen in other vaccines as well as in allergies to ingredients such as egg protein and gelatin.[95] Gardasil doesn't seem to increase patients' risk of getting the disorder. Lingering pain at the injection site[96] is also common with many vaccines. Fainting and hyperventilating are more serious and suggest a need for extended monitoring of patients after injection to prevent injury from falling.[97] Potential paralysis and blood clots could potentially be deeply worrying, but so far these conditions haven't been definitively tied to the shot (in several deaths, Merck has been quick to point out that patients were also on oral contraceptives, a more likely culprit for clotting and cardiac events). Still, even the hint of a connection to these life-threatening conditions makes it worthwhile to ask how serious the cancer risk is to begin with if patients are already participating in an annual program of cervical screening. Until we are sure what problems the shot can cause, it is always valuable to use precaution in making decisions for our own health and the health of our children.

One of the major issues to emerge from the conversation about compulsory Gardasil vaccination concerns the power of parents to decide what is right, medically and socially, for their children. In fact, when public health is in the balance, US states are well within their rights to require vaccination. Alexandra M. Stewart, a lawyer with George Washington University Medical Center, notes that early in the twentieth century the Supreme Court granted the states "police power" with which to enforce vaccinations thought to "protect the public health and the public safety."[98] At issue, of course, is the difference between HPV and other infectious diseases that can be prevented with shots. As I noted before, the key difference is how the infections are spread. While measles, for example, can be spread through casual contact, HPV transmission requires intimate contact. This makes the public health threat, from a traditional perspective, much less compelling.

Parental objections to Gardasil are often framed by other cultural conversations. One group that particularly opposes the idea of forced vaccinations is the growing number of parents who object more generally to state enforcement of shots. This movement has gained momentum in past years because of unproven beliefs that vaccines cause autism (a claim that all recent science suggests is unfounded) and fear that chemicals and metals used to increase vaccine uptake, like aluminum hydroxide, may lead to degenerative diseases like Alzheimer's or Parkinson's.[99] One study found that parental willingness for children to receive Gardasil in any context, not simply in mandatory programs, was considerably informed by their more general attitude toward childhood vaccination programs.[100]

Another major group predictably objects to HPV vaccination out of the worry that promoting it prematurely forces a conversation about sexuality with young children. As one expert editorialized in the *New England Journal of Medicine*, "Opposition seems to be based on the concern that to recognize the reality of teenage sexual activity is implicitly to endorse it."[101] An inability to communicate complicated ideas about this part of adult life to children is also a source of anxiety. One British mother writes, "Of course we need to tell our kids about sexually transmitted disease, but I'm not sure I want them, at a tender and impressionable age, to equate sex with disease."[102] She adds more pointedly about school immunization programs, "We're constantly told we should be responsible parents, but I'm coming to think that this is a euphemism for compliant."[103]

If the right of parents to determine whether their daughters will be vaccinated is important, it is equally valid to ask what an individual girl's rights to self-determination should be in the context of HPV prevention. Catherine DeAngelis addresses this problem, noting, "Consider the information a clinician can honestly provide to a twelve-year-old girl to obtain her assent: 'the three injections will probably protect you from an infection that you can only get from sexual contact, but research has not shown how long the protection will last or whether it might have bad effects on your health.'"[104] The *Lancet*, one of Britain's top medical journals, comes to a similar conclusion: "It is worrying that most girls being offered vaccination against HPV might have no concept of what the virus does, and certainly therefore no understanding of the benefits of immunity."[105]

Concerns about children and sexuality pose serious threats to access for young women who might decide later in their teen years to be vaccinated before becoming sexually active. As one British mother explains, "If the decision is left up to the girl, is she really going to go to her parents when she is fifteen and say: 'I think it's time to have this vaccination'?"[106] If going to parents is an admission of intent, it is difficult to imagine most teen girls paying a minimum of $360 (most likely closer to $500 or $600 once doctors fees are factored in) out of pocket to avoid parental detection. So most girls will either get the vaccine when they are too young to be informed consumers, or they will wait until they are financially independent—and by then, statistically speaking, they will already be sexually active.

If there are serious ethical problems with giving the shot to young girls, there are practical concerns as well, particularly the lack of extensive clinical data on that age group. While thousands of women received Gardasil shots as part of approval studies, very few women under fifteen—less than two thousand—received the vaccine in advance of approval. So while it was found safe in many women, the age group most likely to receive the shot was left out. Efficacy studies, which show near 100 percent effectiveness for women sixteen to twenty-six, are lacking in younger girls.[107] Canadian Women's Health Network representative Madeline Boscoe spoke to the age gap in trial evidence saying, "It's scary to think of vaccinating a whole generation of nine-year-old girls in this country based on a hundred [people] . . . The duty around evidence here should be so much higher."[108]

For feminists and women's health activists, the Gardasil experience raises a different set of ethical and historical problems. While Gardasil is most likely as efficacious in men as it is in women, only female populations were tested for approval of the vaccine. This happened for complicated reasons, among them a desire on the part of the drugmaker to establish the product with as few ties to the term "sexually transmitted infection" as possible. If Gardasil could be sold as an anticancer measure, it stood to gain faster acceptance than as a prophylactic for safer sex.

This singling out of women coupled with the speed and heavy-handedness with which most states attempted to enforce programs raised fears that Gardasil was about to become the next chapter in America's unfortunate history of forcing the burden of STI prevention on female bodies. A particularly dramatic example of this occurred during World War I, even as American attitudes toward contraception were changing and easing. Carole R. McCann notes, "During the war, an adolescent girl could be arrested for public flirting or consorting with military personnel."[109] Once arrested, women could be medically examined to test for STIs, and if the results were positive, they were often incarcerated without trial for indefinite periods of time and subjected to treatment.

Because women in America—particularly poor, immigrant, or non-white women—live with this history, it is little wonder that they are suspicious when government bodies begin mandating medical procedures and threatening the removal of basic rights—such as school admittance—for noncompliance. As Abby Lippman explains, "All the focus on the vaccine makes it seem as if this is only a women's health care issue. Why is it almost always girls' and women's sex lives that are put under scrutiny? Why are they alone made to bear the weight of preventing HPV transmission?"[110]

Despite many very good reasons to reject mandatory programs, it seems likely that such plans failed more because of dubious parental anxiety about sexuality and peripheral vaccine-related illness than out of concern for the individual rights of women. Somehow it has become very complicated to say that HPV vaccination could be a wonderful thing and that women should be able to choose it for themselves. Along the way these two ideas have become mutually exclusive.

But the silver lining in any case is that the vaccination has given parents new confidence as savvy health consumers who can talk back to forces in the medical and political communities who are in the service of drugmakers instead of families. Patients reorganizing such power relationships can be seen as a step in the right direction as long as it can be coupled with good science and informed (rather than frightened) health consumership.

For immigrant girls and young women, there is still no choice when it comes to HPV vaccination. Because of a 1996 law requiring the Citizen and Immigration Services to mandate all suggested shots, all women immigrating to the United States who fall into the CDC's recommended age group must get the vaccine.[111] Most young women must have the first dose before they come to the United States, and they probably pay the huge price out of pocket. Tuyet G. Duong, a lawyer with the Asian American Justice Center in Washington, DC, explains that Gardasil, in part because of its high cost, "is just an additional barrier to coming to America . . . It just adds another layer to what has become a toxic environment for immigrants."[112] Because of steep costs, many girls may not be able to get the second and third shots to make the entire process efficacious. Immigrant advocates point out that it is premature to force Gardasil on such a large population without more conclusive data about side effects and long-term usefulness. Angelica Salas, the director of the Coalition for Humane Immigrant Rights in Los Angeles, says, "We don't want to convey that we don't want individuals to make healthy choices or seek out preventative healthcare . . . We just don't see why it should be linked to immigration."[113] At the time this chapter was being edited, the HPV requirement was being reviewed but had not yet been repealed.

For low-income women in America there are more options. If parents opt to have young daughters vaccinated, they can likely get the majority, if not the entirety, of the shot covered. The Vaccines for Children Program provides the vaccine for children on Medicaid and those who are uninsured or underinsured. While adults must pay entirely out of pocket for any vaccine, "for children, almost 60 percent of vaccine doses are purchased through federal contracts."[114] The government is paying a hefty sum for the shot; despite intense negotiations, federal immunization program administrators received only a 20 percent discount, bringing

Gardasil's price tag to $288 instead of the usual $360. Merck also offers assistance to low-income individuals through the Merck Patient Assistance Program.

According to the *New York Times*, "Health economists estimate that depending on how they are used, the two cervical cancer vaccines will cost society $30,000 to $70,000 or higher, for each year of life they save in developed countries . . . The number will be far higher if a booster is needed."[115] This astronomical amount of money will direct resources away from other health measures, particularly for the uninsured and the underinsured.

How many girls have received the vaccine? Around 25 percent in the United States have been given at least one of the three doses, according to Lance Rodewald, director of immunization services at the Centers for Disease Control and Prevention.[116] Of these, only one fourth have received all three shots. There are significant ethnic, class, and racial differences in the data. For example, only 1 percent of Latina teens have gotten the shot despite the fact that they are at greater risk for contracting dangerous strains of HPV than their white peers.[117] African American teens are also at an increased risk of both HPV and cervical cancer. But despite slower than expected uptake, Merck is making a tremendous amount of money: in 2008, Gardasil had "projected sales of $1.4 billion to $1.6 billion outside Europe" in addition to, of course, "more sales from Europe."[118]

Gardasil for Boys

It was only a matter of time before pharmaceutical companies started imagining the possibilities their vaccine held for men. In November 2008, a Merck-funded study of four thousand boys aged sixteen to twenty-six found that Gardasil had the same antiwart efficacy for men—as much as 90 percent protection—as it offered female populations.[119] In addition, the drugmaker stressed that certain rare but terrible cancers in men were also tied to HPV.

Allan Cassels, a tireless crusader against pharmaceutical company machinations, worries that a desire to market Gardasil to young men will lead to an overstatement of the risks of rare illnesses, such anal and penile cancers, which have been tied to HPV but don't pose the threat seen with cervical cancer: "It strikes me this is the vaccine manufacturer seeking basically more markets . . . In order to sell the vaccine, you've got to sell the size of the problem."[120] A 2007 *New England Journal of Medicine* article authored by Stina Syrjänen (who disclosed receiving consulting fees from Merck) tied certain head and neck cancers to HPV and argued, "It is worth considering the possibility that some oral, oropharyngeal, and laryngeal cancers might be prevented by HPV vaccination."[121]

In early 2009, Merck filed paperwork with the FDA to extend their recommendation to boys ages nine to twenty-six, and in October of that year, the FDA approved the use of Gardasil in men. The approval came only hours after the FDA threw Merck's rival, GSK, a bone by finally green-lighting Cervarix after years of delay.

Women's health groups, family health advocates, and others in the public health world are conflicted about the news. Diana Zuckerman, head of the Washington, DC–based National Research Center for Women and Families, testified against FDA approval. Her concerns, most of which apply to girls as well, include the short length of trials, the uncertainty of the shot's duration of efficacy, and—specifically in the case of boys—the very limited health benefits. "When the vaccine was first approved for girls, we supported it," Zuckerman tells me. "But now that we have examined the data more carefully, we question its value, for women or men."[122]

Media coverage of Gardasil's extension to boys has been limited, and even as Merck moves to publicize the expanded market, government bodies like the CDC's Advisory Committee on Immunization Practices have equivocated. While recommending Cervarix for women ages thirteen to twenty-eight who have not received an HPV vaccine, the committee said its recommendation of Gardasil for boys would remain optional.

What to make of the important distinction between telling women to get vaccinated and making it an optional recommendation for men? As one Canadian journalist wryly observed, "There's a subtle 'dirty girl' air to this campaign—as if guys had nothing to do with it. Hello? You don't get genital warts from the HPV fairy."[123] If, as recent trials suggest, Gardasil works in men as well as it works in women, it may be to everyone's benefit to offer the shot to both sexes.

Many, however, balk at the notion that boys—since they aren't at risk for cervical cancer—have a compelling motive to undergo the expense and discomfort associated with the vaccine. Why would boys want to get the shot? Some argue, "Think altruism. Responsibility. Chivalry, even? Oh, and yes: some explicit details about genital warts and sexual transmission."[124] The prevention of genital warts, long a distasteful and painful outcome of unprotected sex, may indeed prove a compelling reason for men to roll up their sleeves. But a parent of two boys ages eight and twelve provides an alternate perspective: "You don't want to say it's just the girls' problem, but my sons won't contract cervical cancer. And genital warts are treatable. I'm very skeptical. What risks will I expose them to?"[125]

This debate drives home the point that concerns that exist for women don't receive serious consideration until male bodies are at stake. Boys shouldn't be unnecessarily exposed to risks and neither should girls. And if approving the vaccines for boys is what it takes to have a serious conversation about the risks and benefits of this health measure, than the move to extend the shot to men is a good thing.

International Concerns

Even before approval of the vaccine in the United States, doctors' hopes for its usefulness in the developing world were building.[126] Healthy debate about the shot is valuable in America, but the places where it might do the most good—in poor nations around the globe that still list grossly disproportionate rates of cervical cancer diagnosis and death—are the places with little to no access to the shots.

Internationally, there are 500,000 new cases of cervical cancer each year, and somewhere around 274,000 deaths. Writing in the *New England Journal of Medicine* in 2005, authors noted that screening methods that have dramatically reduced rates of both cervical cancer and death from that illness, such as Pap smears, are more difficult to implement in the developing world.[127] Cervical cancer is the second leading cause of cancer death in women, but more than 80 percent of those fatalities are in developing nations, a number expected to rise to 90 percent by 2020.[128] Compare that with America, where cervical cancer fails to make the

American Cancer Society's top ten list of most deadly cancers, and deaths from the disease account for under one tenth of the fatalities caused by cancer of the lung and breast.[129]

Merck has donated large batches of Gardasil to the World Health Organization for use in poorer countries. Unfortunately, these donations are comparatively small; for example, the initial gift—substantial in terms of monetary value at $375 million[130]—was enough to provide 1 million women with full courses of the vaccine. While this is certainly a lot of women and a generous gift, it is not enough to affect the virus's spread in any serious way. In order to be cost effective in a nation where the gross domestic product is less than one thousand dollars per capita, Sue J. Goldie and Jan M. Agosti argue in the *New England Journal of Medicine* that the vaccine would need to cost as little as one dollar.[131] In the meantime, public health experts note, "It is essential . . . for developing countries to allocate their limited resources toward screening, rather than vaccination."[132]

All the existing questions about efficacy, disease change, and safety in America also apply to these populations, and caution in America may ultimately be good for women in the developing world if it turns out that the HPV vaccines aren't effective after a decade or two of use.

To date, close to a hundred countries have approved Gardasil, and forty-four have given Cervarix the green light.[133] Fifteen countries have issued formal recommendations to their populations.[134] Much more information is needed, but the drugs show enormous promise for improving women's lives. The controversies surrounding the vaccine highlight the way that international health care conversations between doctor and patient, government and community, developed and developing nations are emerging and changing. It is important for women to be able to take advantage of this major advance, while still asking serious questions about safety and efficacy.

Chapter Ten

What About the Boys? Or, Why Is There *Still* No Pill for Men?

Revolution . . . Often it is sounded to drama, drums and discussion, but sometimes it just settles over us like a mist.
—Barbara Seaman, *Women and the Crisis in Sex Hormones*

Imagine how America might look a year or two from now: the streets are full of green cars, and everyone carries reusable shopping bags. People read the newspaper on their phone, and everyone is talking about the new health care system. Life is much as it is now with the exception of small but important changes. Oh yeah, and men take the Pill.

"Wait!" I can hear you saying. "That won't happen anytime soon. That's in the distant future."

Maybe. Or perhaps it's right around the corner.

Scientists, doctors, and women have been talking about the possibility of a birth control pill for men since before there was one for women. Gregory Pincus, the father of the Pill, imagined it even as he tinkered with his nascent creation in 1950s America. Feminists in the 1970s, spurred by fears about oral contraceptive dangers, raged that men weren't made or encouraged to bear similar dangers and wondered loudly why the responsibilities of fertility control weren't carried more evenly by the sexes. In the 1990s, the runaway success of Viagra got pharmaceutical companies asking if, despite conventional wisdom, men weren't an enormous untapped market for contraceptive pharmaceuticals.

Today, close to sixty years after the first hormones were given to a male patient with the purpose of curbing sperm production, it's worth returning to what has become an age-old question: Why is there *still* no pill for men? How would drug safety, reproductive policy, and gender relationships change if the other half of the world began using pharmaceutical contraceptives? And why has the road to making and marketing a male pill been such a long one?

The answers to these questions are part of a larger conversation about the way that our society has historically treated male and female bodies differently, and the pathways through which this is (slowly) changing. It is, after all these years, a deeply contemporary topic. The male pill is a technology whose future is as bound up in the economic uncertainties of the current Great Recession as it is in egalitarian approaches to reproductive health and intimate conversation between sexual partners. It teaches us about the changing relationships between pharmaceutical giants and non-governmental organizations in the creation of new pills, and the global nature of drug development. It also illustrates the increasing medicalization of men's bodies and the complicated implications of that process.

Today, the options for male birth control are the same as they have been for a long time: condoms, withdrawal, and vasectomy. Imagining a social world in which birth control is an equal responsibility for men and women is a step toward making it a reality and, in its own way, a radical act.

Always Already: The Long Search for the Male Pill

Alice Wolfson was used to righteous anger, but this time the force of it shocked her. The young Barnard graduate had come into her own as an activist, like so many second-wave feminists, as part of the civil rights and antiwar movements. She had learned firsthand the strategies of fighting for social change and had started, with other young women, to apply those lessons to the long fight for sexual and gender equality. After moving to Washington, DC, with her husband, Wolfson formed a new social circle by making connections with other feminist-minded women and creating the group DC Women's Liberation.

The group decided to attend the Nelson pill hearings after several members relayed that they'd had bad health experiences with the drug. Though the group often staged activism, in this case, their intention was fact-finding. As the young women listened to the testimony, their outrage and disbelief mounted. Although many of them had experienced unpleasant side effects with the Pill—hair loss, in Wolfson's case—they had no idea that the drug was potentially fatal. Why hadn't they been given all the information?

When she could stand it no longer, Wolfson raised her hand to ask questions. After this went ignored, she and the other young women got on their feet and began to yell out their concerns, disrupting the hearing. Years later, health activist Barbara Seaman, whose book had led to the hearings, would recall the scene: "Why are there no patients testifying?" the Wolfson women demanded. "Why is the press whitewashing all the adverse comments against the Pill? *Why is there no pill for men?*"[1]

It was, in its way, one of the foundational questions of the women's health movement. Seaman would personally take up the issue at several points in her long career, most powerfully in her 1977 book *Women and the Crisis in Sex Hormones*, writing, "Although it's a well-known fact that it takes two to make a baby, contraception in general is viewed today as a woman's problem."[2] The mother of the women's health movement thought that this state of affairs, which was due at least in part to greater cultural concern for the health of men, was changing: "Partly as a result of today's egalitarian movement . . . men and women are coming to regard contraception as a shared problem."

Wolfson and Seaman were identifying a fundamental issue in women's health care at that time: the doctor-patient relationship was paternalistic in structure, and unless male patients helped articulate and validate women's complaints, doctors tended to write them off as the result of suggestion (meaning they expected the problem and imagined it in to being) or even something closer to hysteria. Women were denied even basic mechanisms of informed consent, and doctors were trained to avoid telling patients about potential side effects, lest they materialize.[3] If an unbiased evaluation of the Pill's risks and benefits was ever to be obtained, activists reasoned, it would happen only after the chemicals were floating through male veins.

In a larger sense, Margaret Sanger's successful campaign to medicalize contraception had the intended consequence of divorcing birth control and sexuality. Because pregnancy prevention happened in a doctor's office and was therefore a negotiation between a woman and her doctor, the male sexual partner was effectively removed from the conversation. This allowed "women's health," as it was euphemistically called, to be ghettoized and, from a standpoint of medical safety and ethics, to receive less consideration than the already lax standards of the day required.

The women most responsible for the Pill, Margaret Sanger and Katherine McCormick, believed only women should control contraception, and it was for this reason that they chose to focus on hormonal drugs for women instead of other possible approaches that were in the air in the early 1950s, including an antisperm vaccine.[4] Part of the issue was social: women were simply more willing to serve as trial subjects. One scientist observed, "Male volunteers for fertility control studies may be numbered in the low hundreds, whereas women have volunteered for similar studies by the thousands . . . He [the human male] has psychological aversions to experimenting with sexual functions."[5]

In addition, the science on men's bodies and endocrine systems was lagging far behind the science on women's bodies. Scientists had been synthesizing hormonal compounds for use in female patients for decades, but only limited work had been done on men.

These central concerns—social and cultural myths that men are unwilling to take a birth control pill, a lack of fundamental science and chemical recourses for male bodies, and a dearth of infrastructure for executing contraceptive clinical trials—continue to haunt the development of pharmaceutical contraception for men to this day. What was clear at the time and is still true today is that, unlike the female population that historically lobbied for contraceptive access and technological innovation, "the need to develop male contraceptives was never articulated by the potential users of any new technology: men."[6]

Gregory Pincus, to be fair, was always optimistic that men could be included among pill users. By 1957, he was a man in love with his creation and believed that the good results seen in female patients could also be achieved in men. To test his theory, Pincus gave progestin to male prisoners at the Oregon State Penitentiary. While inhumane and unethical by today's standards, pharmaceutical testing on prisoners and mental patients was common in the 1950s, and Pincus speculated that the lowered sperm counts of the men receiving the drug had the potential to prevent pregnancy, lower sexual desire, and even "cure" homosexuality.[7] The side effects experienced by these early male patients, including a loss of libido and feminization, made the idea of marketing the drug to men impractical.

By the mid 1960s, young scientists inspired by the female pill began to pursue further research on a male alternative. The voices of feminists from northern nations were joined by those of political leaders from the southern ones. Governments concerned with population growth, particularly China and India, called for the advancement of the technology.

Gender and technology professor Nelly Oudshoorn studies the path from scientists' first tentative steps to today in *The Male Pill: A Biography of a Technology in the Making*. Oudshoorn identifies several hurdles that had to be overcome before progress could be made on the new drug. Significantly, many of these hurdles aren't related (at least directly) to gender issues, although closer analysis reveals connections. Oudshoorn dismisses the notion that male contraceptive technology has evolved slowly out of happenstance, either because women are more biologically suited to be the subjects of pharmaceutical birth control or because accidents of fate have simply prevented the product from emerging.

The first problem scientists faced was one of basic biology. In considering whether to pursue a hormonal or nonhormonal approach to pregnancy prevention through male bodies, would-be pill makers were at a loss because so many key pieces of information about the male reproductive system simply remained ambiguous. The reproductive systems and cycles of women had been of interest to the medical community since before the 1920s and 1930s, when a generation of groundbreaking scientists mapped the reproductive cycle and began synthesizing female hormones. By the 1950s and 1960s there were many compounds available for testing and many more in development. A lack of equivalent chemicals for male hormones—particularly affordable, practical ones—posed a huge problem for potential drug innovators. Still, because of the success of the female pill, taking a hormonal approach to male contraception seemed to be the most likely path.

One of the early steps, then, was to create more chemical compounds. The male pill, like the female pill before it, struggled at first because there was a lack of interest and financial investment from pharmaceutical makers. Although drug companies got on the contraceptive bandwagon in a big way after Searle's success with Enovid, they played only small roles in the Pill's development, and indeed a female pill would never have been successful without substantial and continued private investment from Katherine McCormick. Pharmaceutical companies have always been reluctant to invest in contraceptive research and development because of concern that there will be a cultural backlash to the drugs and devices produced. They like to play it safe, but as the female pill demonstrated, they are willing to get in the game once it is clear that there will be general acceptance of the drug.

Contraceptive development has always made drugmakers more vulnerable to lawsuits. A male pill promised to be even more risky because men would take it not to prevent health risks to themselves, but theoretically to prevent them in their sexual partners. There was simply no precedent for such a thing: a drug whose physical risks were borne by one population but whose benefits were transferred to another.

Oudshoorn writes that intellectual, financial, social, physical, and scientific supports must be in place to encourage the creation of a new technology. The male pill has suffered the lack of these supports. In the 1970s, in addition to the lack of prior scientific work to draw on and a dearth of serious financial resources, there was no male equivalent for the medical specialty of gynecology or the social networks developed in women's public health clinics—both of which were invaluable buttresses for the research and popularization of female birth control. And even if money and the required chemicals could be found, it would be difficult to mount serious clinical trials, because the networks and resources needed to recruit the appropriate male populations and conduct trials simply didn't exist.

So how do new products, pharmaceutically speaking, come into the world? For drug technologies, one way is by creating a protected space[8] where the scientists involved don't have to play by the usual rules and can think outside the box (or the laboratory, as it were). For Gregory Pincus, this involved the patronage of a wealthy woman who supported his work. For male contraception, it involved the intervention and support of powerful international organizations and foundations, primarily the World Health Organization (WHO), but also to some extent the Population Council.

WHO had been interested in getting involved with global population issues since the early 1950s, when India requested help with natural contraception. Birth control was still deeply controversial business, and WHO backed off involvement when several member states threatened to leave if the group continued to pursue it.[9] By the 1960s, anxieties about global population growth and its relationship to the spread of Communism had made the topic of international contraception fashionable.[10]

Among other projects, WHO—through avenues that included the Male Task Force—made a serious commitment to aiding the development of innovative contraceptives for men. Note that only in the context of global hysteria about the fertility of poor people in the developing world did male birth control become a serious option. That is to say, male bodies became public in this way only by exploiting fears about marginalized communities of men, not through a desire to address the needs and responsibilities of all men. From the beginning interest the male pill was at least somewhat about maintaining inequality, not about creating a more even reproductive playing field.

Whatever the motivation, WHO crossed boundaries when they got into contraceptive research and development. In the past, research and development had always been the terrain of big pharmaceutical firms. Even Pincus had relied on the material support of Syntex and Searle to provide him with steroid compounds. WHO accomplished this task by thinking creatively. One good reason for trying to make drugs without industry involvement was that it allowed WHO to start imagining a world where it would have access to the drugs it wanted without payouts and concessions to big pharmaceutical companies. While they lacked the infrastructure of a large drug company—they didn't have large centralized facilities, for example—they created a new model based in international cooperation. Instead of relying on one or two large laboratories, the Male Task Force established a network of laboratories around the world working to create new chemicals that could be used for future drugs. The success of this program created a model that WHO would return to in the future for the establishment of clinical trials. Bringing several laboratories together had additional benefits. For one thing, it hastened information gathering and brought together the few experts who existed in the field. Second, the broad geographic scope of the laboratory network helped to anticipate ethnic and cultural differences that would prove important in troubleshooting drugs from both a medical and a social standpoint.

While early programs were promising, old problems were not entirely overcome. Doctors proved unwilling to refer male patients for trials, and

no male equivalent of the public health clinic existed, so it was tough finding men willing to give the male pill a go. The media provided one limited
way to convince men to participate. Today, the problem of trial scope and
size remains a significant one for the development of male contraceptives.
The largest trials have been performed in China under authoritarian rule.
In the West there is (thankfully) no comparable means of "encouraging"
participation.

Of course, not all problems with making the male pill are logistical.
Perceptions about gender have always lingered in the foreground of this
debate. A 1999 Canadian documentary on the Pill shows footage from a
1960s news program on contraception. A handsome, thirty-something
male doctor who works for the drugmaker G. D. Searle is being interviewed by a strikingly pretty blonde reporter. He talks to her about
potential innovations in pill technology, including a long-acting contraceptive injection that, he opined, would make the Pill obsolete. Intrigued
but unconvinced, the young woman looks him in the eye and asks, "What
about the Pill for men?" Almost embarrassed, the doctor laughs at the
question and answers with a slightly patronizing tone that "the hormones
or chemicals that might halt sperm production are very toxic," adding that
besides, what woman would trust her husband to take the Pill?[11]

Arguments about masculinity and male character have reappeared at
various points in the past fifty years to suggest that ultimately male contraception is a doomed project. Most of these are based on either
erroneous or outdated stereotypes of male/female relationships and gender ideologies. Some are based on outright mythology. They include the
notions that men (unlike women, of course) don't want to do anything
that would interfere with their reproductive systems; that they (in particular those who are low income or live in the developing world) have no
interest in family limitation and in fact consider large numbers of children to be status symbols; and that they are unreliable and untrustworthy.
According to this reasoning, the physical risks incurred by a woman in
accepting contraceptive responsibility are worth the psychological benefit
of not having to sit up nights worrying whether her partner has remembered to do his part. Finally, some worry that men would never be willing
or tough enough to tolerate the pain and discomfort inherent in pharmaceutical approaches. These old-fashioned ideas about men—they are

tough, virile, and in control while also irresponsible and afraid of pain—are contradictory. This sort of gender kitsch isn't helpful to women and should be insulting to men.

Whatever the perceptions about masculinity, the underlying concern that men simply wouldn't be willing to use contraception has always presented a major stumbling block for potential pill makers. In the 1960s it was clear that cultural perceptions would need to be scientifically and repeatedly proven false if the male pill was to gain any ground.

On Gossypol: The Male Pill Comes of Age in the 1980s and 1990s

If interest in the male pill seemed promising in the late 1960s, it had dimmed by the early 1980s. Backlash against the female pill contributed to a dwindling interest in male methods. Then, without warning, Gossypol entered the public consciousness. A nonhormonal, botanical drug derived from the seed, stem, and roots of the cotton plant using hot alcohol, Gossypol was introduced to the world by Chinese scientists who announced, around 1979, that they had created and were already testing a pill for men.[12] While the reports of this triumph had been announced preemptively, China and male contraception suddenly had the world's undivided attention.

The cotton plant's amazing fertility-curbing properties were first discovered in parts of China where, particularly during droughts, the cakelike substance left over after the plant's fiber and oil had been removed was used as an alternative food source.[13] The plant has a brilliant natural defense system: it contains a chemical that renders bugs that feed on it infertile, strategically limiting future generations of predators. So when men and livestock ate the cotton product, they stopped fathering offspring. By the 1970s, more than eight thousand Chinese men were taking the drug at a clinical dose.

For the most part, men did well on the drug. Unlike hormonal alternatives, it didn't change endocrine function or cause libido problems. It didn't adversely affect blood pressure or cause weight gain like testosterone.

Unfortunately, Gossypol failed in two key respects. It lowered blood potassium (which can cause liver problems), and more importantly, it proved irreversible in a significant group of men.[14] Because of this, initial enthusiasm for the drug petered out, and by 1986, after a WHO- and Rockefeller Foundation–sponsored symposium on the subject, investigators concluded that Gossypol had little promise of becoming a generally accepted method of birth control.[15] What had been accomplished, however, was the revival of organizational enthusiasm, and WHO began pouring money into research in China.

In the 1990s, WHO began conducting larger, multicenter clinical trials of testosterone therapy. This moved hormonal options up the scientific development chain, but didn't advance the drugs to a point where they were ready for marketing. Despite the impressive accomplishments of WHO and other public sector organizations, the fact remains that it is almost impossible to conduct advanced clinical trials (phase 3) and bring a drug to market without the involvement of the pharmaceutical industry.

Women's activists again played a key role in the story of male contraception in the 1990s. By taking key positions at population and public health organizations, such as the Population Council and WHO, women began to slowly change the agenda of international family planning efforts. Journalist Michelle Goldberg points out that "women needed power, not just pills, and population programs could be harnessed to improve their health and status."[16] Shifting the focus from the xenophobic frenzy of fertility control that had driven efforts in the 1960s and 1970s to concerns about "reproductive health and rights,"[17] feminist leaders were able to put reproductive equity at the center of the international agenda. Their agenda at two conferences—the United Nations International Conference on Population and Development held in Cairo in 1994 and the United Nations Fourth World Conference on Women held in Beijing in 1995—characterized birth control as a shared responsibility. Leaders specifically identified the importance of increasing the role of "men as partners" and "male responsibility" in contraception. In this formulation, male contraception became a women's health issue.

Not everyone thought male contraceptives would improve female lives. Feminists also articulated concerns that female power could be reduced if men took control of pregnancy prevention. Some voiced anxieties that after decades of fighting to get women moved to the center of public health agendas, men were back in the spotlight. Might shifting contraceptive priorities to men, who already in general enjoyed a higher standard of health care, simply siphon specialized resources from women? In international contexts, activists argued that contraception provided a small measure of power to those women who still lived in more traditional patriarchal environments.

This bold emerging global health agenda both helped and hurt prospects for male birth control. It helped in that it again revived dying institutional interest in the possibility of male methods, particularly at the Population Council and WHO. It hurt in that this redefinition of goals, at both Cairo and Beijing, marked the moment at which such institutions' financial backing of contraception began to decline. A cynic might point out that as soon as reproducing women in the abstract were removed as a cultural threat, and women in particular were championed and empowered as reproductive actors, cultural urgency to provide family planning fell away.

Hope for the male pill surged again in the late 1990s, when pharmaceutical firms finally got involved with research on male methods. Two European companies, Schering and Organon, were the first to launch research programs, with a small number of American firms, including Wyeth, sticking their toes reluctantly in the water. This change of heart for drugmakers is attributable, at least in part, to the blockbuster success of the anti-impotence drug Viagra, which changed the way that industry thought about drugs and male sexuality.[18] Its runaway success indicated the presence of untapped markets, and for a fleeting moment, drugmakers thought birth control might become hugely profitable. In 1996, an article in the British medical journal the *Lancet* noted that "after 30 years of research, the prospects for a new male contraceptive are at last looking good,"[19] and they estimated that a drug would hit the market within five to seven years. When Nelly Oudshoorn published *The Male Pill* in 2003, prospects for the availability of a male option were excellent. A few hormonal variations had entered later clinical trial phases, and pharmaceutical companies seemed—at last—to be on board.

And then it all went wrong again. In a 2008 article in the journal *Contraception*, Michael J. K. Harper chronicles the retreat of drug companies from contraceptive research and development in general, and research on men in particular.[20] First, the two major industry players in male birth control, Schering and Organon, became the same company when Schering acquired Organon. Then Schering designed a massive merger with drug giant Merck. The American companies, Wyeth (now part of Pfizer) and Johnson & Johnson, both left the birth control development business for the most part. Today, only one large European firm and two American companies, including Teva, continue to develop new birth control options. This, coupled with the serious problems in the global economy, has put the future of male birth control technology, even after all these years, in serious doubt.

Birds, Bees, and Pharmaceuticals: Changing Old Ideas about Men and Women to Make a New Drug

As I have said, some of the biggest obstacles to the development of male methods are mental ones; drug companies, media outlets, and scientists all continue to insist on a set of outdated ideas about men, women, and birth control that have been reiterated—although not substantiated—for fifty years. When you say something often enough, most people will accept that it is true.

One of the greatest surprises to me during the process of writing this book has been how many men have asked me, upon finding out about my project, when a good option for them is coming. "I would be all about it," one twenty-seven-year-old told me. "It would be nice to have a feeling of control about that part of my life. And also responsibility; I feel bad always putting that on my girlfriend." Another newlywed in his early thirties told me that after getting married, his wife had used the Pill. Soon, though, her frequent migraines led them to ditch OCs. Today they use the fertility awareness method, but he wishes there were more choices available to him.

Doctors and social scientists working on male birth control have gone to great efforts to dispel notions about male unwillingness to embrace pharmaceutical options. Nearly every piece of research on male contraception feels the need to initiate reports by reiterating two important points: first, that men want and would use male birth control and second, that their partners would support such drugs and would trust their partners to use them successfully.

One such study, conducted by Edinburgh-based scientist Richard Anderson and colleagues, notes that among men in Scotland, Shanghai, Hong Kong, and Capetown, 44 to 83 percent said that they would welcome a male pill.[21] Anderson also found that men were more likely to be open to trying a contraceptive if their partners encouraged them to do so. A related study found even more support among women for the drug, with 71 percent saying it would be a good idea and only 2 percent expressing concern that their partners weren't up to the job.[22]

Stereotypes about the willingness of men to be primary contraceptive actors are particularly pernicious when applied to men in the developing world. Surveys have been conducted to disprove stereotypes about men in developing nations, particularly the notion that they are generally opposed to birth control and want to have lots of babies. In fact, with the notable exception of Sub-Saharan Africa, research shows that men in the non-Western world desire families similar in size to their American counterparts, an average of two to three children.[23] Researchers found that the greatest limitation on men taking a more active role in contraception is a lack of available options.[24] A 2002 survey of men in Argentina, Brazil, France, Germany, Indonesia, Mexico, Spain, Sweden, and the United States found that 55 percent of respondents said they would be willing to try a hormonal contraceptive,[25] although specific acceptance rates varied by country between 21 and 71 percent.

Of course, as Jacqueline E. Darroch points out, men's responses to potential technologies in the abstract may be different than what they would be if a drug were actually to hit the shelves: "It is very difficult to predict ultimate levels of interest and use of new methods until they are actually introduced."[26] This might be particularly true if, after a few months or years, a nasty side effect were to emerge.

The strangest part of the cultural insistence that men wouldn't be willing to take responsibility for pregnancy prevention is that until the advent of the female pill, that is exactly what they had been doing. Indeed, in 1955, condom use and withdrawal—two male-dependant methods—accounted for 32 percent of total contraceptive use in the United States, and 21 percent used periodic abstinence to limit births.[27] While we can breathe a sigh of relief that more options are now available, it is interesting that with a history of substantial male involvement, we have become convinced that men want nothing to do with mediating the consequences of sex.

Today male involvement is on the decline, despite the rise of HIV/AIDS, which gave condoms a new relevance and prevalence on the world stage as well as increasing their overall use.[28] The percentage of total contraception for which men are responsible has dropped from 37 percent in 1987[29] to 25 percent in 2005.[30] Men cannot necessarily be blamed for this: the last time science offered them an improvement in their options that was truly novel and fully reversible was when the vulcanization of rubber facilitated better condoms in the middle of the nineteenth century.

In a certain way, the AIDS crisis and concerns about sexually transmitted infection have created more than one generation of young men who know that they will use condoms for at least part of their sexual lives. This expectation of involvement provides a good opportunity for changing the balance of the contraceptive burden. If young men are used to taking responsibility for pregnancy prevention through condom use, a transition to injections or pills would seem more natural than for the generations of men who fell, sexually speaking, between the Pill and the advent of HIV/AIDS.

It is conceivable that men protected from pregnancy might worry less about STIs and neglect using barriers for disease prevention. This would put countless people at risk and potentially create problems for partners who felt pressure to engage in sex without protection. With every technological innovation we must be careful not to abandon the wisdom and strengths of former methods in our enthusiasm for new ones.

The first oral contraceptives were offered only to "married" women in the hopes of avoiding a cultural backlash. The first male options were tested only on men in "committed relationships," however dubiously this is defined. In this case the concern is not over morals, but sexual health and informed consent. Early trials of hormonal methods insisted on condom use because of ethical concerns for women. Women would ultimately reap the benefits of a male pill while their partners endured the risks, but during the trial phase, women are the ones at risk of pregnancy if the drugs don't work.

Nelly Oudshoorn points out that the weight we give to side effects and risks varies based on the power and social status of the person facing risk. When it comes to contraception, for better or for worse, science and industry seem to be much more concerned about the potential hazards of drugs for men than they are about comparable drugs for women. For example, there is deep concern over sexual side effects experienced by men in trials of hormonal drugs. While curtailed libido is indeed disturbing, the problem has always been a commonly reported side effect of the female pill. In one case this side effect has been a major factor in keeping potential drugs off the market, and in the other, it is merely a small-type footnote in a patient-package insert. The medical community simply does not consider the loss of sexual desire in women to be as serious a consequence as it is in men. Because stereotypical ideas about sexuality imagine sex drive to be a fundamental part of male identity and less important to females, the problem is given different weight in these two populations.

Some argue that greater weight is given to problems with male pills because of the history of safety issues with female drugs. While it would be deeply encouraging to imagine that science has "learned the lesson" of hormonal contraception in the 1960s—namely, that aggressive marketing and a lack of informed consent are undesirable—problems with other drugs reveal that the matter isn't a simple historical progression to better, more ethical medicine. A look at the course of hormone therapy and estrogen therapy in the 1990s shows that pharmaceutical firms were willing to very aggressively market hormone drugs to healthy populations of women even after serious concerns about the risk of cardiovascular disease and cancer in connection with these drugs had been raised in previous decades. When the issue of testosterone therapy for aging men was raised, many scientists were quick to dismiss the idea, noting, like G. D. Searle's doctor in the 1960s, how dangerous such drugs might be; among other problems, doctors noted that the risks of testosterone replacement therapy included cancer and increased risk of heart disease.[31]

Side effects in a male pill are harder for doctors and drugmakers to justify because men don't face the potential health problems that women do if a pregnancy results. Their risk/benefit analysis is skewed. If a new male method is ever going to be put on the market, Oudshoorn theorizes, then side effects in men can and should be weighed against the health difficulties alleviated in women. Thinking this way requires, to some extent, that birth control be taken out of the doctor's office and placed back in the context of sexuality. If contraception is somehow inherently relational, then it makes sense that two people, not one, should be considered when discussing the benefits and drawbacks of a method. A failure to change this thinking will mean ultimately that no male drug will ever be safe enough. As Oudshoorn writes, "The aim of clinical testing of male hormonal contraceptives has culminated in a quest for zero risk."[32] But as women have learned through experience, every drug and method carries potential problems. Without a certain willingness to endure and address side effects, these essential tools in contraceptive health would never have become available.

Of Tails and Targets: The Male Reproductive System and Contraceptive Options

The male reproductive system, much like the female, relies on a series of chemical reactions among the brain, pituitary gland, and reproductive organs. Remember that female reproductive cycles actually begin not in the pelvis, but in the brain. Men work the same way. Hormonal male contraception functions by manipulating gonadotropins, chemicals that trigger a hormonal chain of events that culminates in sperm production. Like women, men make follicle-stimulating hormone (FSH) and luteinizing hormone (LH). When these chemicals are suppressed in men, sperm counts either seriously decline or disappear.

Because a typical ejaculation contains 100 to 200 million sperm, and men can ejaculate multiple times a day, it is surprising to realize that the journey of a sperm cell from its genesis in the testicle to its exit through the external urethral orifice at the tip of the penis can take about seventy-four days—over two months. This journey starts in the tightly packed cells of the testicle, where coiled tubes house the growing sperm. In between the sperm cells are other cells that produce testosterone. FSH causes the sperm to grow, and LH stimulates testosterone production. The inside of the testicle is carefully protected by the body from outside toxins and dangerous changes in external temperature. This very effective protection system makes this stage of sperm growth hard to disrupt through nonhormonal means.

When the sperm have reached a certain level of maturity, they move slowly into a long and winding tube called the epididymis, up through the ductus deferens (or vas deferens) to the urethra. Key maturation happens in this part of the body, and because of this the epididymis and ductus deferens are one potential target for chemical intervention. As sperm leave the ductus deferens and enter the urethra, they are joined by seminal fluid.

Sperm have three main parts: the head, the midpiece, and the tail. The design of the tail is unique, enabling it to move at astounding speeds when traveling in the female body. The head, which carries DNA, also houses an enzyme essential for breaking into an egg. The midpiece carries mitochondria, which help to power the tail. Seminal fluid is essential to sperm functioning, providing, among other things, chemicals that make the ejaculate alkaline and help sperm survive in the acidic vaginal climate, and fructose to provide energy for the long swim. When scientists think about male contraceptive drugs, they must decide at which point in this system to chemically intervene.

The goal of hormone drugs is to either eliminate sperm or seriously reduce them. When a man stops making sperm he is said to be "azoospermic." If his sperm count is simply rendered low enough to prevent pregnancy, he is said to be "oligozoospermic." Early experiments hoped to completely eliminate sperm, but this proved to be a difficult task, and later scientists readjusted the goal. While most admit that eliminating sperm would be ideal, researchers are also interested in how low sperm volume needs to be to prevent most pregnancies and create a drug with efficacy on par with the female pill.

A major setback to hormonal therapies has been the huge racial and ethnic variation in efficacy. Drug regimens that eliminated sperm in 90 to 100 percent of men in Asian trials had only 60 percent efficacy in white men in North America and Australia.[33] While scientists are baffled by this difference, they acknowledge that it means that geographically specific trials aren't necessarily applicable in other parts of the world. Beyond ethnic and racial differences, scientists struggle to understand why hormonal methods seem to work so well for some men and not for others; an answer to this question remains to be found.

All hormonal therapies require testosterone supplementation. Without it, patients begin to have sexual side effects, including loss of libido. Testosterone therapy that used testosterone enanthate was tested in two large multicenter trials by the World Health Organization in the 1990s. In the first trial, 200 mg of testosterone was administered in weekly injections to 271 men for six months.[34] Of these men, 60 percent became azoospermic, and another 30 percent became oligozoospermic. Only one pregnancy resulted. In the second study, 399 men received 200 mg injections weekly.[35] Ninety-eight became either azoospermic or oligozoospermic. In this case, pregnancies were around 8.1 per one hundred people—an efficacy rate that is similar to actual use rates for the female pill. Adverse health effects included a reduction in high-density lipoprotein (so-called good cholesterol), acne, and reversible shrinking of the testicles. Researchers didn't find significant changes in mood and sexual function or negative impacts on cardiovascular health.

One of the biggest problems with this regimen was practical: weekly injections are simply not a realistic way to deliver birth control to a large population of people in the long term. The high frequency of injections was necessary due to the relative weakness of testosterone enanthate. Other forms of testosterone, including testosterone decanoate (TD)[36] and testosterone undecanoate (TU), have been tested because of their longer life in the body. In theory, these versions could be given by injection every month to every three months, making them more similar from an administrative standpoint to Depo-Provera in women. These drugs have been tested alone[37] and in combination with progestin therapy.[38] Combination therapy, in which testosterone is combined with a variety of progestins, including levonorgestrel, norethisterone, medroxyprogesterone acetate (MPA, the progestin used in Depo-Provera), and desogestrel, has received much preliminary testing. Progestins are administered in a variety of forms, including implants, patch, and gel. Testosterone gel[39] or cream, which could be applied frequently by users, might provide a more acceptable alternative to frequent injections.

So how close are any of these options to hitting pharmacy shelves or becoming available in doctors' offices? It depends who you ask. It has almost become an old joke that the male pill—or more likely injection or implant—is just five years away. In 2005 one group of doctors complained about the modest size and scope of hormone trials, noting, "All trials have been small, and the power to detect clinically important differences has been poor."[40] Additional complaints returned to a problem that has plagued male birth control for decades: a lack of standardization, particularly as it pertains to defining "oligozoospermia." Much will depend, in the next few years, on pharmaceutical involvement and other factors that may be subject to economic twists and turns. Currently, trials of a formula combining TU and progestin seem the closest to moving on to phase 3 clinical testing and, perhaps, FDA approval.

All of the current androgen options are fairly imprecise, and as a result, drug potency is decreased and side effects are more numerous. Hormones bind with target tissues through a mechanism that is somewhat like a lock and key; testosterone is a skeleton key, and despite the fact that it doesn't work as well as we'd like it to, it compensates for the gaps in our steroid knowledge. In future decades new hormonal compounds may allow more specific, finely tuned tools. Selective hormone receptor modulators—drugs that act on certain tissues and not on others—are further along for use in women. The anticancer drug tamoxifen and the menopause drug raloxifene are two female examples. The goal of such medicines is to offer the benefits of hormone therapy—such as increased bone mass in the case of raloxifene—without some of the risks, like breast cancer. The male versions of these drugs are called selective androgen receptor modulators (SARMs).[41]

One early example of this option for men is the compound 7 alpha-methyl-19-nortestosterone (MENT). Championed by the Population Council, the drug is delivered in implants like the female contraceptives Implanon, Norplant, and Jadelle. Unfortunately, it has proved disappointing in the laboratory. The drug has trouble maintaining efficacy over several months.[42] Other SARM options are being explored for the possibility of oral administration, and all of these options are in much more formative stages of development than testosterone therapy.

While androgens and progestins act on FSH and LH, gonadotropin-releasing hormone antagonists (GnRH antagonists) take the process back a step by curtailing the chemicals that trigger FSH and LH.[43] This method has two steps: in the first, a GnRH antagonist works to quickly decrease FSH. The second part, a maintenance step, uses testosterone to keep sperm levels low. Should this approach make it to the market, it would theoretically have a couple of advantages: it would seek to speed up the normally slow onset of azoo- and oligozoospermia, and the testosterone dose needed for maintenance would be lower than testosterone-only therapy, reducing unpleasant side effects.

Hormone treatments have many potential side effects that seem to vary based on the particular androgen or progestin being used. The side effects include acne, weight gain, changes in blood pressure and cardiovascular health, psychological and mood changes, and the potential to increase the risks of certain cancers, most distressingly, prostate cancer. Chemical hormones carry similar risks for women (minus the prostate cancer risk). A significant benefit of hormonal contraception is that in men, as in women, it is entirely reversible for the vast majority of patients.

Nonhormonal Birth Control and the Future of Contraceptive Medicine

All hormonal methods of controlling male fertility draw on previously existing female methods, and while innovative, they don't constitute a truly radical break with older contraceptive medicine. Nonhormonal alternatives, although much further behind scientifically, provide opportunities for scientists to think in truly creative, groundbreaking ways about reproduction.

There are three stages at which sperm can be stopped in its journey toward egg fertilization: during development in the testicle, in maturation in the epididymis, while moving toward the egg and trying to penetrate its surface (the zona pellucida). Think of it this way: you can stop them at the beginning, middle, or end of their journey.

Gossypol is one compound that works at the beginning. Despite obvious problems, some research on the method continues; Elsimar Coutinho, the Brazilian gynecologist who helped to invent Depo-Provera and start the menstrual suppression craze, has been one advocate of continued work in this field. Coutinho argues that later trials have not revealed the potassium reduction problems seen in earlier trials and theorizes that the original results might have been, at least in part, a by-product of the Chinese diet.[44] He also points out that regardless of this, many common drugs can cause potassium reduction. Coutinho thinks that Gossypol might provide a good, more easily reversible alternative to vasectomy for men who have already had the number of children they desire. While permanent infertility for many remains a serious problem with Gossypol, the chance of renewed potency may be higher than it is with vasectomy reversal. In China, scientists continue to tinker with Gossypol, combining lower doses with hormonal therapy that includes either estrogen or progestin.[45]

Chinese men participated in trials of another herbal extract, Tripterygium wilfordii, a chemical used to treat rheumatoid arthritis that had the unexpected effect of inducing infertility.[46] This compound has similar problems to Gossypol, namely, irreversible infertility and has been similarly disregarded by most of the scientific community.

Both botanicals target the sperm cells. Another approach works on other cells that allow the sperm to develop, such as Leydig or Sertoli cells that make testosterone and prevent the exposure of developing sperm to dangerous toxins. Some versions of this approach, at least as it is imagined now, might require testosterone supplementation and therefore do not truly constitute a nonhormonal method. Methods that try to disrupt the sperm while they are still in the testicle are complicated because it is very difficult to penetrate the blood-testes border, a membrane separating the fragile reproductive cells from the bloodstream.

Because of this, targeting sperm while they are maturing in the epididymis is a promising alternative. The idea with this approach is to "shake the tree"—to release sperm that are immature and therefore incapable of fertilization. Although a number of methods have been proposed, "pursuit of these . . . is still a number of years from clinical use."[47]

Finally, sperm can be prevented from fertilizing an egg by introducing chemicals that act on their ability to swim or penetrate the outer coating of the egg. One potentially innovative approach involves blocking unique calcium channels that exist only on the tails of sperm. Discovered only in the last decade, this possible method has shown promise in tests on mice.[48] This sort of therapy still lives in the realm of fantasy, but if realized, it would have the unique advantage of being administered in the form of a pill that either a woman or a man could take before sex to prevent pregnancy.[49] Some scientists believe that it might be possible for women to take it after sex, providing a nonhormonal morning-after pill.

Animal tests often prove promising, but human tests tend to have very different results. *N*-butyldeoxynojirimycin (*N*B-DNJ), a compound that is used to treat Gaucher's disease, a genetic disorder, showed promise in rendering mice reversibly infertile by forcing the production of inferior sperm.[50] However, later tests in humans showed no negative effect on sperm.[51]

Sperm vaccines provide a completely different sort of nonhormonal option. In this approach, the immune system works as a birth control method, responding to the shot by producing antisperm or antiegg proteins. Eppin is a protease inhibitor found on sperm that has become the subject of early efforts in this arena.[52] Tests in monkeys have proved promising, but great concerns exist about moving on to human trials. Vaccine contraceptives are controversial, and there are even greater safety concerns and unknowns than exist with other new methods. Scientists worry about how frequently injections would be required and, more troubling, the failure to restore fertility after discontinuation. A version targeting gonadotropins is in phase 1 trials for women;[53] for males, however, immunocontraception is still in very early testing stages and is being studied mostly for use in animals.

If all of this sounds like science fiction, that's because it essentially is at this point: nonhormonal methods are years behind hormone treatments[54] and may prove more difficult and expensive to advance down the scientific pipeline. Even if they work, they will probably bring new and unimagined safety problems. But this type of creative thinking about fertility control is what has been lacking in the past fifty years since the last truly innovative option, Pincus's pill, was first introduced to the public. Doctors dream of a drug that would encourage male use by offering benefits beyond contraception. Diana Blithe notes, "It would be nice if we could develop methods that also protect the prostate or prevent hair loss."[55] Perhaps changing the context of contraceptive research and development to male bodies will continue to encourage this sort of originality.

During the course of writing this book I attended a friend's birthday party on a warm June night, one of the few in an otherwise wet, dismal summer. When a new acquaintance heard I was researching birth control, her eyes lit up. "Did you hear?" she asked me, excitement building in her voice. "They finally made a male pill. I heard it on the news yesterday!" I didn't want to disappoint her, so I smiled and said, "Yeah—that's great."

I didn't tell her that if you Google "male birth control" or "pill for men" you will get results boasting a breathless story from a major media outlet that has been claiming this same breakthrough for years. Sensing my hesitation, my new friend pressed the point: "I mean, don't you think it will happen?"

"Yes," I said, and I do. It will probably happen when we are least expecting it, when we have stopped looking for stories about it. And when it does, men will have to face the same problems and live with the same caveats that women have struggled with for decades. They will have to decide if the health risks are too great and if they are willing to live with annoying side effects. There will undoubtedly be preventable tragedies and even deaths. Men will have to read between the lines of studies that try to hide risks, and perhaps they will have to argue with doctors who insist that the ailments they complain about are all in their heads. I don't wish these problems on the men in my life. But expanding birth control technologies creates more options for *all* of us and helps us to understand the responsibilities and dilemmas of pregnancy prevention in new ways.

Chapter Eleven

Going Green: The Environmental Burden of Contraception

It's not so much we've got the answers . . . it's that we've got some of the questions.
—Patricia Colsher, West Virginia Cancer Registry

Most people who live in cities don't like pigeons, but they are a fact of urban life, like paying too much money in rent and using public transportation. Still, as the city of St. Paul prepared to host the Republican National Convention in 2008, they wondered if perhaps there wasn't an easy way to limit the bird population. Maybe the prolific pigeons simply needed to be put on the Pill.[1] The summer before the convention, officials placed feeders around the city laced with OvoControl P, a drug that would cause the eggs of the unwanted winged city dwellers to develop incorrectly so that they would be unable to hatch.[2] The contragestational drug, made by a California company called Innolytics, LLC, had already been put into use in other cities including Hollywood, El Paso, and Denver. It was also considered by New York City when the birds invaded the newly renovated $124 million St. George terminal of the Staten Island Ferry. Councilman James S. Oddo was quick to dismiss health concerns, noting, "The reproductive rights of pigeons comes in a distant second to my constituents and their commute."[3]

While some did worry about the health of the birds, this sort of prevention seemed to be a step up from electric fences, spikes designed to impale the birds, and poisons. But the greater worry for many people was, of course, the environmental impact of putting a chemical with such dramatic effects on avian reproduction into general use. Drugs designed to curtail the fertility of wild animals—by preventing conception or disrupting gestation—have been used on geese and even larger animals like deer. It's possible that, as Innolytics claims, the drugs are harmless to humans and not dangerous to other birds and animals. But the great push in recent years to put pigeons on birth control highlights the larger problems of releasing pharmaceuticals and chemicals into the environment without sufficient data on their mechanisms and potential harms. Chemicals used to control wildlife are small potatoes next to the massive quantity of hormones used on farm animals. And, of course, there are the drugs we take on a daily basis, which also end up back in our water.

We are coming to understand the importance of considering the unintended consequences of dumping medicines into our natural environment and the impact of doing it on such a massive scale. We live in a world that is awash in pharmaceuticals. Even if civic engineers and farmers had never schemed to put animals on drugs, the ones taken by people every day would have already caused this problem. Our waterways are full of the residues of drugs that have been taken by patients and peed out or simply dumped unused into the toilet. Our factories use chemicals to process and make products that also find their way into our water. And our farms use them to fatten animals for slaughter.

What danger does this pharmaceutical soup pose to animals and humans? And what is the role of hormone products, such as oral contraceptives and hormone therapy pills, in causing it? As environmental concerns of every manner dominate national and international conversations, has the issue of making birth control green been overlooked?

Something Fishy in the Potomac: Intersex Bass and Prescription Drugs

Scientists around the Potomac River were noticing something strange: male smallmouth bass had started to act like females. Specifically, they were producing a protein that preceded egg development, and in some cases they were actually growing eggs. Vicki S. Blazer, a scientist who works at a fish laboratory in West Virginia, was one of the first to notice the phenomenon in 2003.[4] By 2004 the problem had spread downstream 170 miles to Maryland, very close to the nation's capital.

There had been disturbing evidence of this kind of problem before: in the 1980s and 1990s, scientists observed problems in the reproductive organs of birds in the Great Lakes region and in alligators in the Florida Everglades. Female songbirds in California began singing songs usually reserved for males.[5] In 1995, Arizona scientists observed sexual changes in fish downstream from Las Vegas.⁶ Such problems are caused by chemicals called endocrine disruptors, which, like birth control pills, work by blocking or interfering with a body's hormones in ways that change sexual functioning.

How do chemicals and pharmaceutical agents make their way into the water system? When it comes to prescription drugs, they are usually flushed down the toilet, either in urine or as a way of disposing of unused medicines. A powerful chemical like a synthetic hormone isn't completely broken down by the body and survives in human waste. On the way to sewage treatment plants, the drugs are further dismantled by bacteria and further still by treatment at facilities. Still, some survive and flow into lakes and rivers. Journalist Dawn Fallik explains it this way: "People drink and flush and wash, and the water has to go somewhere—and mostly it goes into the sewer system, into the wastewater treatment plant, and then into a river or stream. Drinking water plants take up water from the rivers and streams, treat it, and send it into the taps."⁷

Part of the problem with figuring out which drugs have been causing occurrences of intersex fish around the world has been that there are so many different chemical contenders. Tests conducted on the St. Lawrence River found a pharmacopeia, including trace amounts of ibuprofen, antibiotics, epilepsy drugs, Alzheimer's drugs, and even caffeine.⁸ While clearly hormonal mechanisms are at work in the fish, what isn't clear is whether industrial or farming chemicals or everyday human pill and product use are responsible. When asked what causes intersex fish, Vicki S. Blazer says, "I feel comfortable saying human activity . . . The question is, which human activity? And is it something we can do anything about?"⁹

When looking at the chemical soups that are US and international waterways, hormones stand out as a particular problem, despite the fact that it is often a matter of pulling apart a consommé, not a chowder. The US Geological Survey noted in the first comprehensive study of chemical contaminants in American waters in 2002 that fish and aquatic wildlife were particularly at risk for health problems in water that showed traces of hormones and hormonelike compounds.¹⁰ For this reason scientists tend to see illnesses or physical changes in fish, frogs, or other animals that live in waterways as warning signs of a bigger problem.

There are three major categories of environmental hormones. The first is synthetic, and it exists because people and farm animals on such drugs either excrete or dump the chemicals into the sewage and water systems. In addition to the many chemicals humans rely on, there are those used to produce our food. Professor and food writer Michael Pollan has chronicled the overuse of agricultural hormones from firsthand experience. Visiting a massive factory farm in 2002, Pollan watched as cows were "funneled into a chute, herded along by a ranch hand wielding an electric prod, then clutched in a restrainer just long enough for another hand to inject a slow-release pellet of Revlar, a synthetic estrogen, in the back of the ear."[11] Pollan noted that approximately two thirds of the 36 million beef cattle raised in the United States receive hormones. The reason, of course, is to get the animals' weight up: humans aren't the only animals who can respond to outside hormones by packing on pounds. Pollan notes that drugs like Revlar can get "a beef calf from 80 to 1,200 pounds in 14 months."[12] Of course, in addition to the hormones entering the ground through the urine of livestock, people who eat meat are often consuming small amounts of the chemicals when they eat beef, pork, or poultry that have been treated with the compounds.

The second category of environmental hormones is natural estrogens—called phytoestrogens—that enter the environment through plants and foods that act like estrogens on the body. Soy, for example, is a popular phytoestrogen. The chemicals in this plant act on estrogen receptors in the body and cause some of the same changes that a pharmaceutical estrogen would.

The third major type comes from industry. It involves compounds and products that release chemicals that act like estrogens. Certain plastics, for example, have fallen under scrutiny in recent years for causing this sort of unintentional pollution. Industrial chemicals such as Bisphenol A—a chemical added to plastic to make it harder, which has recently gotten attention for its presence in some baby bottles, and phthalates—additives used to make plastic flexible and keep chemicals like perfume from evaporating—have been studied for their dangers to humans who come in contact with them. Shanna Swan, director of the Center for Reproductive Epidemiology at the University of Rochester, notes that one study found that children of mothers whose bodies showed high levels of phthalates were more likely to be "undermasculinized."[13]

Pharmaceutical estrogens are one of the most widespread contaminants. A study out of Villanova University tested twenty-one streams in one Pennsylvania county and found that all contained synthetic hormones.[14] Ten of those streams contained ethinyl estradiol (the compound used in most birth control pills) in quantities thirty times greater than those shown to damage fish. Despite this sort of evidence, the sheer volume of different chemicals makes it difficult to assess both which compounds are causing the worst damage and where they're coming from. Christian Daughton, head of the EPA's National Exposure Research Library explains, "No organism is exposed to one toxicant at a time. What's happening here involves multiple chemicals at a time, and naturally occurring toxic chemicals as well."[15] Science works best when it can isolate one variable and test it. This often becomes difficult in real-world contexts and requires scientists to think creatively when designing studies.

In one innovative experiment, a team of Canadian scientists set out to test whether synthetic estrogens could cause male fish to show female characteristics. A team led by Professor Karen Kidd of the University of New Brunswick has spent years observing what happens when chemicals like those in oral contraceptives are released into the environment. Because most waterways are already polluted by different kinds of drugs, Kidd and her colleagues chose a small, isolated lake in northwestern Ontario. The area is so remote and the bodies of water so numerous that the lakes have never been given names. Instead, the target pond, chosen for its purity, is known only by the number 260. Because it is tiny and far away from other bodies of water, 260 was as close as the scientists could come to finding a pristine body of water suited for experimentation; it allowed them to feel with some certainty that if fish started showing female characteristics, it was because of the specific chemicals they were putting into it.[16] The study, called "the most controlled experiment ever to look at the effects of estrogen on ecosystems,"[17] cost a million dollars, provided mostly by the Canadian government but also by funds from the Environmental Protection Agency (EPA). Over the course of seven years, Kidd and her colleagues added synthetic estrogen to the lake at levels lower than or equal to the concentration of the chemicals in many waterways. The experiment used the amount of hormone that would result from six thousand women taking the Pill.[18]

What they found was that within the first year, male minnows had problems developing sex organs and female fish grew eggs too slowly.[19] Minnow populations started to decline dramatically, and in later years the population failed to recover even after Kidd and her team stopped putting hormones in the lake. This fact contradicts those who argue that the variability of estrogen content—and the fact that it can be cleared out of water with haste—means that contamination isn't dangerous. While the minnow population was affected right away because of its short lifecycle, scientists theorize that fish with longer life spans, such as trout, would experience similar problems with more prolonged exposure. In areas where hormone concentrations are sustained, multigenerational exposure may enhance this problem.

It should come as no surprise that synthetic hormones prove particularly impervious to breakdown. When the creators of various hormone compounds were first creating these pharmaceutical wonders, they worked hard to make sure that the chemicals would not be easily destructible. They were designed to be strong, to express gastric durability and withstand the harsh digestive fluids in the stomach.

The Grain of Sand in the Swimming Pool

The levels of all pollutants are said to be small, "trace" amounts of chemicals that could be dangerous in larger quantities but likely have little impact in their diluted states. According to the US Geological Survey and others, this means that most are found in amounts that are less than one part per billion or even trillion, equivalent to a grain of sand in an Olympic-sized swimming pool.[20] But all these little bits of pollution may add up to a larger health hazard for animals: "When all the substances in some streams were tallied, levels were similar to those that in other studies appeared to harm fish and other aquatic life."[21] Herbert T. Buxton, a member of the Survey's toxic substances hydrology program who helped conduct the 2002 study of American waterways, says he hopes research like theirs will "help people understand that the chemicals they use and consume on a daily basis and their behavior can affect our environment and water resources."[22] In this study, 80 percent of sampled waters contained between one and ninety-five of the chemicals scientists were screening for and included not just drugs, but industrial chemicals and detergents, which have been shown to have hormonelike effects as they break down. Michael Thurman of the University of Colorado cautions that even small amounts may yet prove dangerous: "Low concentrations of parts-per-billion or parts-per-trillion generally aren't considered dangerous over the short term, but no one knows about the long-term human and ecological effects."[23]

Some scientists even argue that pollution hasn't gotten worse—it's that we've gotten better at detecting it. They say that the reason we are becoming aware of contaminants is because our ability to test for them has improved. This may be true; just because we lacked the ability to test for chemicals in previous decades doesn't mean they weren't harmful. And while many tests don't reveal a violation of any antipollution or clean water laws, that may be because many potentially harmful substances are not currently subject to regulation.

The blame for this lies in part with the Environmental Protection Agency, which was required by Congress in a 1996 law to begin screening for endocrine disruptors. Close to fifteen years later, little progress has been made. As Barbara Seaman explained in 2003, the EPA and the National Institutes of health "spent several years and several million dollars investigating natural and synthetic chemicals that mimic hormones. Shockingly, both these massive multimillion-dollar studies ignored the proverbial elephant in the room: the pharmaceutical and veterinary estrogens and other hormones that humans and animals have been eating and depositing into the environment for years—hormones that have been proven to be linked to hormone-dependent breast, uterine, ovarian, and testicular cancers."[24] Instead, the EPA spent time giving reasons why more progress had not been made. As Christian Daughton puts it, "The United States is a late bloomer on the issue of these emerging organic wastewater contaminants, particularly pharmaceuticals."[25]

Astoundingly, even as more was being demanded of the EPA in the nineties, less was being asked of drugmakers. In 1997, the Food and Drug Administration slashed the number of drugs required to demonstrate environmental safety.[26] This happened in part because the FDA reviewed hundreds of environmental assessments and found no problems. Of course chemicals like hormones, because they occur in some form naturally in the body, were left out of this review.[27] But by 2005 the FDA was reconsidering this stance, noting that the potential health hazards of various chemicals remain unknown.[28] It is past time to reconsider old ways of thinking that deem synthetic hormones "natural."

While regulatory agencies struggle to catch up, some towns are taking steps to clean up their acts, creating drug collection programs where citizens turn in unused pills rather than flush them.[29] Because many prescriptions are controlled substances, they must be turned in to the police or other law enforcement professionals. In one pilot program in Maine, the police watched in amazement as fifty-two people turned in fifty-five thousand pills.[30]

Not surprisingly, the Vatican has been vocal in promoting the association of oral contraceptives and pollution. Seizing on global interest in the environment, the Vatican newspaper *L'Osservatore Romano* reported in early 2009 that the Pill "has had devastating effects on the environment for some years by releasing tons of hormones into nature."[31] Accusing the drug of causing male infertility in the West, the Vatican in dramatic tones called for people to give up pharmaceutical contraception. It is only fair to point out that church leaders failed to voice active concern for the multitude of other drugs found in waterways whose effects are unknown; there was no cry to give up Advil, for example, or antidepressants, or to stop washing or using sunblock. It is a mistake to isolate the Pill and blame women for using birth control rather than examining the very serious and complicated issues of pharmaceutical pollution facing our society.

Drugmakers, while denying that their products are pollutants, have cautiously offered financial support for efforts to determine the nature of the risks that exist and develop methods to contain them. While this can be viewed as hypocritical, it is also important that scientists working to make pharmaceuticals more environmentally friendly have the support of funders with deep pockets.

Taking the First Step: The Long Journey to Understanding Environmental Carcinogens

It is clear that all of these hormones and hormonelike chemicals are caus-ing problems for wildlife, but the effect on humans remains unknown. As the *Washington Post* notes, "For now, no connections to human ail-ments have been proved. But some studies have provided hints that people might be affected by crossed hormones, and activists wonder if this kind of pollution could contribute to diabetes, birth defects, and infertil-ity."[32] Many activists are concerned that, especially in areas of high population concentration, women are, in essence, taking the Pill simply by drinking water.[33] As scientists contemplate the quadrupling of infertil-ity rates since the 1960s, such possibilities seem particularly poignant and worthy of exploration.

One person who is trying to navigate the murky waters of the phar-maceutical and chemical contamination of our world is Devra Davis. Davis was the founding director of the world's first center for environ-mental oncology at the University of Pittsburgh and she now heads the Environmental Health Trust, a nonprofit dedicated to conducting research on preventable environmental causes of cancer. I first met Davis in 2007 while she was promoting her groundbreaking and terrifying book *The Secret History of the War on Cancer*. In the book, Davis argues that cancer research in the United States has been tragically slowed by an approach that overemphasizes treating the disease while not working hard enough to prevent it. In chronicling the history of this ongoing "war," Davis argues compellingly that when it comes to cancer and our envi-ronment, we know less than we should: powerful political and industrial players have worked to ensure that scientific challenges are not the only barriers to our knowledge.

Davis explains that a radical reexamination of what causes cancer is necessary to begin making real progress in research on prevention. We know that estrogen can cause cancer, so whether small exposures, such as those to trace amounts in water supplies, can cause the dreaded disease is a subject worthy of further scientific research, especially given the dra-matic rise in reproductive cancers in recent decades that point to hormonal culprits. She notes that until something can be shown beyond the shadow of a doubt to cause certain cancers, the companies that make potentially dangerous products will continue to deny that they cause problems, brandishing doubt "like a cross in front of a vampire."[34] It is very difficult to collect the sort of data that can stand up against these protests for a number of reasons, the biggest of which is the difficulty of studying chemicals and their dangers individually.

Davis stresses the importance of looking at all the pollutants and potential carcinogens together in real-world contexts; we encounter multiple chemicals every day, and they can impact or compound each other. Cumulative exposures are part of reality. And she insists we can't wait for perfect evidence before taking action: "Requiring proof of sick or dead people before acting to prevent harm is a fundamentally wrong approach to public health."[35]

This can seem like an overwhelming dilemma. We have a host of potential pollutants, limited science, and companies with vested interests in concealing known dangers and inhibiting the discovery of new ones. Davis recommends taking a cue from an old Chinese proverb: "A long journey begins with the first step." For consumers, this can mean making sensible changes when you suspect a certain chemical or product of harboring dangers. Making these changes is not about overreacting or becoming paranoid that every drug or chemical will kill you; it is about making smart decisions based on the best information we have. It's about not waiting so long for proof that you become it.

Going Green: What Can We Do?

Synthetic hormones are an important piece of the larger problem of chemical omnipresence. For women who care strongly about this issue or for those who don't like hormonal contraception, the environmental burden of the Pill is a great reason to try another method.

For those who choose to stay on the Pill, an important step toward going green will need to be technological: our current sewage treatment systems aren't designed to screen out hormones and so are relatively ineffective at doing so. Some water treatment plants are responding to the demands of a chemical-infused world. Others balk at the high cost of testing water for such contaminants—around $1,000 per sample—and note that until the EPA requires such screening, it simply doesn't make sense.[36]

But the cost of doing nothing may prove higher still. Joel A. Tickner of the University of Massachusetts points to cautionary tales: in cases of health hazards like asbestos and lead, America waited too long to take action.[37] The reason, of course, was that it can take many years and much experimentation to prove conclusively that a certain pollutant causes, or even exacerbates, a deadly health problem. By the time this happens, both the financial cost of undoing the damage and the social cost of unnecessary suffering and death are inevitable.

Lest you suppose that you can avoid this problem by simply drinking packaged water, think again. One German study found that the majority of tested bottled water contained estrogen, probably from chemicals in the plastic container.[38] And again, while contaminated water is a major problem, it is only one of many hormonal exposures. Day-to-day interaction with cleaners, beauty products, foods, supplements, pesticides, plastics, and other products that act as estrogen on our bodies compound the potential danger. Birth control pills and hormone replacement drugs are part of an environmental problem that affects us all, and even if giving them up isn't the answer, having conversations about their impact is an important way to start finding the right questions.

Scientists at Sweden's Goteborg University are worried that newer hormonal contraceptives—namely the contraceptive patch and the vaginal ring—may be even bigger polluters than the Pill if not disposed of properly. When a woman throws away her monthly patches, each one still contains around 600 µg of ethinyl estradiol.[39] If that patch is then flushed down the toilet, it continues to release hormones into the environment at rates higher than they occur in urine as by-products or in discarded pills. While most women don't flush their old patches, scientist Joakim Larsson figures that even a few could cause big problems for fish and pollute water supplies: "Just a single patch flushed every 3 days into the catchments of a Swedish sewage plant serving 3,500 people would release enough hormone to impair fish downstream."[40]

The vaginal ring may be even worse: NuvaRing has around 2.4 milligrams of estrogen by the time it is thrown away, 33 percent more than three discarded patches and six times more than a full cycle of oral contraceptives.[41] Even though package instructions advise women not to flush the rings down the toilet, sometimes it happens anyway, either because the instructions are ignored or because the device is accidentally expelled because of muscle straining (for example, during a bowel movement). While women should, of course, avoid throwing either rings or patches into the sewage system, other solutions need to be developed. One might be encouraging device makers to distribute disposal bags or creating collection programs through pharmacies where used devices could be returned for more environmentally friendly discarding.

Many women are choosing to go green in the bedroom, eschewing hormones and opting for less polluting birth control options like an IUD or a barrier. But barriers, too, have an environmental impact. Because condoms are the only effective method besides abstinence in preventing sexually transmitted infections, giving them up is not a good option for anyone at risk of these problems. Environmental organizations including the EPA are concerned about improper condom disposal. The Ocean Conservancy, a nonprofit group based in Washington, DC, estimates that 30,252 condoms are picked up on beaches each year, and the devices are among the many pollutants making up the growing amount of sea trash disrupting coral reefs and ocean ecosystems.

Most condoms are made of latex. Because this is a natural product, they will (in theory) biodegrade with time. But since a condom isn't entirely made of latex (there are other chemicals and material components involved), it does not happen very quickly. Polyurethane condoms, an important alternative for people with latex allergies, won't break down because this material is a type of plastic. Female condoms are also made of polyurethane or equally unbiodegradable synthetic rubber. Lambskin condoms, literally made from animal skin, are completely biodegradable, but they don't offer protection against sexually transmitted infections (however, if you are in a fluid-bonded relationship, this can be an option for you).

There is currently no way to recycle condoms. The paper box that the prophylactics are packaged in can be put in the recycling bin, but the foil or plastic wrappers and the condoms themselves cannot be. Health educators at Columbia University note that because of this, the best thing to do is to wrap condoms in a biodegradable material—like tissues or a paper bag—and throw them into the trash can[42] (wrapping them in plastic and other indestructible materials can prevent the already slow breakdown of the latex). The worst thing to do is to flush them down the toilet: this can clog your plumbing, and even rubber-based latex won't biodegrade if it is underwater.

Some environmentalists argue that the environmental burden created by contraceptives, including estrogens and condoms, is offset by the prevention of many births. They insist that nothing creates more pollution than the birth of new people. A 2009 *Washington Post* article chronicles this movement, noting, "Every new life . . . is a guarantee of new greenhouse gasses,"[43] adding that "birth control could be one of the world's best tools for fighting climate change." A report published in 2009 out of Oregon State University estimates that one baby born in the United States will create 1,644 tons of carbon dioxide in his or her life, five times that of a child born in China and ninety-one times the amount of a baby born in Bangladesh.[44] This sort of thinking—get rid of polluters rather than pollution—is obviously problematic. The suggestion of incentive programs to encourage family limitation smacks of older government efforts in the service of eugenics and social engineering. Research from the London School of Economics suggests that if governments offered free contraception, they could more effectively reduce carbon dioxide than by using alternative energy like solar and wind power. While making contraception accessible and affordable is, in itself, an admirable project, trying to limit or encourage births on the population level should not be the work of government. History tells us that these efforts generally create more problems than they solve. Instead, empowering and educating individuals to make informed choices and offering them the resources to do so is a more ethical course for leaders with respect to the reproductive lives of their citizens.

Luckily, leaders of most environmental groups don't endorse this sort of thinking. The Sierra Club's David Hamilton says, "I don't want to rain on anybody's parade, but the primary solutions to climate change have to deal with what we do with the people who are here,"[45] noting that encouraging renewable energy and reducing greenhouse gases should be chief among these efforts.

So what can a woman do if she wants to be green and also avoid pregnancy? Considering a reusable barrier, like a diaphragm or a cervical cap, might be a start. While a condom must be thrown out after each use, a diaphragm is good for one to two years. This means saving money as well as preventing pollution and pregnancy. And for the committed environmentalist, particularly if she is in a committed relationship, the fertility awareness method offers the ultimate green birth control. This method requires education and dedication, but has no chemical or material waste. Many FAM educators emphasize that the method seeks to bring practitioners in synch with the rhythms of the natural world around them and with their own bodies.

We have much to learn about the environmental impact of our contraceptive choices, but including birth control chemicals and devices in our conversations about creating a greener world is a start. The effects of our choices on the natural world is a subject that touches on many intimate parts of our daily lives: how we get from place to place, what we eat, how we use the basic resources in our lives like water and heat. It should come as no surprise, then, that the massive project of environmental responsibility has moved into the bedroom.

Chapter Twelve

Around the World in Twenty-eight Days: International Issues in Reproductive and Contraceptive Health

Americans are used to thinking of birth control and abortion as thoroughly domestic issues, but reproductive politics have been global from the start.
—Michelle Goldberg

The ground didn't actually shake under John D. Rockefeller III as he spoke to a crowd of several hundred onlookers on a hot day in Bucharest, Romania, in 1974, but it might as well have. The occasion was a talk he gave at the United Nations' first international conference on population. Rockefeller, a longtime supporter of population control initiatives, had been influential in establishing decades of American policy dealing with global fertility. During the height of Cold War hysteria about burgeoning third-world births, the grandson of the legendary industrialist had helped create the Population Council, a massive organization that remains active around the globe to the present day. Once a stalwart believer in plans to curb births in the developing world at all costs, Rockefeller announced to an astonished crowd that he had "changed his mind."[1]

It wasn't that he felt any less passionate about achieving this outcome; as one commentator would later summarize, he would come to feel that "people's socioeconomic status, especially women's, must improve before they will want to limit their families."[2] Instead of creating massive programs that sought to provide birth control to faceless masses by any means, Rockefeller had come to believe that a better method lay in empowering women. "In my opinion," he explained, "if we are to make genuine progress in economic and social development, if we are to make progress in achieving population goals, women increasingly must have greater freedom of choice in determining their roles in society."[3]

The speech, besides enraging the more traditionally minded sects of the population movement, signaled the start of a new chapter in the story of American involvement in global reproductive politics. While the thirty years that followed the Bucharest conference would prove as tumultuous as those that preceded it, they charted a different course, one that was increasingly set by women. The government of the United States played a part in both leading and derailing global efforts to help women control their fertility and their lives. As the United States alternated between Republican and Democratic administrations, funding for women's health became a ball in an increasingly raucous match of political tennis. Domestic politics were negotiated in an international arena, and women (often poor and with limited access to health care) were the losers.

When American feminists look at issues of reproduction and contraception, they tend to be preoccupied with domestic problems; abortion rights, insurance coverage for birth control, and the availability of new contraceptive methods often dominate discussions. While a comprehensive look at the particularities of international contraceptive access is beyond the scale of this chapter, it is important to understand the ways in which our social and political battles at home have impacted women abroad in complex and often dangerous ways.

The Most Dangerous Bomb: The Cold War and Population Fears

For the men who brought the population control movement to the forefront of American life, uncontrolled population growth was a threat far more tangible than the atom bomb or the other bogeymen of the anti-Communist United States in the 1950s. Eugenics, the pseudoscientific movement that had dominated early the twentieth-century contraceptive conversation, melted away, tainted by the revelations of Nazi atrocities and the Holocaust. But the ideas of Thomas Malthus, the eighteenth-century thinker on whose work many eugenic ideas were based, still carried currency. Malthus argued, among other things, that growing populations would eventually lead to a world without enough food to sustain its swelling throngs. After World War II it became apparent that fertility in the developed world had slowed, and that the developing world was for the first time showing higher rates of population growth. The social and political figures tracking this change saw it as a cause for alarm. Certainly, part of their concern was attributable to simple racism and nationalism. The burgeoning population in Asia, Africa, and Latin America posed a potential threat to both white and American power. Many believed that if these growing groups ran out of resources, they would turn to Communism as a possible solution to their problems. On the other hand, some population control advocates were driven by humanitarian concerns. They believed that growing numbers would lead to starvation, suffering, and violence. The answer, thought men like Rockefeller, Dixie cup creator Hugh Moore, and others, was to provide poor countries with the means to limit fertility. Perhaps, they reasoned, waging a battle from within resource-strapped nations would prevent the need for one from without.

All these ideas were in the air when veteran journalist Arthur Krock published an October 1959 newspaper column called "The Most Dangerous Bomb of All,"[4] in which he summarized the impending peril for the general public. Concern about population control went mainstream. The idea of exporting contraceptives was radical at a time when birth control was still illegal in certain parts of the United States, and politicians avoided the issue, afraid of alienating powerful Catholic supporters. President Eisenhower, bowing to Catholic pressure and a general distaste for confronting sexual subject matter, insisted at a December 1959 press conference that the United States government was not, and would not be, in the birth control business.[5] By 1963 the former president had come to regret this stance, and as domestic politics shifted under the weight of the approval and popularity of the birth control pill and the official legalization of contraception, exporting modern family planning methods seemed increasingly possible. By 1965, President Johnson officially announced the intention of the United States to "use our knowledge to help deal with the explosion in the world's population and the growing scarcity in world resources" in his State of the Union address.

Early efforts were at best simplistic and at worst coercive. Journalist Michelle Goldberg explains that "in one shameful instance" Johnson used "food aid as leverage to pressure India to adopt both agricultural reforms and family planning."[6] Richard Nixon continued and expanded on Johnson's work, buying the classic population control arguments lock, stock, and barrel. In the same year that Nixon was elected, a scientist named Paul Ehrlich published a best-selling book called *The Population Bomb* that assured the public in grim and fatalistic tones that "in the 1970s, the world will undergo famines; hundreds of millions of people are going to starve to death."[7] During these years, many organizations continued or initiated programs to help spread the contraceptive gospel, including the Population Council, Planned Parenthood, the Ford Foundation, the United Nations Population Fund (UNFPA), and the US Agency for International Development (USAID). Ironically, in later decades conservative presidential administrations would work to inhibit the work of groups that earlier Americans had fought so hard to create.

During the early decades of population control, many people got involved out of an earnest desire to help people in distant lands. There was tremendous contraceptive creativity in these early years. For example USAID workers, concerned that plain, dry condoms would prove distasteful to users, switched to colorful lubricated models. In another innovation, seven iron tablets (the equivalent of the seven sugar pills in most birth control packs) were added to the twenty-one-pill regimen to streamline the transition between months for female patients who didn't have calendars. An added bonus, of course, was that the iron supplements helped treat anemia.[8] Thousands of people began to receive reproductive technologies as a result of these early efforts.

The biggest problem was that the (mostly male) members of the population control movement were only concerned with big picture issues. They worried about women in the abstract, not understanding the realities and specificities of individual lives, cultures, and families. They were concerned with outcomes and numbers, not with helping women change their lives for the better. By the mid 1970s, as birth control was moving from mainstream acceptance to outright respectability, a group of women was beginning to change the course of the movement from the inside. In her important chronicle of the history of modern reproductive justice struggles, *The Means of Reproduction*, Michelle Goldberg documents how, energized by the growth of second-wave feminism, these women began to ask questions that sought to reprioritize the international birth control business.

The Road to Cairo: Feminism and the Transformation of International Family Planning

It wasn't easy to be a woman in the population movement during those early decades. Adrienne Germain, a young graduate student who had moved to New York from California to be with her husband, applied to the Ford Foundation for a job doing research. She was well qualified for such a position, having been active in the Zero Population Growth movement during her years at Berkeley. Ford turned her down, noting that because she was married, she would most likely leave in a short space of time to have children. Two years later, after Germain had logged some important time with the Population Council, Ford reconsidered and offered her a job.

At the same time, an expatriate Englishwoman named Joan Dunlop endured five months of interviews to get a job working for John D. Rockefeller III. Rockefeller's wife told Dunlop that she was delighted: "I'm very glad to see you here," the older woman said. "I've wanted him to have a woman on his staff for many, many years, for a long time. But I want to say to you that you must tell him the truth. He's not being told the truth."[9]

The truths that women like Germain and Dunlop were being called on to tell were hard for many of the movement's veterans to hear. First, international family planning groups had some serious image problems. Led nearly exclusively by Americans and Europeans, population control organizations were suspected in many parts of the world of being players in a larger colonial plan to prevent poorer nations from gaining power. In many cases, this was a difficult claim to dispute. Second, the sometimes well-meaning intentions of many in the movement were confounded by misplaced priorities. When it came to helping female patients, programs focused almost entirely on preventing births, ignoring other crucial aspects of women's health. Particularly in populations where such clinics constituted the only available health care for many women, the fact that they would provide contraception, but not help with infertility, sexually transmitted infections, children's health, and other serious problems seemed evidence of a lack of care for women's total well-being and of an obsessive interest in controlling and limiting fertility at all costs. And offering contraceptives with dubious health profiles, such as high-dose oral contraceptives and older IUDs, seemed like proof of disrespect for female lives.

What separated women like Germain and Dunlop from others in the population movement was their belief that the best way to achieve the goal of family limitation was through empowering women. They understood that instead of trying to force contraceptives down the throats of sometimes unwilling, often bewildered women, organizations should be working to provide women with options that extended beyond the home and childbed. If women were given greater knowledge of their bodies, better health care, and greater financial control over their lives, they would willingly *choose* to have smaller families. According to this way of seeing, overpopulation is evidence of women's oppression, a sign that their rights are being undervalued. This combated the common perspective that overpopulation was a crisis of such proportions that the rights of individuals didn't matter. As she set out to change people's minds, Germain reckoned that there was a lot of work to be done in a field that frequently referred to women as "contraceptive acceptors" instead of people and that was headed by cavalier and often sexist leaders (one, Reimert Ravenholt of USAID, enraged an audience of feminists at a conference on abortion by suggesting that the proper anesthetic for a first trimester abortion was two martinis "because that's the way she got pregnant in the first place"[10]).

In some ways, these women were gaming the system. While certainly concerned about population growth, Adrienne Germain had also realized early in her graduate work that the only health care monies reaching poor women were coming through population control channels. After six months in Peru, where Germain saw women beaten, raped by husbands, and subjected to botched abortions, she became convinced that getting resources to such women was necessary by any means. The only large-scale infrastructure for doing so at that time was family planning groups.

Shifting the focus from demographics to women's rights and reproductive justice was an uphill battle, but Dunlop, Germain, and women like them had powerful friends. Foremost among them was John D. Rockefeller III, who laid out the new family planning agenda in his 1974 speech in Bucharest. At the same conference, activists from developing nations protested population programs arguing that "development was the best contraceptive" and pointing out that "simply encouraging the use of birth control without taking any additional efforts to address problems with development was not a sufficient solution to the overpopulation problem."[11] The *New England Journal of Medicine* explains, "Western nations advocated the implementation of programs aimed at controlling the high rates of population growth then prevalent in resource-poor countries in Africa, Asia and Latin America. Most leaders from these countries, however, saw this as an inappropriate, imperialist goal . . . when the real problems were related to poverty."[12] Such critiques were similar to the feminist ones in that they spoke to a need to make international health care programs dynamic and to understand the problem of overpopulation as the product of complicated factors deserving of similarly sophisticated solutions. They were different in that they pointed away from women: If the real problem was development, then why throw money at female health? Wouldn't it be better spent in economic initiatives? Such arguments appealed to conservative forces in the United States who were becoming increasingly wary of throwing government dollars into sexual health programs, particularly those that had any connection with abortion rights. Within a decade, many leaders in developing nations would change their minds, coming to the conclusion that indeed, high population growth was hindering economic progress, but by that time, representatives of the Reagan administration were using development arguments to try to defund and derail global women's health programs.[13]

In 1981, Adrienne Germain put her precepts into practice, moving to Bangladesh to head the Ford Foundation's office there. In addition to broadening health care funding away from the contraceptives-only model, she also worked to secure a huge grant for the Grameen Bank, a financial institution founded in part to increase the number of women participating in the financial system. Started at a time when women made up less than 1 percent of bank creditors, the Grameen Bank worked to extend resources to female clients. Muhammad Yunus, the Bangladeshi economist and Nobel Peace Prize–winner who created the bank, explains, "Once they have increased their incomes through self-employment, Grameen borrowers show remarkable determination to have fewer children, educate the ones they have, and participate actively in our democracy."[14]

Even as women were transforming "population control" into "reproductive rights," controversy over abortion began to threaten their tenuous gains. For centuries, the distinction between contraception and abortion was semantic. Most women saw them as part of a common process, an effort to prevent a birth from happening. In the United States, the federal legalization of both birth control and pregnancy termination happened within ten years, although both had been gradually decriminalized[15] and eventually legalized in many states before becoming a part of national law. In 1965 *Griswold v. Connecticut* made contraception legal everywhere in the United States. In 1973 *Roe v. Wade* did the same thing for abortion. The relationship between the population control movement and the legalization of abortion in America is interactive: the effective activism of organizations such as Zero Population Growth convinced President Nixon to sign a program of contraceptive funding that included abortion with birth control as a population limitation strategy into law. Although Republican politicians and other conservatives would come to be associated with the anti-choice movement, in the 1970s there was nothing inconsistent in the president's support of certain varieties of pregnancy termination. Historian Rickie Solinger explains that at that time, many "Republicans quite fervently supported legal abortion on a variety of grounds, from population control to women's rights." She adds, "Unquestionably, the population controllers helped cultivate the ground for *Roe v. Wade*."[16]

After *Roe*, everything changed. Solinger notes, "As long as abortion was illegal, Americans did not protest against the vast number of abortion procedures carried out in the United States each year."[17] Although the estimated number of terminations performed in the United States each year remained consistent before and after legalization, the case marked a momentous change in the political significance of ending a pregnancy in America. Coming as it did amid the political and social upheaval of the 1960s and 1970s, abortion rights became a tangible symbol of women's shifting social power. For those who were mourning the loss of a more traditional way of life or who were scared and uncomfortable with the many fundamental social changes in the second half of the twentieth century, abortion was a concise symbol of multiple grievances. For the first time, women in America had the legal right to reject motherhood—the social role that had historically defined them. For people who wanted to go back to the "way things were," this was an ideal place to begin.

Politicians who were comfortable with a nameless, faceless woman in a third-world country terminating a pregnancy in the name of saving public dollars were much less at home with the process when it involved affluent American women claiming the right to undergo the procedure.

By the time that Ronald Reagan was elected, in part due to the fierce support of anti-choice forces in the religious right, growing domestic controversy over both abortion and feminism was about to go global. Reagan wanted to appease abortion foes, but also to stop spending massive amounts of money on women's reproductive health abroad. In addition to hostility toward abortion, the new administration targeted contraceptive funding. In a nod to powerful Catholic groups, in 1984 the government gave a million-dollar grant to the Family of the Americas Foundation (FAF), a group promoting natural family planning. FAF used the money to promote the Billings method (which monitors changes in cervical fluids to prevent pregnancy) internationally. In the same year, another United Nations conference on population took place, this time in Mexico City. Held just days before the Republican National Convention, the conference provided the Reagan administration with the perfect theater for introducing its new anti-abortion strategies and proving its credibility on the issue.

The global gag rule was certainly one of the most enduring policies from this agenda. In a reversal of former strategies, it was announced that the United States would cease to offer USAID monies to any organization that promoted or offered abortions alongside other family planning strategies. This meant that organizations couldn't council patients about pregnancy termination and couldn't perform the procedure even if they were relying on separate funds to do so. So an organization like Planned Parenthood, which was receiving one fourth of its monies ($11 million each year) from USAID, suddenly lost a significant part of its budget.[18] The policy is, to this day, a piece of political table tennis. When Bill Clinton came to office in 1993, he reversed the policy, and George W. Bush reinstated it in 2001.[19] Both presidents issued the change on the anniversary of *Roe v. Wade*.[20]

The other important precedent set at the Mexico City conference was the threat to withdraw or freeze American contributions to UNFPA if it was found to be bankrolling abortion or coercive reproductive policies.

Two years later, claiming that the organization was supporting coercive Chinese abortion policies, the administration made good on their promise and blocked promised monies. Like the gag rule, the UNFPA freeze was undone by Clinton and reaffirmed by George W. Bush.[21] The UNFPA had, unfortunately, made itself an easy target. Michelle Goldberg explains that while the organization didn't agree with China's one-child policy, it had provided computers for tallying birth statistics. They also gave the architect of the policy, Qian Xinzhong, its first population award. Qian shared the honor with Indira Gandhi, the Indian prime minister who had initiated a campaign of forced sterilization during a time of martial law in the mid-1970s. These choices—both the cowardly (failing to stand up for Chinese women) and the stupid (prioritizing population issues over human rights)—provided the pretext for stripping UNFPA of tens of millions of dollars in American contributions each year.

The various batterings and bruisings that the population movement underwent in the 1980s created enough instability to allow women like Adrienne Germain and Joan Dunlop to finally wrestle control. When Bill Clinton came to the White House in 1993, the stage was set for another important period of international family planning, this time led by women.

The Unfinished Agenda: Cairo and Beijing

If 1974 marked the beginning of the transformation from population control to reproductive rights, 1994 announced the completion of this change and a new ambitious agenda for the revamped movement. While Rockefeller's 1974 speech sent shock waves through the domestic community, the effect of the UN International Conference on Population and Development in Cairo was felt around the world. The most important result was the official acknowledgment by 179 countries that reproductive rights are human rights. As Adrienne Germain and Jennifer Kidwell would reflect in 2005, ten years after the historic meeting, the groundbreaking consensus statement "also recognized that the most pressing international problems—poverty, hunger, disease, environmental degradation and political instability—can be solved only by securing women's sexual and reproductive health and rights."²² The idea that providing health care and education to women was the key to alleviating world poverty was no longer a fringe notion; it had become dogma.

Even as conference leaders prepared for the massive event, they were getting ready for problems. There was, of course, right-wing opposition to the event, particularly from foes of abortion. The Catholic Church, alarmed by what it saw as a nascent alliance on contraception and abortion issues among the United States, European leaders, and the United Nations, rushed to form coalitions of its own. Approaching Muslim organizations like the World Muslim League, World Muslim Conference, and the Organization of the Islamic Conference and contacting governments in predominantly Islamic countries, the Vatican began to form tenuous alliances. What conservative Muslims and traditional Catholics had in common was their concern over an emerging agenda that placed the rights of individual women—of which reproductive rights were a powerful metonym—over the claims of traditional religious and social power structures. What they did not have in common (and would to some extent undermine the alliance) was a stalwart opposition to birth control and even abortion. While the Catholic Church has consistently opposed both, contraception isn't illegal in most Muslim countries, and some therapeutic abortions—those conducted to save the life of the mother—are allowed even in Iran and Saudi Arabia.

There were left-wing opponents of the conference and its goals as well. At another massive international meeting—the Earth Summit in Rio de Janeiro in 1992—a group of feminist women condemned population control advocates as coercive imperialists and also criticized contraceptive methods as dangerous drugs.²³ These sorts of critiques would lead to an even more dramatic desertion of demographic targets in the Cairo Consensus.

The Consensus, created after ten days of painstaking negotiations, delighted international feminists and enraged traditionalists the world over. The document insisted that reproductive rights were human rights and called for signing nations to work toward universal access to reproductive health care. It also outlined a broad plan that included reducing maternal and infant mortality, increasing life expectancies, and closing educational gaps between male and female students by ensuring that everyone could get at least a primary education. It was an enormous checking of the influence of powerful religious groups to dictate important global reproductive positions, and it had profound implications on reproductive law and justice. Months later the United Nations International Women's Conference in Beijing would reaffirm that the official position of the UN was now that women's reproductive rights were human rights, a stance soon adopted by groups like Amnesty International and Human Rights Watch. Then First Lady Hillary Clinton energized an international crowd in China, proclaiming, "If there is one message that echoes forth from this conference, let it be that human rights are women's rights and women's rights are human rights, once and for all."[24]

While these agreements were groundbreaking, the next fifteen years would challenge optimism about reproductive justice and globalism. Big ideas take big money, and while many nations made generous promises during Cairo, they weren't always able or willing to make good on their commitments. The United States always plays an important financial role in any massive international initiative, and this was no exception. But in 2001, with the election of George W. Bush, international reproductive funding faced unprecedented challenges.

With Strings Attached: The Legacy of George W. Bush

First, of course, Bush reinstated the global gag rule, making its revival nearly his first act as president. This came as no surprise to anyone, and yet the effects were dire for many organizations, including Planned Parenthood and Marie Stopes International. Such groups, it should be noted, provide an array of services for underserved women that go beyond contraception and abortion to include Pap smears, prenatal care, childhood vaccinations, and treatment of sexually transmitted infections. Bush's reinstatement of the gag rule was particularly devastating in light of the global AIDS pandemic. But for a while, it looked as though the bleeding might stop there. Colin Powell, secretary of state and a powerful voice in Bush's ear, was a friend of UNFPA, and the administration asked Congress to put aside $25 million for the agency. Congress did better, and $34 million was appropriated. Within days, fifty-four Republican congresspeople demanded that the money be frozen, again raising old charges of collusion with China to commit reproductive coercion. If these accusations had limited traction in the 1980s, they were completely unjustified at this point. Bush set up a State Department investigation of the charges, and they eventually concluded that, in fact, UNFPA was trying to convince the Chinese government to loosen the strictness of their one-child policy and was not engaged in any kind of coercive activity. Despite these findings, Bush bowed to conservative pressure and withheld the $34 million.[25] UNFPA estimates that the results of not releasing these funds has been devastating: "$34 million could have been used to prevent 2 million unintended pregnancies, 800,000 induced abortions, 4,700 maternal deaths, and 77,000 infant and child deaths."[26] Such numbers boggle the mind, and it is hard to understand how such losses were justified in the name of *preserving* life.

The Bush administration also began to try to convince other countries not to honor the Cairo agreement because it used language that supported abortion rights. An editorial in the journal *Contraception* notes, "In addition to funding cutbacks, the US has also taken a series of diplomatic actions that have called into question its support for reproductive health and family planning programs."[27] It wasn't that the United States wasn't pouring large sums of money into family planning; indeed, America was still the largest international donor to such efforts. It was that they were supporting only certain kinds of work. In other venues, such as large international conferences, they attacked language they felt was too supportive of pro-choice values. Offending phrases included "reproductive health services" (at the UN Special Session on Children) and "reproductive rights" (the UN Population Conference in Bangkok).[28] In 2004 the United States was the only dissenter in a resolution to reaffirm the commitments of Cairo.[29]

Some members of the population movement felt that the fundamental shifts in values within the movement had allowed such things to happen. By taking the focus off things that were easily measured—like demographic targets—they had blurred the focus of their agenda. By removing the crisis mentality they had taken away some of the incentives for powerful governments to assure funds. In this context, as Steven W. Sinding of the Guttmacher Institute argues, "family planning, which had been seen as a global imperative," had morphed at Cairo and become "one among many desirable but nonessential public services."[30] As evidence, Sinding cites an enormous funding decline for programs since 1995.

Of course there were other reasons that this might have happened. First, in the fifty years since many programs were initiated, fertility rates had declined in most parts of the world—in other words, family planning programs had worked. Second was a shift in interest from preventing births to stopping the spread of HIV/AIDS.

Adrienne Germain argues that whatever changes family planning had undergone in terms of its status in international development work, the evidence of their success spoke for itself. Since Cairo, the percentage of couples using some form of contraception has gone up from 55 to 61 percent, and even Africa, the part of the world with the lowest rates of contraceptive use in the world, had seen rates rise from 15 percent in the early 1990s to 25 percent.[31] Other positive changes included reduction in maternal deaths in parts of South America, increased antenatal care in Asia, and a rise in female life expectancy. Reflecting on the conference goals on its ten-year anniversary in 2004, Germain identified four areas for continued work: to provide young women with comprehensive rights-based sexual education, to stop unsafe abortion, to help slow the spread of HIV/AIDS, and to try to align the UN's Millennium Development Goals (a major statement of international development objectives that did not include reproductive rights) with the Cairo statement.[32]

The election of Barack Obama was seen by many in the reproductive rights community as a hopeful sign that American funding might return to important programs, and the ambitious agendas of Cairo and Beijing could be put back on track. There are indeed reasons to hope but also signs that caution is necessary. Obama quickly lifted the global gag rule, and in March 2009 released $50 million in UNFPA funds. At the same time, Obama chose to lift the gag rule the day *after* the anniversary of *Roe*, a gesture of goodwill to abortion foes. Given the president's reluctance to take stands on issues of reproductive justice, this choice is not heartening.

Moving Forward

The future of American funding for international initiatives remains, of course, unwritten. While today programs are able to take advantage of funds to work on behalf of women, it is always possible that a new administration could again undo these gains. Regardless of the position of politicians on abortion, it is time to stop making international women pawns in nasty domestic battles. It is hypocritical to deny women in the most economically disadvantaged parts of the world essential health services because an organization offers—or simply acknowledges and councils—women on a procedure that is legal in the United States. While it is not surprising that politicians would choose to make statements about issues concerning the bodies of women who cannot vote against them, it is both unfair and unwise.

One of the most astounding facts about international population trends in the twenty-first century is that, according to the United Nations, the use of modern contraceptives in less developed regions of the world is now nearly equal to that of the more developed, around 56 percent.[33] More couples in more developed regions use contraception in general, but that greater percentage comes from the use of traditional methods (such as withdrawal, timed abstinence, and fertility awareness). Family planning organizations and proponents of international economic development have both claimed this change as a personal victory, and while certainly both have played a role, it would be reductionary to see the massive global shift in fertility as the product of one movement or social force.

Within the neat average of 56 percent lies a massive diversity of lives and cultures, desires and realities. Around the world, the average number of couples who use modern contraceptives ranges from 3 percent in Chad, where men still say they want close to twenty children, to 90 percent in China, where restrictive government regulation limits families to between one and three children. In defiance of simplistic early attitudes about population control, which assumed that fewer children was better, the past fifty years have seen both coercive governmental and international efforts that forced women through horrifying measures to limit family size, as well as movements within countries all over the world to defend larger families. There has also been profound change both on the national and individual level. When developing nations attended the United Nations population summit in Bucharest in 1974, they articulated concern that population control movements were really Western imperialist efforts to control poor nations. Within a decade, many of these nations had come to believe that limiting population was in their countries' economic as well as environmental interest. Beyond government efforts, in nearly every part of the world today expect for Sub-Saharan Africa, couples themselves express the desire for significantly smaller families. In Europe, declining populations have created a new panic, and some worry that such changes will bring new political instability.

In all places, the old debates linger: What is the point of family planning programs? Do they exist to accomplish a larger international goal of driving down population to avoid political and environmental problems? Or are they there to try to provide individuals with options, to help them build better lives on their own terms? And are programs that function on the latter set of principles as successful as those governed by the former? As hunger and resource shortages, temporarily put at bay by agricultural practices of the 1970s and 1980s, return, so do advocates of the former perspective. Without diminishing the true challenges faced by the global community today, the main focus must always be on the latter.

This difference of opinion, though, makes it difficult to measure how many people want contraception and don't have it. Public health workers use the term "unmet need," but it is not always clear whose need we are talking about. A pregnancy is not, for many women, an undesired outcome, even when it is unplanned. Generally, "unmet need" refers to women who want to avoid or postpone having a baby but who lack any form of contraception.[34] The World Health Organization (WHO) estimates that around 123 million women worldwide want birth control and don't have access to it.[35] Other estimates put the number higher, at around 137 million.[36] Approximately 38 percent of all pregnancies around the globe are unplanned and 50 to 60 percent of these end in abortion.[37] Unmet need is, according to research, highest in Sub-Saharan Africa (23 percent), followed by Latin America (19.4 percent) and Northern Africa and the Middle East (19.4 percent).[38]

A lack of cultural sensitivities on the part of those offering family planning services plays a role in many places. For example, methods that require insertion or application by an often male provider are objectionable to women in certain cultures. Differing perceptions of who should be responsible for contraception are also influential in how well a given method will be adopted.

Just because a woman begins using a method doesn't mean she will continue: as in the United States, international studies in developing nations have found that contraceptive discontinuation is high for all methods,[39] with a third of patients deserting their method within a year and half and giving it up within two. The most common reason for discontinuing modern methods, including the Pill and IUD, is concern about side effects and safety. For natural methods, accidental pregnancy is the main cause of stopping method use. Importantly, *lacking* access to a contraceptive method is not as frequent a reason for discontinuation as researchers had anticipated.[40]

Forty-three percent of people in the world today live in countries that have finished the "demographic transition"—that is, they live in places where the average number of births is at or below replacement levels.[41] This means that the population has stabilized and isn't growing significantly or at all. Another 43 percent live in countries where population growth has slowed significantly but is still ultimately expanding, and 16 percent live in countries where growth is still high.

It is important to note that the risks of carrying a baby to term are markedly different in various parts of the world. Some estimates suggest that the risk of dying during pregnancy and childbirth in many parts of the developing world is "several hundred times higher"[42] than in North America. The majority of deaths from unplanned pregnancy around the world results from unsafe abortion practices.

While certainly the risk/benefit analysis of contraceptive use changes dramatically for women living with inadequate access to health care and safe living conditions, the right to be an informed patient should be international. Greater risk of maternal or infant mortality is not an excuse for not providing patients with complete information about the safety profiles of their contraceptive methods.

Today, when it comes to anxiety about the global population, the old is new again. As food and energy get more expensive, previous fears about outstripping the planet's resources find new currency. Food riots in over a dozen countries in 2008[43] seemed like proof of impending disaster to those predicting Malthusian chaos.

While populations have declined in most parts of the world and fertility in the developing world has fallen by half in the last fifty years,[44] overall, the global population continues to grow. In the developing world, the size of the average family has fallen from around six children to three, but this number is still above replacement fertility (two children), and that means that the globe continues to swell by 75 million people each year.[45] People are now living longer, which can compound the pressure being placed on the earth's resources. This has led some to argue that family planning initiatives are more relevant than ever.

Increasing contraceptive access globally is a valuable goal as long as it is part of a broader program of improving health care access. The problem with the return to neopopulationist ideologies is that they seek to fix bigger problems of global inequality and injustice in women's bodies.

Nearly all of the major population growth that demographers predict in the next forty years will happen in the developing world. Resource shortages don't happen simply because poor women have babies. In fact, overconsumption in developed nations and unequal distribution of global resources that allocate more to fewer people play a much bigger role. Overpopulation is a symptom of these injustices, not the cause.

As the old saying goes, "Hope for the best and prepare for the worst." Many people hope that recent gloom and doom scenarios of food and energy crisis will be averted by technological or agricultural innovation. Just as the dire predictions of the 1950s, 1960s, and 1970s proved significantly overstated, perhaps today's population worries will be prevented. In the meantime, those who are concerned about ballooning human numbers should put their efforts into empowering women. Part of this project entails improving contraceptive access and making sure that women can have the number of children that they want. It also means making sure that women have access to education, jobs, and economic autonomy.

Michelle Goldberg writes, "Emancipated women become a symbol of everything maddening and unmooring about modernity. To tame them seems a first step to taming an unruly world. But the oppression of women doesn't create order; it creates profound social deformities."[46] As we move toward the problems of the future, let's hope that we can apply the lessons of the past half century without having to painfully relearn them.

Resource Guide

General Resources for Women's Health

The Center for Menstrual Cycle and Ovulation Research, http://www.cemcor
.ubc.ca, founded by Dr. Jerilynn C. Prior.
Feminist Women's Health Center, http://www.feministcenter.org
Mayo Clinic, http://www.mayoclinic.org
Medline Plus, http://medlineplus.gov
National Women's Health Network, http://www.nwhn.org
Our Bodies Ourselves, also known as the Boston Women's Health Book Collec-
tive, http://www.ourbodiesourselves.org
Parker, William H., with Rachel Parker. *A Gynecologist's Second Opinion*. New
York: Plume, 2003.
Planned Parenthood, http://www.plannedparenthood.org
RH Reality Check, http://www.rhrealitycheck.org
Sanson, Gillian, http://www.gilliansanson.com, an Australian's women's health
writer and activist with an excellent website.
Scarlateen, http://www.scarlateen.com, a great website with information on con-
traception and sexual health.

On Contraceptive History

Gordon, Linda. *The Moral Property of Women: A History of Birth Control Politics
in America*. Urbana and Chicago: University of Illinois Press, 2007.
Jütte, Robert. *Contraception: A History*. Cambridge, UK, and Malden, MA: Polity
Press, 2008.
McCann, Carole R. *Birth Control Politics in the United States, 1916–1945*. Ithaca,
NY, and London: Cornell University Press, 1994.
Roberts, Dorothy. *Killing the Black Body: Race, Reproduction and the Meaning of
Liberty*. New York: Vintage Books, 1999.
Silliman, Jael, Marlene Gerber Fried, Loretta Ross, and Elena R. Gutierrez. *Undi-
vided Rights: Women of Color Organize for Reproductive Justice*. Cambridge,
MA: South End Press, 2004.

Solinger, Rickie. *Pregnancy and Power: A Short History of Reproductive Politics in America*. New York and London: New York University Press, 2005.

Tone, Andrea. *Devices and Desires: A History of Contraceptives in America*. New York: Hill and Wang, 2001.

On the Pill and the History of the Pill

Read

Bennett, Jane, and Alexandra Pope. *The Pill: Are You Sure It's for You?* Crows Nest, NSW, Australia: Allen & Unwin, 2008.

Dickey, Richard P. *Managing Contraceptive Pill Patients*. 13th ed. Dallas, TX: EMIS Medical Publishers, 2007.

Djerassi, Carl. *The Man's Pill: Reflections on the 50th Birthday of the Pill*. Oxford and New York: Oxford University Press, 2001.

Grigg-Spall, Holly. Sweetening the Pill. www.sweeteningthepill.blogspot.com.

Marks, Lara V. *Sexual Chemistry: A History of the Contraceptive Pill*. New Haven and London: Yale University Press, 2001.

May, Elaine Tyler. *America and the Pill: A History of Promise, Peril, and Liberation*. New York: Basic Books, 2010.

Seaman, Barbara. *The Doctors' Case Against the Pill*. Alameda, CA: Hunter House, 1995.

Watkins, Elizabeth Siegel. *On the Pill: A Social History of Oral Contraceptives, 1950–1970*. Baltimore and London: Johns Hopkins University Press, 1998.

Watch

The Pill. Directed by Erna Buffie and Elise Swerhorne. Montreal: National Film Board of Canada, 1999.

The Pill. Directed by Chana Gazit. Steward/Gazit Productions, Inc., for *American Experience*, 2003. See http://www.pbs.org/wgbh/amex/pill/.

On Menstruation

Buckley, Thomas, and Alma Gottlieb, eds. *Blood Magic: The Anthropology of Menstruation*. Berkeley and Los Angeles: University of California Press, 1988.

Delaney, Janice, Mary Jan Lupton, and Emily Toth. *The Curse: A Cultural History of Menstruation*. New York: E. P. Dutton & Co, 1976.

Houppert, Karen. *The Curse: Confronting the Last Unmentionable Taboo, Men-struation*. New York: Farrar, Straus and Giroux, 1999.

Kipnis, Laura. *The Female Thing: Dirt, Envy, Sex and Vulnerability*. New York: Vintage, 2007.

Kissling, Elizabeth Arveda. *Capitalizing on the Curse: The Business of Menstrua-tion*. Boulder and London: Lynne Rienner Publishers, 2006.

Laws, Sophie. *Issues of Blood: The Politics of Menstruation*. London: MacMillan Press, 1990.

Martin, Emily. *The Woman in the Body: A Cultural Analysis of Reproduction*. Boston: Beacon Press, 1987.

Muscio, Inga. *Cunt: A Declaration of Independence*. Berkeley, CA: Seal Press, 2002.

Museum of Menstruation, http://www.mum.org.

On Menstrual Supression

Rako, Susan. *The Blessings of the Curse: No More Periods?* Lincoln, NE: Backin-print.com, 2006.

On Fertility Awareness Method (FAM)

Singer, Katie. *The Garden of Fertility*. New York: Avery, 2004. See http://www.gardenoffertility.com.

Weschler, Toni. *Cycle Savvy: The Smart Teen's Guide to the Mysteries of Her Body*. New York: HarperCollins, 2006.

―――. *Taking Charge of Your Fertility: The Definitive Guide to Natural Birth Control and Pregnancy Achievement*. New York: HarperCollins, 2006.

On the Male Pill:

Oudshoorn, Nelly. *The Male Pill: A Biography of a Technology in the Making*. Durham, NC, and London: Duke University Press, 2003.

On Hormones and the Environment

Davis, Devra. *The Secret History of the War on Cancer*. New York: Basic Books, 2007.

On Global Reproductive Justice

Goldberg, Michelle. *The Means of Reproduction: Sex, Power and the Future of the World*. New York: Penguin Press, 2009.

Kristof, Nicholas D., and Sheryl WuDunn. *Half the Sky: Turning Oppression into Opportunity for Women Worldwide*. New York: Alfred A. Knopf, 2009.

Acknowledgments

First, I want to thank Dan Simon and Seven Stories Press for understanding the enduring importance of Barbara Seaman's work and for having confidence in my ability to carry on some small piece of it. Theresa Noll has been much more than an editor; indeed, she is the co-parent of this project, imagining it with me so many months ago and being there at every step to make sure that it became a reality. Her patience and guidance have been invaluable to me and her wisdom and enthusiasm illuminate each page. Crystal Yakacki and Ruth Weiner went above and beyond the call of duty in promoting the book and I am so grateful for their efforts and enthusiasm on this project. I would also like to thank Veronica Liu, Mary Taveras, and Caitlin Thompson for their hard work readying the book for publication.

There are many people who have been generous with their knowledge, time, and advice. For taking the time to answer my questions, guide my research, and help me understand their work, I am grateful to Cynthia Pearson, Amy Allina and the National Women's Health Network, Judy Norsigian, Andrea Tone, Toni Weschler, Katie Singer, Leonore Teifer, Cynthia Graham, Jennifer Baumgardner, Jacques Rossouw, Susan Love, Alice Wolfson, William Parker, Gillian Sanson, Devra Davis, Susan Rako, Sybil Shainwald, Shere Hite, Susan Wood, Barbara Zuckerman, and Gillian Sanson.

For their books, which informed and inspired me during the writing process, I am grateful to Elizabeth Siegel Watkins, Lara V. Marks, Michelle Goldberg, Nelly Oudshoorn, Jane Bennett, Alexandra Pope, Dorothy Roberts, Rickie Solinger, and Karen Houppert.

I owe a great debt of gratitude to the many women who shared their personal stories. Their accounts inform and enrich this book and remind me for whom I am writing.

Lauren Porsch has been my dear friend for well over a decade, and her weekly counsel and willingness to help me find important information strengthened this book. Her tireless efforts as a health activist continue to inspire me. Irene Xanthoudakis also generously shared her years of experience and knowledge in this field. Helen Lowery gave me an early forum to present my research and ideas, which was invaluable to the development of the project. I am lucky to have her as a friend. Marlo Dublin kindly read chapter drafts at a key moment, and Katie Walker helped with organizing interviews and provided constant enthusiasm and support. Much love and many thanks are also due to the family of choice that sustains me: Rebecca Kraut, Rachel Fisher, Molly Barry, April Timko, Stephanie Kirk, Nicole Richman, Chi Kim, Rumela Mitra, and Rob Tennant. Rabbi Lisa Grushcow, Rabbi Sari Laufer, and Emily Huber provided necessary spiritual guidance, and my Philly women's group provided professional support.

I feel lucky each day to be a part of the Weinberg family. Beth, Sheldon, Josh, Marnie, and Zachary Weinberg are always in my heart, and thanks and love is due as well to Lisa, Stu, and Michelle Alperin and Stephanie and Eric Biderman. Ray Josell-Metz is not only a fantastic grandmother and constant cheerleader, but a marvelous friend.

The Seaman family has been a tremendous source of love and support since the death of my dear friend Barbara. Noah, Elana, and Shira Seaman are like family to me, and I feel lucky to have them in my life.

This book, quite simply, would not have happened without the love, interest, and faith of the Eldridge family. During its writing, my grandfather, Paul W. Eldridge Sr., passed away, and his loss is a constant sorrow. Everyone who met Gea was impressed by his humor and charm, and it was from him that I learned how to tell stories. My brothers David, Reed, and Peter are always my best friends, and I would not know what to do without them. David in particular has been a huge help with this book, offering his knowledge and research assistance and reading chapter drafts. My parents, Susan and Paul, make my work possible. They provide an amazing model of parenting, and although they don't always agree with my conclusions, they teach me how to be a person of conviction and conscience.

Finally, I must say thank you to my husband, Jeremy Weinberg. Jeremy basically acted as a research assistant for this book despite the fact that he was amply occupied finishing his law degree. He was willing to run to the library or find an article or read a chapter, even with only a small amount of advance notice. Jeremy always put my work first, and for this I don't know how to thank him. He is also a brave companion in navigating the sometimes-convoluted world of contraceptive decision making. His kindness, intelligence, and good humor enrich my life, and I feel lucky every day that he is my partner.

The work of Barbara Seaman continues to impact and inform women's health. I was fortunate to learn from her over the course of ten years. While I have tried in this project to honor her work, I want to pay tribute here to Barbara as a person. There is not a day that I don't think about her and miss her. A picture of Barbara and me taken in 2007 sits over my computer, and I hear her voice still advising, correcting, encouraging, and chiding as I write. In the photo we are laughing, as we did so often, and I am reminded of the countless conversations we used to have in which she treated me as an equal in our work despite the fact that she was clearly the senior partner. I was one of many, many young women who Barbara not only inspired, but helped in tangible ways to begin careers as health writers and activists. In our words and work, as well as in the countless changes in women's lives that she made real, her legacy continues. Still, most days, I don't know how we continue without her.

Notes

Introduction

1. Jael Silliman, Marlene Gerber Fried, Loretta Ross, and Elena R. Gutierrez, *Undivided Rights: Women of Color Organize for Reproductive Justice* (Cambridge, MA: South End Press, 2004), 11.
2. Bonnie Scott Jones and Michelle Movahed, "Lesson One: Your Gender Is Your Destiny—The Constitutionality of Teaching Sex Stereotypes in Abstinence-Only Programs," American Constitution Society for Law and Policy issue brief, September 10, 2008, http://www.acslaw.org/node/7096.

Chapter One: Past Tense

1. Elizabeth B. Connell, "Contraception in the Prepill Era," *Contraception* 59, no. 1 (January 1999): 7S–10S.
2. Bernard Asbell, *The Pill: A Biography of the Drug That Changed the World* (New York: Random House, 1995).
3. Connell, "Contraception," 7S.
4. Aine Collier, *The Humble Little Condom: A History* (Amherst, NY: Prometheus Books, 2007), 11.
5. Ibid., 11–32.
6. Angus McLaren, *A History of Contraception: From Antiquity to the Present Day* (Cambridge, MA: Blackwell, 1990).
7. Eric Chevallier, *The Condom: Three Thousand Years of Safer Sex* (London: Puffin, 1995).
8. John M. Riddle, *Contraception and Abortion from the Ancient World to the Renaissance* (Cambridge, MA: Harvard University Press, 1992). See also, by the same author, *Eve's Herbs: A History of Contraception and Abortion in the West* (Cambridge, MA: Harvard University Press, 1997).
9. Ghislaine Lawrence, "Condoms and Contraception: Tools of the Trade," *Lancet* 360, no. 9327 (July 13, 2002): 178.
10. Andrea Tone, *Devices and Desires: A History of Contraceptives in America* (New York: Hill and Wang, 2001), 51.
11. Ibid.
12. Connell, "Contraception," 7s.
13. Tone, *Devices and Desires*, 56.
14. Ibid.
15. Ibid., 54.

16. Ibid., 55.
17. Leslie J. Reagan, "'About to Meet Her Maker': Women, Doctors, Dying Declarations, and the State's Investigation of Abortion, Chicago, 1867–1940," in *American Sexual Histories*, ed. Elizabeth Reis, 228–45 (Malden, MA, Oxford, and Victoria: Blackwell Publishing, 2001).
18. Quoted in James Reed, *From Private Vice to Public Virtue: The Birth Control Movement and American Society Since 1830* (New York: Basic Books, 1978), 16.
19. Rickie Solinger, *Pregnancy and Power: A Short History of Reproductive Politics in America* (New York and London: New York University Press, 2005), 70.
20. Ibid., 71.
21. Anthony Comstock, *Second Annual Report of the New York Society for the Suppression of Vice* (New York, 1876), 5.
22. Comstock Law, *US Statutes at Large* 17 (1873), chap. 258, 598.
23. Tone, *Devices and Desires*, 40.
24. Solinger, *Pregnancy and Power*, 79–83.
25. Janet Farrell Brodie, *Contraception and Abortion in Nineteenth-Century America* (Ithaca, NY: Cornell University Press, 1994), 7.
26. "People & Events: Eugenics and Birth Control," supplementary information provided about *The Pill*, a film that aired on the PBS program *American Experience*, www.pbs.org/wgbh/amex/pill/peopleevents/e_eugenics.html.
27. Linda Gordon, *The Moral Property of Women: A History of Birth Control Politics in America* (Urbana and Chicago: University of Illinois Press, 2007), 141.
28. Peter Neushul, "Marie C. Stopes and the Popularization of Birth Control Technology," *Technology and Culture* 39, no. 2 (April 1998): 249.
29. Ibid., 251.
30. Solinger, *Pregnancy and Power*, 104.
31. Dorothy Roberts, *Killing the Black Body: Race, Reproduction and the Meaning of Liberty* (New York: Vintage Books, 1999), 81.
32. Ibid., 58–59.
33. Ibid., 88.
34. *Buck v. Bell*, 274 US 200 (1927).
35. Tone, *Devices and Desires*, 93.
36. Many African-American women continue to struggle with perceptions, both in and outside the black community, that contraceptives and other reproductive services—and the organizations that provide them—are in the service of racist agendas. These toxic ideas prevent many women from receiving care and further complicate the issue of reproductive health disparities between black women and their white counterparts. In early 2010, an anti-abortion group put up dozens of billboards in metropolitan Atlanta proclaiming that black babies are "an endangered species," in reference to the higher rate of abortion among black women compared to other racial and ethnic groups. See Guttmacher Institute, "No conspiracy theories needed: Higher abortion rates among women of color reflect higher rates of unintended pregnancy," news release, August 13, 2008, http://www.guttmacher.org/media/nr/2008/08/13/index.html; and Shani O. Hilton, "Black Women Don't Need Billboards," *American Prospect*, February 24, 2010, http://www.prospect.org/cs/articles?article=black_women_dont_need_billboards.

The campaign specifically targeted Planned Parenthood and sought to exploit Margaret Sanger's problematic history with race to suggest that the modern organization is pursuing a racist agenda. Whatever eugenic ideas Margaret Sanger truly embraced—and as we saw there is good evidence that she never truly bought in to a eugenic program—Planned Parenthood as a modern organization has worked tirelessly and heroically to provide a range of reproductive health services to all women who need them, including contraception, abortion, adoption referrals, and prenatal care.

37. Barbara Seaman, *The Greatest Experiment Ever Performed on Women: Exploding the Estrogen Myth* (New York: Hyperion, 2003).

38. Carl Djerassi, *This Man's Pill: Reflections on the 50th Birthday of the Pill* (Oxford and New York: Oxford University Press, 2001), 16.

39. Seaman, *Greatest Experiment*, 13.

40. Ibid., 37–44.

41. Lara V. Marks, *Sexual Chemistry: A History of the Contraceptive Pill* (New Haven and London: Yale University Press, 2001), 64.

42. Ibid., 70.

43. Ibid.

44. Ibid., 92.

45. Katherine McCormick to Margaret Sanger, May 31, 1955, Margaret Sanger Papers, Sophia Smith Collection, Smith College, Northampton, MA.

46. Barbara Seaman, "The Pill and I: 40 Years On, the Relationship Remains Wary," *New York Times,* June 25, 2000, 15–19.

47. Marks, *Sexual Chemistry*, 115.

48. Solinger, *Pregnancy and Power*, 171.

49. John Rock, transcript of a lecture to the Planned Parenthood Federation of America meeting, 1954.

50. Seaman and Wolfson, together with other women's health activists, went on to found the National Women's Health Network (a grassroots organization that continues to advocate for women's health causes and refuses funding from drug or device makers) and continued to write prescient critiques of other drugs, most notably those used in hormone and estrogen treatments for menopause.

Chapter Two: A Pill Primer

1. *The Pill*, Erna Buffie and Elise Swerhone, directors, National Film Board of Canada, 1999.

2. Ibid.

3. Jon Zonderman and Laurel Shader, *Birth Control Pills* (New York: Chelsea House, 2006).

4. Kate Lunau, "Ditching the Pill For Good," November 23, 2009, *Macleans,* http://www2.macleans.ca/2009/11/23/ditching-the-pill-for-good.

5. Virginia Hopkins, "Truthiness in Advertising: Is Qlaira Really a 'Natural' Birth Control," http://www.virginiahopkins.com/qlairabirthcontrol.html.

6. Progestins are sometimes referred to as Progestogens. Frank Z. Stanczyk and Milan R. Henzl, "Use of the name 'Progestin,'" *Contraception* 64, no. 1 (2001): 1–2.

7. Zonderman and Shader, *Birth Control Pills*, 21.

8. Rachel E. D'Souza and John Guillebaud, "Risks and benefits of oral contraceptive pills," *Best Practice & Research Clinical Obstetrics and Gynaecology* 16, no. 2 (2002): 133–54 (135).

9. Family Health International, "Using Progestin-only Pills Correctly," http://www.fhi.org/NR/Shared/edFHI/PrinterFriendly.asp.

10. R. D. Blackburn, J. A. Cunkelman, and V. M. Zlidar, "Oral contraceptives—an update," *Population Reports*, ser. A, no. 9 (2000): 1–40.

11. Jane Bennett and Alexandra Pope, *The Pill: Are You Sure It's For You?"* (Crow's Nest, NSW, Australia: Allen and Unwin, 2008), 61.

12. Family Health International, "Using Progestin-only Pills Correctly," http://www.fhi.org/NR/Shared/edFHI/PrinterFriendly.asp.

13. Barbara Seaman, *The Doctors' Case Against the Pill* (New York: Peter H. Wyden, Inc., 1969), 83.

14. Jean-Patrice Baillargeon, Donna K. McClish, Paulina A Essah, and John E. Nestler, "Association between the current use of the low-dose oral contraceptives and cardio-vascular arterial disease: A meta-analysis," *Journal of Clinical Endocrinology & Metabolism* 90, no. 7 (2005): 3863–70.

15. Richard P. Dickey, *Managing Contraceptive Pill Patients*, 13th ed. (Dallas, TX: EMIS Medical Publishers, 2007), 192.

16. "Advisory on Contraceptives," *Journal of the American Medical Association* 284, no. 8 (August 23–30, 2000): 951.

17. Barbara A. Frempong, Madia Ricks, Sabyasachi Sen, and Anne E. Sumner, "Effect of Low-Dose Oral Contraceptives on Metabolic Risk Factors in African-American Women," *Journal of Clinical Endocrinology & Metabolism* 93, no. 6 (June 2008): 2097.

18. It is important to mention that this particular study was not comparing African American women with women of other races. It wasn't arguing that the Pill posed a greater risk to black women; rather, that it was worth asking what discrete risks it posed to that community.

19. T. M. Farley, O. Meirik, J. Collins, "Cardiovascular disease and combined oral contraceptives: reviewing the evidence and balancing the risks," *Human Reproduction Update* 5, no. 6 (November–December 1999): 721–35.

20. Ibid.

21. Ibid.

22. H. C. Pymar and M. D. Creinin, "The risks of oral contraceptive pills," *Seminars in Reproductive Medicine* 19, no. 4 (2001): 305–12.

23. A. M. Walker, "Newer oral contraceptives and the risk of venous thromboembolism," *Contraception* 57, no. 3 (1998): 169–81.

24. Cheryl A. Frye, "An overview of oral contraceptives," *Neurology* 66, no. 6, suppl. 3 (March 28, 2006): S29–S36.

25. Jean-Patrice Baillargeon, Donna K. McClish, Paulina A. Essah, and John E. Nestler, "Association between the Current Use of Low-Dose Oral Contraceptives and Cardiovascular Arterial Disease: A Meta-Analysis," *Journal of Clinical Endocrinology & Metabolism* 90, no. 7 (2005): 3863–70.

26. The Associated Press, "Some Birth Control Pills Linked to Blood Clots," *MSNBC*, Wednesday February 7, 2007, http://www.msnbc.msn.com/id/17005448/.

27. American College of Obstetricians and Gynecologists, "ACOG committee revises recommendations on OCs with third-generation progestins," *ACOG Today* 42, no. 6 (July 1998): 5.

28. Ojvind Lidegaard, Ellen Lokkegaard, Anne Louise Svendsen, and Carsten Agger, "Hormonal Contraception and the Risk of Venous Thromboembolism: National follow-up study," *British Medical Journal* 339 (2009): b2890.

29. Natasha Singer, "Health Concerns Over Popular Contraceptives," *New York Times,* September 26, 2009, B1.

30. Ibid.

31. L. M. Lopez, A. A. Kaptein, and F. M. Helmerhorst, "Oral contraceptive containing drospirenone for premenstrual syndrome," *Cochrane Database of Systematic Reviews* 2 (2009); Faustino R. Perez-Lopez, "Clinical experiences with drospirenone: From reproductive to postmenopausal years," *Maturitas* 60, no. 2 (2008): 78–91.

32. Conversation with the author, March, 31, 2010.

33. Dickey, *Managing Contraceptive Pill Patients*, 205.

34. American College of Obstetricians and Gynecologists, "The use of hormonal contraception in women with coexisting medical conditions," *ACOG Practice Bulletin* (2006): 73.

35. Rachel E. D'Souza and John Guillebaud, "Risks and benefits of oral contraceptive pills," *Best Practice & Research Clinical Obstetrics and Gynaecology* 16, no. 2 (2002): 140–41.

36. World Health Organization (WHO), *Cardiovascular disease and steroid hormone contraception: Report of a WHO scientific group*, Geneva: World Health Organization, Technical Report Series, no. 877 (1997): 90; Practice Committee of the American Society for Reproductive Medicine, "Hormonal contraception: recent advances and controversies," *Fertility and Sterility* 90, no. 3 (November 2008): S103–S113 (S108).

37. Practice Committee of the American Society for Reproductive Medicine, "Hormonal contraception: Recent advances and controversies," *Fertility and Sterility* 90, no. 3 (November 2008): S108.

38. Salynn Boyles, "Low Dose Birth Control Pills May Up Heart Risk," WebMD Health News, July 7, 2005, http://www.webmd.com/sex/birth-control/news/20050707/low-dose-birth-control-pill-may-up-heart-risk.

39. Ibid.

40. Leslie Allison Gillum, Sai Kumar Mamidipudi, S. Claiborne Johnston, "Ischemic Stroke Risk With Oral Contraceptives: A Meta-analysis," *Journal of the American Medical Association* 284, no. 1 (July 5, 2000): 72–78.

41. Cheryl D. Bushnell, "Stroke in Women: Risk and Prevention Throughout the Lifespan," *Clinical Neurology and Neurosurgery* 26, no. 4 (November 2008): 1161–76.

42. Gianni Allais, Ilaria Castagnoli Gabellari, and Ornella Mana, et al., "Migraine and stroke: the role of oral contraceptives," *Journal of the Neurological Sciences* 29 (2008): S12–S14.

43. C. Chang, M. Donaghy, and N. Poulter, "Migraine and stroke in young women: a case-control study," *British Medical Journal* 318 (1999): 13–18.

44. Some doctors believe that POP use is safer than combined use for women with aura-including migraines.

45. Bushnell, "Stroke in Women: Risk and Prevention Throughout the Lifespan," 1161–76.

46. Deanne Stein, "Birth Control and Stroke," MyHeartCentral.com, June 23, 2006, http://www.healthcentral.com/heart-disease/c/19/1812/birth-stroke/pf/.

47. K. Rexrode, C. Hennekens, W. Willett, et al., "A prospective study of body mass index, weight change, and risk of stroke in women," *Journal of the American Medical Association* 277 (1997): 1539–45.

48. Bushnell, "Stroke in Women: Risk and Prevention Throughout the Lifespan," 1161–76.

49. The American Cancer Society, "Global Cancer Facts and Figures, 2007," www.cancer.org.

50. One meta-analysis estimated that women who don't take the Pill have a 2.4 percent risk of developing the disease through age seventy-four, and those who use OCs for twelve years have a 1.4 percent risk. Another study thought the benefit would be greater, positing that eight years of use could prevent nearly 1,900 cases of the disease in the United States alone. Still other studies insist that the benefit would be smaller: an estimate published in the *Lancet* reckoned that if 100,000 women between the ages of sixteen and thirty-five used the Pill, only ten lives would be saved.

51. J. J. Schlesselman, "Net effect of oral contraceptive use on the risk of cancer in women in the United States," *Obstetrics & Gynecology* 85, no. 5 (1995): 793–801; J. J. Schlesselman, "Risk of endometrial cancer in relation to use of combined oral contraceptives: A practitioner's guide to metanalysis," *Human Reproduction* 12, no. 9 (1997): 1851–63.

52. D. B. Petitti and D. Porterfield, "Worldwide variations in the lifetime probability of reproductive cancer in women: Implications of best case and worst case assumptions about the effect of oral contraceptive use," *Contraception* 45, no. 2 (1992): 93–104.

53. The American Cancer Society, "Cancer Statistics 2009 Presentation," www.cancer.org.

54. Royal College of General Practitioners Oral Contraceptive Study, "Further analysis of mortality in oral contraceptive users," *Lancet* 1 (1981): 541.

55. A. L. Coker, S. Harlap, and J. A. Fortney, "Oral contraceptives and reproductive cancers: Weighing the risks and benefits," *Family Planning Perspectives* 25 (1993): 17–21.

56. "Pill has stopped 100,000 deaths," *BBC News*, January 28, 2008, http://news.bbc.co.uk/1/hi/health/7207812.

57. "Ovarian cancer and oral contraceptives: collaborative reanalysis of data from 45 epidemiological studies including 23,257 women with ovarian cancer and 87,303 controls," *Lancet* 371, no. 9609 (January 2008): 303–14.

58. Ibid.

59. Jon Zonderman and Laurel Shader, *Birth Control Pills* (New York: Chelsea House, 2006), 38.

60. D'Souza, "Risks and benefits of oral contraceptive pills," 137.

61. J. F. Fraumeni Jr., J. W. Lloyd, E. M. Smith, and J. K. Wagoner, "Cancer mortality among nuns: Role of marital status in etiology of neoplastic disease in women," *Journal of the National Cancer Institute* 42 (1969): 445–68.

62. Cristina Bosetti, Francesca Bravi, Eva Negri, and Carlo La Vecchia, "Oral contraceptives and colorectal cancer risk: a systematic review and meta-analysis," *Human Reproduction Update* 1, no. 1 (2009): 1–10.

63. D'Souza and John Guillebaud, "Risks and benefits of oral contraceptive pills," 138.

64. The American Cancer Society, "Cancer Statistics 2009 Presentation," 2009, www.cancer.org.

65. Schlesselman, "Net effect of oral contraceptive use on the risk of cancer in women in the United States," 793-801.

66. A. L. Coker, S. Harlap, J. A. Fortney, "Oral Contraceptives and reproductive cancers: Weighing the risks and benefits," *Family Planning Perspectives* 25 (1992): 17–21.

67. Dickey, *Managing Contraceptive Pill Patients*, 180.

68. Barbara Seaman, *The Greatest Experiment Ever Performed on Women: Exploding the Estrogen Myth* (New York: Hyperion, 2003).

69. Barbara Seaman and Laura Eldridge, *The No-Nonsense Guide to Menopause* (New York: Simon and Schuster, 2008), 152.

70. L. A. G. Ries, M. P . Eisner, and C. L. Kosary, et. al., *SEER Cancer Statistics Review,* 1975-2000, (Bethesda, MD: National Cancer Institute, 2003).

71. Collaborative Group on Hormonal Factors in Breast Cancer, "Breast cancer and hormonal contraceptives: collaborative reanalysis of individual data on 53,297 women with breast cancer and 100,239 women without breast cancer from 54 epidemiological studies," *Lancet* 347 (1996): 1713–27.

72. Petra M. Casey, James R. Cerhan, and Sandhya Pruthi, "Oral Contraceptive Use and the Risk of Breast Cancer," *Mayo Clinic Proceedings* 83, no. 1 (January 2008): 86–91.

73. Tara Parker Pope, *The Hormone Decision* (New York: Rodale, 2007), 68.

74. Practice Committee of the American Society for Reproductive Medicine, "Hormonal contraception: Recent advances and controversies," *Fertility and Sterility* 90, no. 3 (November 2008): S106.

75. C. Giersig, "Progestin and Breast Cancer: The Missing Piece of the Puzzle," *Bundesgesundheitsbl—Gesundheitsforsch—Gesundheitsschutz* 51 (2008): 782–86 (784).

76. Allison Gandey, "Sudden Decline in Breast Cancer Could Be Linked to HRT," *Medscape Medical News*, December 14, 2006, www.medscape.com.

77. Christina A. Clarke, et. al., "Recent declines in Hormone Therapy Utilization and Breast Cancer Incidence: Clinical and Population-Based Evidence," *Journal of Clinical Oncology* 24, no. 33 (November 20, 2006): e49–e50.

78. Jacques Rossouw, e-mail to author, October 7, 2009.

79. Dawn M. Grabrick, Lynn C. Hartmann, and James R. Cerhan, et al., "Risk of Breast Cancer with Oral Contraceptive Use in Women With a Family History of Breast Cancer," *Journal of the American Medical Association* 284, no. 14 (October 11, 2000): 1791–98; Wylie Burke, "Oral contraceptives and breast cancer: A note of caution for high-risk women," *Journal of the American Medical Association* 284, no. 14 (October 11, 2000): 1837–38.

80. L. A. Brinton, M. P. Vessey, R. Flavel, and D. Yeates, "Risk factors for benign breast disease," *American Journal of Epidemiology* 113 (1981): 203–14.

81. Dickey, *Managing Contraceptive Pill Patients*, 184.

82. Ibid.

83. L. Rosenberg, "The Risk of liver neoplasia in relation to combined oral contraceptive use," *Contraception* 43 (1991): 643–52.

84. Jane Bennett and Alexandra Pope, *The Pill: Are You Sure It's For You?"* (Crow's Nest, NSW, Australia: Allen and Unwin, 2008), 40–41.

85. Jerilynn C. Prior, "Choices for Effective Contraception in 2006," CEMCOR, http://www.cemcor.ubs.ca/print/110.

86. Kirsten A. Oinonen and Dwight Mazmanian, "To what extent do oral contraceptives influence mood and affect?" *Journal of Affective Disorders* 70 (2002): 299–40 (229).

87. Susan Rako, conversation with the author, October 5, 2009.
88. The World Health Organization, "Mental Health Report," December 13, 2006, www.who.org.
89. Oinonen, "To what extent do oral contraceptives influence mood and affect?" 230.
90. Ibid., 234.
91. Liane Will-Shahab, Steffen Bauer, and Ullrich Kunter, et. al., "St. John's Wort extract (Ze 117) does not alter the pharmacokinetics of a low-dose oral contraceptive," *European Journal of Clinical Pharmacology* 64 (2009): 287–94.
92. Jonathan Schaffir, "Hormonal Contraception and Sexual Desire: A Critical Review," *Journal of Sex & Marital Therapy* 32, no. 4 (September 2006): 305.
93. Lorraine Dennerstein, interviewed on Catalyst, "Women's Libido," May 20, 2004, http://www.abc.net.au/catalyst/stories/s1112389.htm.
94. Ibid.
95. Cynthia Graham, interview with author, October 7, 2009.
96. Stephanie A. Sanders, Cynthia A. Graham, Jennifer L. Bass, and John Bancroft, "A prospective study of the effects of oral contraceptives on sexuality and well-being and their relationship to discontinuation," *Contraception* 64 (2001): 51–58.
97. Teri Greco, Cynthia A. Graham, and John Bancroft, et al., "The effects of oral contraceptives on androgen levels and their relevance to premenstrual mood and sexual interest: A comparison of two triphasic formulations containing norgestimate and either 35 or 25 ug of ethinyl estradiol," *Contraception* 76 (2007): 8–17.
98. Ray Moynihan, "FDA Panel Rejects Testosterone Patch for Women on Safety Grounds," *British Medical Journal* 329 (December 11, 2004): 1363.
99. Schaffir, "Hormonal Contraception and Sexual Desire: A Critical Review," 305–14.
100. Mary A. Ott, Marcia L. Shew, Susan Ofner, "The Influence of Hormonal Contraception on Mood and Sexual Interest among Adolescents," *Archives of Sexual Behavior* 37 (2008): 605–13.
101. Schaffir, "Hormonal Contraception and Sexual Desire: A Critical Review," 305–14.
102. C. A. Graham, R. Ramos, and J. Bancroft, et al., "The effects of steroidal contraceptives on the well-being and sexuality of women: A double-blinded, placebo-controlled, two-centre study of combined and progestogen-only methods," *Contraception* 53 (1995): 363–69.
103. Raphaelle Chaix, Chen Cao, and Peter Donnelly, "Is Mate Choice in Humans MHC-Dependent?," *PLOS Genetics* 4, no. 9 (September 8, 2008): e1000184, doi:10.1371/journal.pgen.1000184.
104. Melinda Wenner, "Birth Control Pills Affect Women's Taste in Men," *Scientific American*, December 5, 2008.
105. Alexandra Alvergne and Virpi Lummaa, "Does the Contraceptive Pill Alter Mate Choice in Humans?" *Trends in Ecology and Evolution*, October 6, 2009.
106. "The pill 'gives women a taste for boyish men like Zac Efron,'" *Daily Telegraph*, October 8, 2009.
107. Ibid.
108. M. F. Gallo, L. M. Lopez, and D. A. Grimes, et. al., "Combination contraceptives: effects on weight," *Cochrane Database of Systematic Reviews* 2 (2009).
109. Salynn Boyles, "The Pill Won't Add Extra Pounds, Study Shows," January 24, 2006, WebMD Health News, http://www.webmd.com/sex/birth-control/news/20060124/pill-wont-add-pounds-study-shows.

110. Anahad O'Connor, "The Claim: The Pill Can Make You Put On Weight," *New York Times*, January 27, 2007.

111. M. Lofthouse, "Depot medroxyprogesterone acetate for contraception causes weight and fat gain in women," *Nature, Clinical Practice and Metabolism* 1, no. 2 (2005): 69

112. L. M. Lopez, D. A. Grimes, and K. F. Schulz, "Steroidal contraceptives: effect on carbohydrate metabolism in women without diabetes mellitus (Review)," *Cochrane Database of Systematic Reviews* 2 (2009).

113. James Trussell, Eleanor Bimla Schwarz, and Katherine Guthrie, "Obesity and oral contraceptive failure," *Contraception* 79 (2009): 334–38.

114. Bennett, *The Pill: Are You Sure It's For You?*, 56.

115. "Oral Contraceptives Impair Muscle Gains in Young Women," American Physiological Society, April 17, 2009, http://www.the-asp.org/press/releases/09/16.htm.

116. D'Souza, "Risks and benefits of oral contraceptive pills," 146–47.

117. "Taking Birth Control Pills May Place Diabetic Women at Risk for Kidney Disease," American Diabetes Association, http://www.diabetes.org.

118. S. B. Ahmed et al., "Oral Contraceptives, angiotensin-dependent renal vasoconstriction, and the risk of diabetic nephropathy," *Diabetes Care* 28 (2005): 1988–94.

119. World Health Organization (WHO), *Improving access to quality care in family planning: Medical eligibility criteria for contraceptive use* (Geneva: WHO, 2001).

120. Jerilynn C. Prior and Christine L. Hitchcock, "Manipulating Menstruation with Hormonal Contraception—what does the Science say?" CeMCOR, http://www.cemcor.ubc.ca; J. C. Prior, S. Kirkland, L. Joseph, et al., "Oral contraceptive agent use and bone mineral density in premenopausal women: cross-sectional, population-based data from the Canadian Multicentre Osteoporosis Study," *Canadian Medical Association Journal* 165 (2001): 1023–29.

121. Franco Polatti, Francesca Perotti, and Nadia Filippa, et al., "Bone Mass and Long-Term Monophasic Oral Contraceptive Treatment in Young Women," *Contraception* 51 (1995): 221–24.

122. C. Cooper, P. Hannaford, and P. Croft, et al., "Oral contraceptive pill use and fractures in women: A prospective study," *Bone* 14 (1993): 41–45; M. Vessey, J. Mant, R. Painter, "Oral contraception and other factors in relation to hospital referral for fracture—findings in a large cohort study," *Contraception* 57 (1998): 231–35.

123. Ibid.

124. Victoria, interview with author, July 2009.

125. Susan Rako, *No More Periods?* (New York: Harmony Books, 2003), 45–54.

126. D'Souza, "Risks and benefits of oral contraceptive pills," 135–36.

127. Jerilynn Prior, *Estrogen's Storm Season* (Vancouver, BC: Centre for Menstrual Cycle and Ovulation Research, 2005).

128. Dickey, *Managing Contraceptive Pill Patients*, 158; M. J. Rosenberg, and M. S. Waugh, "Oral contraceptive discontinuation: A prospective evaluation of frequency and reasons," American *Journal of Obstetrics & Gynecology* 179 (1998): 577–82.

129. M. F. Gallo, K. Nauda, D. A. Grimes, K. F. Schulz, "20 mcg versus > 20 mcg estrogen combined oral contraceptives for contraception," *Cochrane Database of Systematic Reviews* 2 (2005).

130. Dickey, *Managing Contraceptive Pill Patients*, 160.

131. M. J. Rosenberg, M. S. Waugh, and C. M. Stevens, "Smoking and cycle control among oral contraceptive users," *American Journal of Obstetrics and Gynecology* 174 (1996): 628–32.

132. Jerilynn C. Prior, "Choices for Effective Contraception in 2006," The Center for Menstrual Cycle and Ovulation Research, http://www.cemcor.ubc.ca/print/110.

133. Ibid.

134. Ibid.

135. J. Guillebaud, "Combined oral contraception," in *Handbook for Family Planning*, A. Glasier and A. Gebbie, eds. (London: Churchill Livingstone, 2000).

136. Kurt T. Barnhart, Courtney A. Schreiber, "Return to fertility following discontinuation of oral contraceptives," *Fertility and Sterility* 91, no. 3 (March 2009): 659–63.

137. D'Souza, "Risks and benefits of oral contraceptive pills," 135–36.

138. M. A. M. Hassan and S. R. Killick, "Is previous use of hormonal contraception associated with a detrimental effect on subsequent fecundity?" *Human Reproduction* 19, no. 2 (2004): 344.

139. Dickey, *Managing Contraceptive Pill Patients*, 44.

140. Pope and Bennett, *The Pill: Are You Sure It's For You?*, 99–100.

141. Holly Grigg-Spall, conversation with author, March 31, 2010.

142. Pope and Bennett, *The Pill*, 99.

143. Ibid.

Chapter Three: Hidden in Plain Sight

1. Robert Jütte, *Contraception: A History* (Cambridge, UK, and Malden, MA: Polity Press, 2008), 134.

2. Quoted in Andrea Tone, *Devices and Desires: A History of Contraceptives in America* (New York: Hill and Wang, 2001), 57.

3. Ibid., 117.

4. William D. Mosher, et al., "Use of Contraception and Use of Family Planning Services in the United States: 1982–2002," Advance Data from Vital and Health Statistics, no. 350, December 10, 2004, http://www.cdc.gov/nchs/data/ad/ad350.pdf.

5. "IUDs: Not Scary After All?" October 18, 2005, www.feministing.com.

6. Nancy S. Padian et al., "Diaphragm and Lubricant Gel for Prevention of HIV Acquisition in Southern African Women: A Randomised Controlled Trial," *Lancet* 370, no. 9583 (July 21, 2007): 251–61.

7. "Facts on Contraceptive Use," Guttmacher Institute, January 2008, www.guttmacher .org/pubs/fb_contr_use.html.

8. Quoted in David Crary, "Health Advocates Tout New Model of Female Condom," *TriCity Herald*, April 16, 2009.

9. Ibid.

10. Ibid.

11. Jütte, *Contraception*, 121.

12. William Parker with Rachel L. Parker, *A Gynecologist's Second Opinion* (New York: Plume, 2003), 45.

13. Tone, *Devices and Desires*, 61.

14. Jütte, *Contraception*, 155.
15. Tone, *Devices and Desires*, 263.
16. Jütte, *Contraception*," 207.
17. Tone, *Devices and Desires*, 264.
18. Ibid.
19. Ibid., 265, 266.
20. Private conversation with the author.
21. Tone, *Devices and Desires*, 269.
22. Susan Wood, speech delivered to Law Students for Reproductive Justice (American University School of Law, Washington, DC, February 8, 2009).
23. Tone, *Devices and Desires*, 283.
24. Jacqueline Darroch Forrest, "US Women's Perception of and Attitudes about the IUD," *Obstetrical & Gynecological Survey* 51, no. 12 (December 1996): 30S–34S.
25. Adam Sonfield, "Popularity Disparity: Attitudes about the IUD in Europe and the United States," *Guttmacher Policy Review* 10, no. 4 (Fall 2007): 19–26.
26. "Facts on Contraceptive Use," Guttmacher Institute.
27. Jütte, *Contraception*, 47.
28. Parker, *Gynecologist's Second Opinion*, 46.
29. "IUD," Planned Parenthood, February 10, 2008, www.plannedparenthood.org/health-topics/birth-control/iud-4245.htm.
30. Jerilynn C. Prior, *Estrogen's Strom Season* (Vancouver, BC: CeMCOR, 2005).
31. Mirena package insert, Bayer HealthCare Pharmaceuticals, 2008.
32. Mosher et al., "Use of Contraception," http://www.cdc.gov/nchs/data/ad/ad350.pdf.
33. Parker, *Gynecologist's Second Opinion*, 47.
34. Sonfield, "Popularity Disparity," 19–26.
35. Centers for Disease Control, "About DES," http://www.cdc.gov/DES/consumers/about/index.html.
36. Mirena package insert.
37. Sonfield, "Popularity Disparity," 19–26.
38. Cynthia Pearson, interview by the author, October 19, 2009.
39. Email to the author, October 20, 2009.
40. James Trussell et al., "Cost Effectiveness of Contraceptives in the United States," *Contraception* 79, no. 1 (January 2009): 5–14.
41. Email to the author, June 2008.
42. Tracy Clark-Flory, "Oops, I Accidentally Pulled Out Your IUD!" January 22, 2009, http://www.salon.com/life/broadsheet/index.html?story=/mwt/broadsheet/feature/2009/01/22/iud_abortion.
43. Dorothy Roberts, *Killing the Black Body* (New York: Vintage Books, 1997), 66.
44. Ibid., 89.
45. Ibid., 92.
46. Ibid., 93.
47. Karenna Gore Schiff, *Lighting the Way* (New York: Hyperion, 2005), 372.
48. Ibid., 375.
49. Ibid., 375.

Chapter Four: By Any Other Name

1. Dorothy Roberts, *Killing the Black Body* (New York: Vintage Books, 1999), 139.
2. Ibid.
3. Technically, there are two Norplants: Norplant I, called Norplant, and Norplant II, called Jadell. In this chapter I refer to Norplant I as Norplant and Norplant II as Jadell.
4. Richard P. Dickey, *Managing Contraceptive Pill Patients*, 13th ed. (Dallas, TX: EMIS Medical Publishers, 2007), 100.
5. Andrea Tone, *Devices and Desires: A History of Contraceptives in America* (New York: Hill and Wang, 2001), 288.
6. Conversation with the author, 2000.
7. "Poverty and Norplant: Can Contraception Reduce the Underclass?" *Philadelphia Inquirer*, December 12, 1990, A18.
8. Ibid.
9. Columbia University Mailman School of Public Health, "Issues and Answers—Norplant: Reality Check," *Public Health Magazine* 4, no. 1 (Spring 1996).
10. Barbara Kantrowitz and Pat Wingert, "The Norplant Debate," *Newsweek*, February 15, 1993, 40–41.
11. Sheldon J. Segal, "Norplant Developed for All Women, Not Just the Well-to-Do," *New York Times*, December 29, 1990, A18.
12. Roberts, *Killing the Black Body*, 108.
13. Julia R. Scott, "Norplant and Women of Color," in *Dimensions of New Contraceptives: Norplant and Poor Women*, ed. Sarah E. Samuels and Mark D. Smith (Menlo Park, CA: Henry J. Kaiser Family Foundation, 1992), 39–52.
14. Andrew R. Davidson and Debra Kalmuss, "Topics for Our Times: Norplant Coercion—An Overstated Threat," *American Journal of Public Health* 87, no. 4 (April 1997): 550–51.
15. Ibid.
16. Tone, *Devices and Desires*, 288.
17. Ibid.
18. In other contexts, high-income women and those with good health care coverage are most at risk for the dangers of new drugs. As the line between preventative care and "lifestyle" drugs continues to blur, those with more money are often given unnecessary and potentially dangerous new pills at much higher rates than their low-income peers.
19. Dickey, *Managing Contraceptive Pill Patients*, 100.
20. Sidney Funk et al., "Safety and Efficacy of Implanon, a Single-Rod Implantable Contraceptive Containing Etonogestrel," *Contraception* 71, no. 5 (May 2005): 319–26.
21. Lee P. Shulman and Helena Gabriel, "Management and Localization Strategies for the Nonpalpable Implanon Rod," *Contraception* 73, no. 4 (April 2006): 325–30.
22. Diana Mansour et al., "The Effects of Implanon on Menstrual Bleeding Patterns," *European Journal of Contraception & Reproductive Health Care* 13, suppl. no. 1 (2008): 13–28.
23. Ibid.

24. Practice Committee of the American Society for Reproductive Medicine, "Hormonal Contraception: Recent Advances and Controversies," *Fertility and Sterility* 90, no. 5 (November 2008): S104.

25. Paul D. Blumenthal, Kristina Gemzell-Danielsson, and Maya Marintcheva-Petrova, "Tolerability and Clinical Safety of Implanon," *European Journal of Contraception & Reproductive Health Care* 13, suppl. no. 1 (2008): 29–36.

26. Elsimar M. Coutinho with Sheldon J. Segal, *Is Menstruation Obsolete?* (Oxford and New York: Oxford University Press, 1999), 8–11.

27. Ibid., 9.

28. Rickie Solinger, *Pregnancy and Power: A Short History of Reproductive Politics in America* (New York and London: New York University Press, 2005), 175.

29. Sayed Bakry et al., "Depot-Medroxyprogesterone Acetate: An Update," *Archives of Gynecology and Obstetrics* 278, no.1 (July 2008): 1.

30. Depo-Provera is an intramuscular injection, meaning the shot goes right into the muscle. A subcutaneous injection enters a layer of the skin beneath the dermis and epidermis.

31. Tim Cundy et al., "Menopausal Bone Loss in Long-Term Users of Depot Medroxyprogesterone Acetate Contraception," *American Journal of Obstetrics & Gynecology* 186, no. 5 (May 2002): 978–83.

32. "Black Box Warning Added Concerning Long-Term of Depo-Provera Contraceptive Injection," FDA Talk Paper, Food and Drug Administration, US Department of Health and Human Services, http://www.fda.gov (accessed November 17, 2004).

33. Depo-Provera, patient package insert, 2002.

34. Kathryn M. Curtis and Summer L. Martins, "Progestogen-only Contraception and Bone Mineral Density: A Systematic Review," *Contraception* 73, no. 5 (May 2006): 470–87.

35. Brandon J. Orr-Walker et al., "The Effect of Past Use of the Injectable Contraceptive Depot Medroxyprogesterone Acetate on Bone Mineral Density in Normal Postmenopausal Women," *Clinical Endocrinology* 49, no. 5 (November 1998): 615–18.

36. Andrew M. Kaunitz, Raquel Arias, and Michael McClung, "Bone Density Recovery After Depot Medroxyprogesterone Acetate Injectable Contraception Use," *Contraception* 77, no. 2 (February 2008): 67–76.

37. Edith R. Guilbert et al., "The Use of Depot-Medroxyprogesterone Acetate in Contraception and Its Potential Impact on Skeletal Health," *Contraception* 79, no. 3 (March 2009): 167–77.

38. Dickey, *Managing Contraceptive Pill Patients*, 71.

39. Abbey B. Berenson and Mahbubur Rahman, "Changes in Weight, Total Fat, Percent Body Fat, and Central-to-Peripheral Fat Ratio Associated with Injectable and Oral Contraceptive Use," *American Journal of Obstetrics & Gynecology* 200, no. 3 (March 2009): 329.e1–329.e8.

40. Depo-Provera, patient package insert, 2002.

41. Depo-SubQ Provera 104, physician package insert, 2005.

42. Berenson and Rahman, "Changes in Weight," 329.e1–329.e8.

43. Sharon A. Mangan, Pamela G. Larsen, and Suzanne Hudson, "Overweight Teens at Increased Risk for Weight Gain While Using Depot Medroxyprogesterone Acetate," *Journal of Pediatric and Adolescent Gynecology* 15, no. 2 (April 2002): 79–82.

44. Bakry et al., "Depot-Medroxyprogesterone Acetate," 3.

45. Berenson and Rahman, "Changes in Weight," 329.e1–329.e8.

46. Laura L. Moore et al., "A Comparative Study of One-Year Weight Gain among Users of Medroxyprogesterone Acetate, Levonorgestrel Implants, and Oral Contraceptives," *Contraception* 52, no. 4 (October 1995): 215–19.

47. Berenson and Rahman, "Changes in Weight," 329.e1–329.e8.

48. Bakry et al., "Depot-Medroxyprogesterone Acetate," 4.

49. Dickey, *Managing Contraceptive Pill Patients*, 74.

50. Depo-Provera, patient package insert, 2002.

51. Maria F. Gallo et al., "Combination Injectable Contraceptives for Contraception," *Cochrane Database of Systematic Reviews*, no. 4 (2008), DOI: 10.1002/14651858 .CD004568.pub3.

52. The fifth day of the four-week cycle that patients measure on the calendar, not the fifth day of the menstrual period.

53. George W. Creasy, Larry S. Abrams, and Alan C. Fisher, "Transdermal Contraception," *Seminars in Reproductive Medicine* 19, no. 4, (2001): 374.

54. Dickey, Managing *Contraceptive Pill Patients*, 86.

55. Creasy, Abrams, and Fisher, "Transdermal Contraception," 373–80.

56. Laureen M. Lopez et al., "Skin Patch and Vaginal Ring Versus Combined Oral Contraceptives for Contraception," *Cochrane Database of Systematic Reviews*, no. 3 (2008), DOI: 10.1002/14651858.CD003552.pub2.

57. Ronald T. Burkman, "Transdermal Hormonal Contraception: Benefits and Risks," *American Journal of Obstetrics & Gynecology* 197, no. 2 (August 2007): 134.e1–134.e6.

58. Wolfgang Urdl et al., "Contraceptive Efficacy, Compliance and Beyond: Factors Related to Satisfaction with Once-Weekly Transdermal Compared with Oral Contraception," *European Journal of Obstetrics & Gynecology and Reproductive Biology* 121, no. 2 (August 2005): 202–10.

59. Marie-Claude Audet et al., "Evaluation of Contraceptive Efficacy and Cycle Control of a Transdermal Contraceptive Patch vs. an Oral Contraceptive: A Randomized Controlled Trial," *Journal of the American Medical Association* 285, no. 18 (May 9, 2001): 2347–54.

60. Miriam Zieman et al., "Contraceptive Efficacy and Cycle Control with the Ortho Evra/Evra Transdermal System: The Analysis of Pooled Data," *Fertility and Sterility* 77, suppl. 2 (February 2002): 13–18.

61. Lopez, "Skin Patch and Vaginal Ring."

62. Urdl et al.,"Contraceptive Efficacy," 202–10.

63. US Food and Drug Administration Center for Drug Evaluation and Research, Ortho Evra (norelgestromin/ethinyl estradiol) information, www.fda.gov/NewsEvents/ Newsroom/PressAnnouncements/2005/ucm108517/htm.

64. Susan S. Jick et al., "Risk of Nonfatal Venous Thromboembolism in Women Using a Contraceptive Transdermal Patch and Oral Contraceptives Containing Norgestimate and 35 µg of Ethinyl Estradiol," *Contraception* 73, no. 3 (March 2006): 223–28.

65. Tricia C. Elliott and Cathy C. Montoya, "How Does VTE Risk for the Patch and Vaginal Ring Compare with Oral Contraceptives?" *Journal of Family Practice* 57, no. 10 (October 2008): 680–85.

66. US Food and Drug Administration, "FDA Approves Update to Label on Birth Control Patch," news release, January 18, 2008, www.fda.gov/NewsEvents/Newsroom/ PressAnnouncements/2008/ucm116842.htm.

67. Stephanie Mencimer, "Is NuvaRing Dangerous?" *Mother Jones*, May/June 2009.
68. Associated Press, "Group Asks U.S. to Pull Birth-control Patch from Market," *USA Today*, May 8, 2008, http://www.usatoday.com/news/health/2008-05-08-birth-control_N.htm.
69. See www.orthoevra.com/isi.html (accessed October 5, 2009).
70. Dickey, *Managing Contraceptive Pill Patients*, 82.
71. A. Novák et al., "The Combined Contraceptive Vaginal Ring, NuvaRing: An International Study of User Acceptability," *Contraception* 67, no. 3 (March 2003): 187–94.
72. Jeffery T. Jensen et al., "Effects of Switching from Oral to Transdermal or Transvaginal Contraception on Markers of Thrombosis," *Contraception* 78, no. 6 (December 2008): 451–58.
73. Mencimer, "Is NuvaRing Dangerous?"
74. Ibid.
75. Ibid.
76. Mousumi Bhaduri et al., "The Vaginal Ring: Expelled or Misplaced?" *Journal of Ultrasound in Medicine* 28 (2009): 259–61.
77. Email to the author, June 2008.
78. Bhaduri et al., "The Vaginal Ring," 259–61.
79. Novák, "Combined Contraceptive Vaginal Ring," 187–94.
80. Ragnheidur I. Bjarnadóttir, Marjo Tuppurainen, and Stephen R. Killick, "Comparison of Cycle Control with a Combined Contraceptive Vaginal Ring and Oral Levonorgesterl/Ethinyl Estradiol," *American Journal of Obstetrics & Gynecology* 186, no. 3 (March 2002): 389–95.
81. Email to the author, August 2008.
82. Frans J. M. E. Roumen, "The Contraceptive Vaginal Ring Compared with the Combined Oral Contraceptive Pill: A Comprehensive Review of Randomized Controlled Rrials," *Contraception* 75, no. 6 (June 2007): 420–29.
83. Novák, "Combined Contraceptive Vaginal Ring," 187–94.

Chapter Five: Of Tides and Phases

1. Thomas Buckley and Alma Gottlieb, "A Critical Appraisal of Theories of Menstrual Symbolism," in *Blood Magic: The Anthropology of Menstruation*, ed. Thomas Buckley and Alma Gottlieb (Berkeley and Los Angeles: University of California Press, 1988).
2. Elismar M. Coutinho with Sheldon J. Segal, *Is Menstruation Obsolete?* (Oxford and New York: Oxford University Press, 1999), 17.
3. Gabrielle Hiltmann, "Menstruation in Aristotle's Concept of the Person," in *Menstruation: A Cultural History*, ed. Andrew Shail and Gillian Howie (New York: Palgrave Macmillan, 2005), 27.
4. Quoted in Coutinho with Segal, *Is Menstruation Obsolete?* 18.
5. *Secreta Mulierum*, quoted in Bettina Bildhauer, "The *Secrets of Women* (c. 1300): A Medieval Perspective on Menstruation" in *Menstruation: A Cultural History*, ed. Andrew Shail and Gillian Howie (New York: Palgrave Macmillan, 2005), 66.
6. Ibid.

7. Michael Stolberg, "Menstruation and Sexual Difference in Early Modern Medicine," in *Menstruation: A Cultural History*, ed. Andrew Shail and Gillian Howie (New York: Palgrave Macmillan, 2005), 92.

8. Ibid., 94.

9. Julie-Marie Strange, "'I Believe It to Be a Case Depending on Menstruation': Madness and Menstrual Taboo in British Medical Practice, c. 1840–1930," in *Menstruation: A Cultural History*, ed. Andrew Shail and Gillian Howie (New York: Palgrave Macmillan, 2005), 102.

10. Ibid., 106.

11. Ibid., 103.

12. Anne E. Walker, *The Menstrual Cycle* (London: Routledge, 1997), 30.

13. Ibid., 33.

14. Hubbard, quoted in Walker, *Menstrual Cycle*, 33.

15. James Totherick, quoted in Strange, "'I Believe It to Be a Case Depending on Menstruation,'" 111.

16. Erica Kinentz, "Is Hysteria Real? Brain Imaging Says Yes," *New York Times*, September 26, 2006. www.nytimes.com/2006/09/26/science/26Hysteria.html.

17. Strange, "'I Believe It to Be a Case Depending on Menstruation,'" 113.

18. Sharra L. Vostral, "Masking Menstruation: The Emergence of Menstrual Hygiene Products in the United States," in *Menstruation: A Cultural History*, ed. Andrew Shail and Gillian Howie (New York: Palgrave Macmillan, 2005), 244.

19. Karen Houppert, *The Curse: Confronting the Last Unmentionable Taboo, Menstruation* (New York: Farrar, Straus and Giroux, 1999), 62.

20. Mary Wood-Allen, *Almost a Woman* (Cooperstown, NY: Arthur H. Crist Co., 1915), 5–8.

21. Houppert, *The Curse*, 64.

22. Ibid., 116.

23. Ibid., 95.

24. Buckley and Gottlieb, "A Critical Appraisal," 20.

25. Nelson Soucasaux, "Menstrual Toxin: An Old Name for a Real Thing?" The Museum of Menstruation and Women's Health, 2001, http://www.mum.org/menotox2.htm.

26. Sophie Laws, *Issues of Blood: The Politics of Menstruation* (London: Macmillan Press, Ltd, 1990), 36.

27. Inga Muscio, *Cunt: A Declaration of Independence* (Emeryville, CA: Seal Press, 2002), 35.

28. Margaret Lock, "Cultivating the Body: Anthropology and Epistemologies of Bodily Practice and Knowledge," *Annual Review of Anthropology* 22 (October 1993): 134.

29. Ibid., 135.

30. Buckley and Gottlieb, "A Critical Appraisal," 13.

31. Ray Moynihan and Alan Cassels, "A Disease for Every Pill," *Nation*, September 29, 2005.

32. Laws, *Issues of Blood*, 43.

33. Ibid., 30.

34. Ibid., 64.

35. Ibid., 190.

36. Elizabeth Arveda Kissling, *Capitalizing on the Curse: The Business of Menstruation* (Boulder, CO, and London: Lynne Rienner Publishers, 2006), 1.

37. Houppert, *The Curse*, 8.
38. Nina Darnton and Patrick Rogers, "How Kids Grow: The End of Innocence," *Newsweek*, June 1, 1991.
39. Emily Martin, *The Woman in the Body: A Cultural Analysis of Reproduction* (Boston: Beacon Press, 1987), 49.
40. Houppert, *The Curse*, 77.
41. Laura Kipnis, *The Female Thing: Dirt, Envy, Sex, Vulnerability* (New York: Pantheon, 2006), 120–21.
42. Ibid.

Chapter Six: Spotless

1. Clarissa Kripke, "Cyclic vs. Continuous or Extended-Cycle Combined Contraceptives," Cochrane for Clinicians, *American Family Physician* 73, no. 5 (March 1, 2006): 804.
2. Malcolm Gladwell, "John Rock's Error," *New Yorker*, March 13, 2000, 54.
3. Ibid., 55.
4. Quoted in Deborah Kotz, "FDA Approves Lybrel, a Pill Designed to Stop Menstruation," *U.S. News and World Report*, May 22, 2007.
5. Elsimar M. Coutinho with Sheldon J. Segal, *Is Menstruation Obsolete?* (Oxford and New York: Oxford University Press, 1999), 9.
6. R. V. Short, "The Evolution of Human Reproduction," in *Contraceptives of the Future: A Royal Society Discussion* (London: Royal Society, 1976), 3–24.
7. Ibid., 19
8. R. V. Short, "Reproduction and Human Society," in *Artificial Control of Reproduction*, ed. C. R. Austin and R. V. Short (Oxford: Alden, 1972), 124.
9. Karen Houppert, *The Curse: Confronting the Last Unmentionable Taboo, Menstruation* (New York: Farrar, Straus and Giroux, 1999), 147.
10. Zahra Meghani, "Of Sex, Nationalities and Populations: The Construction of Menstruation as a Patho-Physiology," in *Menstruation: A Cultural History*, ed. Andrew Shail and Gillian Howie (New York: Palgrave Macmillan, 2005), 132.
11. Ibid., 131–32.
12. Coutinho with Segal, *Is Menstruation Obsolete?* xiv.
13. Kathleen O'Grady, review of *Is Menstruation Obsolete?* by Elsimar M. Coutinho with Sheldon J. Segal, *Herizons* (Winter 2000).
14. Elisabeth Beausang, "Childbirth in Prehistory: An Introduction," *European Journal of Archaeology* 3, no. 1 (April 2000): 70.
15. Coutinho with Segal, *Is Menstruation Obsolete?* 15.
16. Zahra Meghani, "Of Sex, Nationalities and Population," 130-45.
17. Coutinho with Segal, *Is Menstruation Obsolete?* 63.
18. Ibid., 71.
19. Ibid., 71.
20. Michael Stolberg, "The Monthly Malady: A History of Premenstrual Suffering," *Medical History* 44, no. 3 (July 2000): 301–22.
21. Ibid., 303.

22. Marni Kwiecien et al., "Bleeding Patterns and Patient Acceptability of Standard or Continuous Dosing Regimens of a Low-Dose Oral Contraceptive: A Randomized Trial," *Contraception* 67, no. 1 (January 2003): 9–13.

23. Susan Rako, *No More Periods?* (New York: Harmony Books, 2003), 46.

24. Meghani, "Of Sex, Nationalities and Populations," 136.

25. Ibid.

26. A. F. Glasier et al., "Amenorrhea Associated with Contraception—An International Study on Acceptability," *Contraception* 67, no. 1 (January 2003): 1–8.

27. Ibid.

28. Linda C. Andrist et al., "Women's and Providers Attitudes Toward Menstrual Suppression with Extended Use of Oral Contraceptives," *Contraception* 70, no. 5 (November 2004): 359–63.

29. F. D. Anderson, Howard Hait, and the Seasonale-301 Study Group, "A Multicenter, Randomized Study of an Extended Cycle Oral Contraceptive," *Contraception* 68, no. 2 (August 2003): 89–96.

30. Kay A. Chitale, Consumer Promotion Analyst and Regulatory Review Officer at the FDA's Division of Drug Marketing, Advertising and Communications, to Joseph Carrado, Senior Director of Regulatory Affairs at Barr Research, Inc., December 29, 2004, http://www.fda.gov/downloads/Drugs/GuidanceComplianceRegulatoryInformation/EnforcementActivitiesbyFDA/WarningLettersandNoticeofViolationLetterstoPharmaceuticalCompanies/ucm054665.pdf.

31. Ibid.

32. Ibid.

33. The study was supported by a grant from Wyeth, and of the scientists performing it, "Drs. David F. Archer, Jeffery T. Jensen and Julia V. Johnson were investigators for this study and received research funding from Wyeth Research." The article notes that "other sources of research funding and/or financial relationships include" a list of over a dozen drug companies and pharmaceutical divisions. Only one of the study's six authors had "no financial affiliations." While such relationships are not uncommon, they are not insignificant.

34. David F. Archer et al., "Evaluation of a Continuous Regimen of Levonorgestrel/Ethinyl Estradiol: Phase 3 Study Results," *Contraception* 74, no. 6 (December 2006): 439–45.

35. Christian Nordqvist, "FDA Does Not Approve Wyeth Contraceptive, Lybrel," *Medical News Today*, June 29, 2006, http://www.medicalnewstoday.com/articles/46224.php.

36. US Food and Drug Administration, "FDA Approves Contraceptive for Continuous Use," news release, May 22, 2007, http://www.fda.gov/NewsEvents/Newsroom/PressAnnouncements/2007/ucm108918.htm.

37. Glasier et al., "Amenorrhea Associated with Contraception," 1.

38. Leslie Miller, Carole H. J. Verhoeven, and Johanna in't Hout, "Extended Regimens of the Contraceptive Vaginal Ring: A Randomized Trial," *Obstetrics & Gynecology* 106, no. 3 (September 2005): 473–82; Fernando Augusto Barreiros et al., "Bleeding Patterns of Women Using Extended Regimens of the Contraceptive Vaginal Ring," *Contraception* 75, no. 3 (March 2007): 204–8.

39. Quoted in Kotz, "FDA Approves Lybrel."

40. Kripke, "Cyclic vs. Continuous or Extended-Cycle," 804.

41. Ibid.

42. Anne R. Davis et al., "Return to Menses After Continuous Use of a Low-Dose Oral Contraceptive," *Obstetrics & Gynecology* 107, suppl. 4 (April 2006): 3S.

43. Society for Menstrual Cycle Research, "Menstruation Is Not a Disease," position statement, June 8, 2007, http://menstruationresearch.org/position-statements/menstrual-supression-2007/.

44. "FDA Black Box Warning" in Richard P. Dickey, *Managing Contraceptive Pill Patients*, 13th ed. (Dallas, TX: EMIS Medical Publishers, 2007), 70.

45. US Food and Drug Administration, "FDA Approves Contraceptive."

46. Rako, *No More Periods?* 20.

47. William H. Parker et al., "Ovarian Conservation at the Time of Hysterectomy for Benign Disease," *Obstetrics & Gynecology* 106, no. 2 (August 2005): 219–26.

48. Society for Menstrual Cycle Research, "Menstruation Is Not a Disease."

49. Ibid.

50. Tracy Clark-Flory, "The End of Menstruation," Salon.com, February 4, 2008, www.salon.com/mwt/feature/2008/02/04/menstruation/print.html.

51. Jaclyn Geller, *Here Comes the Bride: Women, Weddings and the Marriage Mystique* (New York: Four Walls Eight Windows, 2001), 54–63.

52. Society for Menstrual Cycle Research, "Menstruation Is Not a Disease."

53. Clark-Flory, "The End of Menstruation."

54. William Saletan, "Bloodless Revolution: The Abolition of Menstruation," Slate.com, May 26, 2007, http://www.slate.com/id/2166983/.

Chapter Seven: Like Candy

1. L. L. Wynn and James Trussell, "The Social Life of Emergency Contraception in the United States: Disciplining Pharmaceutical Use, Disciplining Sexuality, and Constructing Zygotic Bodies," *Medical Anthropology Quarterly* 20, no. 3 (September 2006): 297.

2. Susan Wood, "Women's Health and the FDA," *New England Journal of Medicine* 353, no. 16 (October 20, 2005): 1650–51.

3. The two morning-after pills would eventually be purchased by the same drugmaker, Barr Pharmaceuticals, and Preven taken off the market.

4. Albert Yuzpe et al., "Post Coital Contraception—A Pilot Study," *Journal of Reproductive Medicine* 13, no. 2 (August 1974): 53–58.

5. W. David Hanger's ex-wife has since accused him, in a notorious *Nation* article, of raping and sodomizing her during their marriage. So perhaps his dark fantasies about sexual offenders stockpiling Plan B for nefarious purposes began at home (Ayelish McGarvey, "Dr. Hager's Family Values," *Nation*, May 30, 2005).

6. Wynn and Trussell, "Social Life of Emergency Contraception," 303.

7. Richard Cohen, "The Doctor Who Didn't Know When to Quit," *Washington Post*, July 17, 2007, A19.

8. Susan Wood, speech delivered to Law Students for Reproductive Justice (American University School of Law, Washington, DC, February 8, 2009).

9. Wynn and Trussell, "Social Life of Emergency Contraception," 304; Government Accountability Office, "Decision Process to Deny Initial Application for Over-the-

Counter Marketing of the Emergency Contraceptive Drug Plan B Was Unusual," Washington, DC, November 2005, report no. GAO-06-109, http://www.gao.gov/new.items/d06109.pdf.

10. Marc Kaufman, "FDA Commissioner Steps Down after Rocky Two-Month Tenure," *Washington Post*, September 24, 2005, A7.

11. Wood, speech delivered to Law Students for Reproductive Justice.

12. Quoted in Kaufman, "FDA Commissioner Steps Down," A7.

13. Wood, "Women's Health and the FDA," 1650–51.

14. Susan Okie, "A To-Do List for the New FDA Commissioner," *New England Journal of Medicine* 360, no. 14 (April 2, 2009): 1373–78.

15. Quoted in Lyndsey Layton, "FDA Commissioner Faces Formidable To-Do List," *Washington Post*, June 17, 2009.

16. Wynn and Trussell, "Social Life of Emergency Contraception," 315 n. 3.

17. Rebekah E. Gee, "Plan B, Reproductive Rights, and Physician Activism," *New England Journal of Medicine* 355, no. 1 (July 6, 2006): 4.

18. Ibid., 5.

19. Ibid., 4.

20. David Crary, "Sales Soar for Morning-After Pill," *Washington Post*, August 22, 2007.

21. Wynn and Trussell, "Social Life of Emergency Contraception," 306.

22. Elisa S. Wells, Mitchell D. Creinin, and Pablo Rodriguez, "From American Idol to Plan B: A Call for a Shift in Priorities," *Contraception* 76, no. 5 (November 2007): 337–38.

23. Cynthia C. Harper et al., "Over-the-Counter Access to Emergency Contraception for Teens," *Contraception* 77, no. 4 (April 2008): 230–33.

24. See http://www.plannedparenthood.org/health-topics/pregnancy/how-pregnancy-happens-4252.htm.

25. Quoted in David G. Savage, "'Conscience' Medical Rule to Take Effect: The Last-Minute Bush Administration Declaration Lets Any Health Worker Refuse to Provide Care," *Los Angeles Times*, December 19, 2008, A18.

26. Robert Pear, "Protests Over a Bush Rule to Protect Health Providers," *New York Times*, November 18, 2008, A14.

27. Ibid.

28. Savage, "'Conscience' Medical Rule," A18.

29. Quoted in Robert Pear, "Abortion Proposal Sets Condition on Aid," *New York Times*, July 15, 2008, A17.

30. Farr A. Curlin et al., "Religion, Conscience, and Controversial Clinical Practices," *New England Journal of Medicine* 356, no. 6 (February 8, 2007): 593–600.

31. Nancy Northup, president of the Center for Reproductive Rights in New York City, letter to the editor, *New York Times*, March 16, 2009.

32. R. Alta Charo, "The Celestial Fire of Conscience—Refusing to Deliver Medical Care," *New England Journal of Medicine* 352, no. 24 (June 16, 2005): 2471–73.

33. Rob Stein, "'Pro-Life' Drugstores Market Beliefs: No Contraceptives for Chantilly Shop," *Washington Post*, June 16, 2008, A01.

34. S. Rovi and N. Shimoni, "Prophylaxis Provided to Sexual Assault Victims Seen at US Emergency Departments," *Journal of the American Medical Women's Association* 57, no. 4 (Fall 2002): 204–7.

35. Valerie Ulene, "Rape's Treatment Gap," *Los Angeles Times*, October 6, 2008, F5.

36. Jennifer Medina, "Connecticut Legislators Approve Contraceptive Pill for Rape Victims," *New York Times*, May 3, 2007, B4.

37. Quoted in Angela Couloumbis, "Bill: Hospitals Must Offer Plan B in Rapes," *Philadelphia Inquirer*, October 3, 2007, B01.

38. Quoted in ibid.

39. Dorothy Roberts, *Killing the Black Body* (New York: Penguin, 1997), 23.

40. Noam N. Levey, "Bush-Era 'Conscience' Rule Gets Another Look; Policy That Lets Health Workers Deny Abortion Care May Be Revoked," *Los Angeles Times*, February 27, 2009, A10.

41. Ibid.

42. Ellen Goodman, "The Endless Game of Family Planning Ping-Pong," *Boston Globe*, January 30, 2009, A17.

43. Ibid.

44. Quoted in Marie McCullough, "Judge Rebukes FDA on Plan B Contraceptive," *Philadelphia Inquirer*, March 24, 2009, A03.

45. Elisa S. Wells, Mitchell D. Creinin, and Pablo Rodriguez, "From American Idol to Plan B: A Call for a Shift in Priorities," *Contraception* 76, no. 5 (November 2007): 337–38.

46. http://www.planbonestep.com/plan-b-prescribers/what-plan-b-is.aspx.

47. John Knowles, "Emergency Contraception," Birth Control Series, Planned Parenthood Federation of America, February 2008.

48. Bhaswati Ghosh et al., "Ectopic Pregnancy Following Levonorgestrel Emergency Contraception: A Case Report," *Contraception* 79, no. 2 (February 2009): 155–57.

49. Rebecca H. Allen and Alisa B. Goldberg, "Emergency Contraception: A Clinical Review," *Clinical Obstetrics and Gynecology* 50, no. 4 (December 2007): 927–36.

50. Quoted in Bridget M. Kuehn, "Group Backs Emergency Contraception," *Journal of the American Medical Association* 295, no. 23 (June 21, 2006): 2708–9.

51. Ibid.

52. Anita L. Nelson and Cindy M. Jaime, "Accuracy of Information Given by Los Angeles County Pharmacies about Emergency Contraceptives to Sham Patient in Need," *Contraception* 79, no. 3 (March 2009): 206–10.

53. Good news for a city where a 2008 Health Department report found that 40 percent of those with multiple partners failed to use a condom during last intercourse and more than one third of women between the ages of eighteen and forty-four neglected to use contraception during their most recent sexual encounter (Kathleen Lucadamo, "Poll: New Yorkers Not Having Safe Sex," *Daily News*, June 25, 2008, 8).

54. Quoted in Jordan Lite, "94% of City Drugstores Have Plan B," *Daily News*, May 21, 2007, 19.

55. Mindelle Jacobs, "Hassle Not over for Plan B Girls," Opinion, *Toronto Sun*, June 24, 2008, 20.

56. Rebekah E. Gee et al., "Behind-the-Counter Status and Availability of Emergency Contraception," *American Journal of Obstetrics and Gynecology* 199, no. 5 (November 2008): 478.e1.

57. Tina R. Raine et al., "Direct Access to Emergency Contraception Through Pharmacies and Effect on Unintended Pregnancy and STIs," *Journal of the American Medical Association* 293, no. 1 (January 5, 2005): 54.

58. Iris F. Litt, "Placing Emergency Contraception in the Hands of Women," *Journal of the American Medical Association* 293, no. 1 (January 5, 2005): 98–99.

59. James Trussell et al., "Emergency Contraceptive Pills: A Simple Proposal to Reduce Unintended Pregnancies," *Family Planning Perspectives* 24, no. 6 (November–December 1992): 269–73.

60. Wells, Creinin, and Rodriguez, "From American Idol to Plan B," 337–38.

61. James Trussell et al., "No Such Thing as an Easy (or EC) Fix," *Contraception* 78, no. 5 (November 2008): 351–54.

62. Mitchell H. Katz et al., "Impact of Highly Active Antiretroviral Treatment on HIV Seroincidence among Men Who Have Sex with Men: San Francisco," *American Journal of Public Health* 92, no. 3 (March 2002): 388–94.

63. Raine et al., "Direct Access to Emergency Contraception," 55; Chelsea B. Polis et al., "Advance Provision of Emergency Contraception for Pregnancy Prevention," *Cochrane Database of Systematic Reviews* (2008), DOI: 10.1002/14651858.cd005497.pub2.

64. Elizabeth G. Raymond and Mark A. Weaver, "Effect of an Emergency Contraceptive Pill Intervention on Pregnancy Risk Behavior," *Contraception* 77, no. 5 (May 2008): 333–36.

65. Tracy Hampton, "Study Examines Effects of Advance Access to Emergency Contraception," *Journal of the American Medical Association* 297, no. 19 (May 16, 2007): 2067–68.

66. Raine et al., "Direct Access to Emergency Contraception," 59.

67. Wynn and Trussell, "Social Life of Emergency Contraception," 315 n. 3.

68. Hampton, "Study Examines Effects," 2067–68.

69. Elizabeth G. Raymond, Jennifer Liku, and Eleanor Bimla Schwarz, "Feasibility of Recruitment for an Efficacy Trial of Emergency Contraceptive Pills," *Contraception* 77, no. 2 (February 2008): 118–21.

70. Lisa M. Williamson, Katie Buston, and Helen Sweeting, "Young Women's Perceptions of Pregnancy Risk and Use of Emergency Contraception: Findings from a Qualitative Study," *Contraception* 79, no. 4 (April 2009): 310–15.

71. Svetlana Osadchuk, "Simply an Issue of Control," *Moscow Times*, April 16, 2008.

72. Colin Brown, "Over-the-Counter Pill Plan," *Independent*, December 13, 2007.

73. Cathy O'Leary, "Call for No-Script Contraceptive Pills Boosted by British Trial," *West Australian*, December 11, 2008, 55.

74. "The Case for Preventing Ovarian Cancer," *Lancet* 371, no. 9609 (January 26, 2008): 275.

75. Ibid.

76. Quoted in Cathy O'Leary, "Push to Sell Pill Over the Counter," *West Australian*, January 26, 2008, 1.

77. Amy Allina, interview with author, October 2, 2009.

78. Quoted in Lucy Cockcroft, "Easy Access to Pill 'Will Not Cut Teen Pregnancies,'" *Daily Telegraph*, December 24, 2008, 8.

79. Ibid.

80. Amy Allina, interview with author, October 2, 2009.

81. Guttmacher Institute, "State Policies in Brief as of July 1, 2008, Insurance Coverage of Contraceptives," www.guttmacher.org/statecenter/spibs/spib_ICC.pdf. July 14, 2008.

82. "Contraception," Law Students for Reproductive Justice: Fact Sheet, 2008.

83. Guttmacher Institute, "State Policies in Brief."

84. Rachel Benson Gold, "Stronger Together: Medicaid, Title X Bring Different Strengths to Family Planning Effort," *Guttmacher Policy Review* 10, no. 2 (Spring 2007): 13–18, http://guttmacher.org/pubs/gpr/10/2/gpr100213.html.

85. Gretchen Borchelt, speech delivered to Law Students for Reproductive Justice at the 2009 DC/South Regional Conference (Washington College of Law, Washington, DC, February 8, 2009).

Chapter Eight: Running in Cycles

1. J. Lindholm and E. Husted Nielsen, "Pituitary-Gonadal Axis: Historical Notes," *Pituitary* 12, no. 3 (September 2009): 227.

2. Helen Blackman, "Embryological and Agricultural Constructions of the Menstrual Cycle, 1890–1910," in *Menstruation: A Cultural History*, ed. Andrew Shail and Gillian Howie (New York: Palgrave Macmillian, 2005), 119–20.

3. Janet Farrell Brodie, *Contraception and Abortion in 19th-Century America* (Ithaca, NY: Cornell University Press, 1994), 80–81.

4. Robert Jütte, *Contraception: A History* (Cambridge, UK, and Malden, MA: Polity, 2008), 204.

5. Katie Singer, *The Garden of Fertility* (New York: Avery, 2004), 226–27.

6. The descriptions I offer of each method are not comprehensive. Before using any method of birth control—natural or otherwise—you should always talk to your doctor or health care professional. This chapter is not intended to serve as a guide to these practices.

7. Marianne C. Burkhart et al., "Incidence of Irregular Cycles among Mayan Women Who Reported Having Regular Cycles: Implications for Fertility Awareness Methods," *Contraception* 59, no. 4 (April 1999): 271.

8. Ibid., 274.

9. Marcos Arévalo, Irit Sinai, and Victoria Jennings, "A Fixed Formula to Define the Fertile Window of the Menstrual Cycle as the Basis of a Simple Method of Natural Family Planning," *Contraception* 60, no. 6 (December 1999): 357–60.

10. James N. Gribble, "The Standard Days Method of Family Planning: A Response to Cairo," *International Family Planning Perspectives* 29, no. 4 (December 2003): 188–91.

11. Quoted in Alison Stein Wellner, "A New Bead on Birth Control," *Washington Post*, July 13, 2004, HE01.

12. Marcos Arévalo, Victoria Jennings, and Irit Sinai, "Efficacy of a New Method of Family Planning: The Standard Days Method," *Contraception* 65, no. 5 (May 2002): 336.

13. Irit Sinai, Victoria Jennings, and Marcos Arévalo, "The Importance of Screening and Monitoring: The Standard Days Method and Cycle Regularity," *Contraception* 69, no. 3 (March 2004): 201–6.

14. Wellner, "New Bead on Birth Control," HE01.

15. Toni Weschler, interview with author, March 19, 2009.

16. Feminist Women's Health Center, "Fertility Awareness," http://www.birth-control-comparison.info/fam.htm.

17. Katie Singer, *Honoring Our Cycles: A Natural Family Planning Workbook* (Winona Lake, IN: New Trends Publishing, 2006), 24.

18. D. B. Dunson, I. Sinai, and B. Colombo, "The Relationship between Cervical Secretions and the Daily Probabilities of Pregnancy: Effectiveness of the TwoDay Algorithm," *Human Reproduction* 16, no. 11 (November 2001): 2278–82.

19. Marcos Arévalo et al., "Efficacy of the New TwoDay Method of Family Planning," *Fertility and Sterility* 82, no. 4 (October 2004): 885.

20. Ibid.

21. Katie Singer, "Cycles of Hot and Cold: Trying to Learn Fertility Awareness in North America," in *For Women Only!* ed. Gary Null and Barbara Seaman (New York: Seven Stories Press, 2000), 1115.

22. Ibid., 1117.

23. Toni Weschler, *Taking Charge of Your Fertility: The Definitive Guide to Natural Birth Control and Pregnancy Achievement* (New York: HarperCollins, 2000).

24. Richard J. Fehring, Kathleen Raviele, and Mary Schneider, "A Comparison of the Fertile Phase as Determined by the Clearplan Easy Fertility Monitor and Self-Assessment of Cervical Mucus," *Contraception* 69, no. 1 (January 2004): 9–14.

25. Weschler, interview with author.

26. Weschler, *Taking Charge of Your Fertility*, 78.

27. P. Frank-Herrmann et al., "The Effectiveness of a Fertility Awareness Based Method to Avoid Pregnancy in Relation to a Couple's Sexual Behaviour During the Fertile Time: A Prospective Longitudinal Study," *Human Reproduction* 22, no. 5 (May 2007): 1310–19.

28. Quoted in "Natural Family Planning Method as Effective as Contraceptive Pill, New Research Finds," *ScienceDaily*, February 21, 2007, http://www.sciencedaily.com/releases/2007/02/070221065200.htm (accessed February 16, 2009).

29. James Trussell, "Contraceptive Failure in the United States," *Contraception* 70, no. 2 (August 2004): 90.

30. David A. Grimes et al., "Fertility Awareness-Based Methods for Contraception: Systematic Review of Randomized Controlled Trials," *Contraception* 72, no. 2 (August 2005): 85–90.

31. Weschler, *Taking Charge of Your Fertility*, 128.

32. Toni Weschler, *Cycle Savvy: The Smart Teen's Guide to the Mysteries of Her Body* (New York: Collins, 2006).

33. Quoted in Maia Szalavitz, "Girls Fertility Chartbook Stirs Debate," *Washington Post*, March 20, 2007.

34. Catherine Price, "Fertility Charting 101," Salon.com, March 20, 2007, www.salon.com/mwt/broadsheet/2007/03/20/cycle_savvy/print.html.

35. Beth Roth, "Fertility Awareness as a Component of Sexuality Education: Preliminary Research Findings with Adolescents," *Nurse Practitioner* 18, no. 3 (March 1993): 47.

36. Marcos Arévalo, "Expanding the Availability and Improving Delivery of Natural Family Planning Services and Fertility Awareness Education: Providers' Perspectives," *Advances in Contraception* 13, nos. 2–3 (June 1997): 278.

37. Singer, *Garden of Fertility*, xxvi.

Chapter Nine: One Less?

1. Alan K. Cassels, letter, *Canadian Medical Association Journal* 177, no. 12 (December 4, 2007): 1526.
2. Victoria Stagg Elliott, "Dr. Pap's Smear: The Test and Its Times," *American Medical News*, September 3, 2007, http://www.ama-assn.org/amednews/2007/09/03/hlsa0903.htm.
3. George N. Papanicolaou and Herbert F. Traut, "The Diagnostic Value of Vaginal Smears in Carcinoma of the Uterus," *American Journal of Obstetrics and Gynecology* 42, no. 2 (August 1941); 193–206.
4. Quoted in Elliott, "Dr. Pap's Smear."
5. Ibid.
6. "Cervical Cancer Statistics," Centers for Disease Control and Prevention, http://www.cdc.gov/cancer/cervical/statistics/.
7. Jenny Johnston, "Our Very Modern Dilemma," *Daily Mail*, April 16, 2007, 26.
8. Kerry Gillespie, "Girls to Get Cancer Vaccine; McGuinty to Announce Cervical Cancer Program for Up to 84,000 Grade 8 Students across Ontario," *Toronto Star*, August 2, 2007, A01.
9. Catherine Boyle, "Reports Grow of Adverse Reactions to Cancer Vaccine," *Business*, October 20, 2007.
10. Carolyn D. Runowicz, "Molecular Screening for Cervical Cancer—Time to Give Up Pap Tests?" *New England Journal of Medicine* 357, no. 16 (October 18, 2007): 1650.
11. Jan M. Agosti and Sue J. Goldie, "Introducing HPV Vaccine in Developing Countries—Key Challenges and Issues," *New England Journal of Medicine* 356, no. 19 (May 10, 2007): 1909.
12. Sigrid Fry-Revere, "The Rush to Vaccinate," *New York Times*, March 25, 2007, Opinion section, 17, http://www.nytimes.com/2007/03/25/opinion/25Clfry-revere.htm.
13. Marie-Hélène Mayrand et al., "Human Papillomavirus DNA versus Papanicolaou Screening Tests for Cervical Cancer," *New England Journal of Medicine* 357, no. 16 (October 18, 2007): 1579–1588.
14. American Cancer Society, "Thinking about Testing for HPV?" revised January 18, 2008,www.cancer.org/docroot/CRI/content/CRI_2_6x_Thinking_About_Testing_for_HPV.asp.
15. James Morgan, "'This Is a Great Thing for Women'; The Scottish Biochemist Who Discovered a Vaccine against Cervical Cancer Talks to James Morgan," *Herald* (Scotland), July 3, 2007, 11.
16. Laura A. Koutsky et al., "A Controlled Trial of a Human Papillomavirus Type 16 Vaccine," *New England Journal of Medicine* 347, no. 21 (November 21, 2002): 1645–51; Food and Drug Administration, Gardasil (quadrivalent human papillomavirus [types 6, 11, 16, 18] recombinant vaccine), package insert, Whitehouse Station, NJ: Merck & Co; 2006, http://www.fda.org/BiologicsBloodVaccines/Vaccines/ApprovedProducts/UCM094042.
17. FDA, "FDA licenses new vaccine for prevention of cervical cancer and other diseases in females caused by human papaloma virus," June 8, 2006, http://www.fda.gov/NewsEvents/Newsroom/PressAnnouncements/2006/ucm108666.htm.
18. André Picard, "How Politics Pushed the HPV Vaccine," *Globe and Mail* (Toronto), August 11, 2007, Health section, A1.
19. Thomas Ginsberg, "Glaxo Asks Cervarix Approval," *Philadelphia Inquirer*, March 30, 2007, C01.

20. Karen Attwood, "Glaxo Wins EU Approval for Cervical Cancer Vaccine," *Independent* (London), September 25, 2007, 42.
21. Bridget M. Kuehn, "CDC Panel Backs Routine HPV Vaccination," *Journal of the American Medical Association* 296, no. 6 (August 9, 2006): 640.
22. Ibid.
23. Walter A. Orenstein and Alan R. Hinman, "The Immunization System in the United States—The Role of School Immunization Laws," *Vaccine* 17, suppl. 3 (October 1999): S22.
24. Quoted in Gregory Lopes, "HPV Vaccine Concerns Give Legislatures Pause," *Washington Times*, April 25, 2007, A01.
25. "Texas' Perry Allows Ban of HPV Order," *Wall Street Journal*, May 9, 2007, 2.
26. Elisabeth Rosenthal, "Drug Makers' Push Leads to Cancer Vaccines' Rise," *New York Times,* August 20, 2008, A1.
27. Ibid.
28. Pam Belluck, "In New Hampshire, Soft Sell Eases Vaccine Fears," *New York Times,* May 12, 2007, 1.
29. Gillespie, "Girls to Get Cancer Vaccine," A01.
30. Quoted in Picard, "How Politics Pushed the HPV Vaccine," A1.
31. Paul Stokes, "Nine-Year-Olds Offered Cervical Cancer Vaccine," *Daily Telegraph* (London), December 28, 2007, 10.
32. Tory Shepherd, "Warning on Cancer Screening Myth," *Advertiser* (Adelaide, Australia), January 4, 2008, 11.
33. Lopes, "HPV Vaccine Concerns," A01.
34. Rosenthal, "Drug Makers' Push," A1.
35. Ibid.
36. Antonia Zerbisias, "Pap Smears Are First Line of Defense," *Toronto Star*, August 23, 2007, L01.
37. Angela Cullen, Bloomberg News, "An Anti-Cancer Bonanza for Merck," *International Herald Tribune*, October 5, 2007, 15.
38. André Picard, "Why Politics and Public Health Don't Mix," *Globe and Mail* (Toronto), February 21, 2008, L6.
39. Ibid.
40. Janelle Miles, "Academic Ordered to Apologise—Free Speech under Attack, Say Doctors," *Courier-Mail* (Queensland), April 8, 2008, 19.
41. "Gardasil Now Approved in 80 countries," *Pharma Marketletter*, July 30, 2007.
42. Rosenthal, "Drug Makers' Push," A1.
43. Abby Lippman et al., "Human Papillomavirus, Vaccines and Women's Health: Questions and Cautions," *Canadian Medical Association Journal* 177, no. 5 (August 28, 2007): 485.
44. Clare Masters, "Gardasil Inventor Breaks Silence," *Daily Telegraph* (New South Wales), May 26, 2007, 5.
45. Kate Sikora, "Bulletproof Girls—Cervical Cancer Vaccine Hailed a Success," *Daily Telegraph* (New South Wales), July 23, 2008, 5.
46. Tracy Hampton, "Attacking Cervical Cancer," *Journal of the American Medical Association* 269, no. 4 (July 26, 2006): 384.

47. Lawrence O. Gostin and Catherine D. DeAngelis, "Mandatory HPV Vaccination: Public Health vs. Private Wealth," *Journal of the American Medical Association* 297, no. 17 (May 2, 2007): 1921–23.

48. Fry-Revere, "Rush to Vaccinate," 17.

49. FUTURE II Study Group, "Quadrivalent Vaccine against Human Paillomavirus to Prevent High-Grade Cervical Lesions," *New England Journal of Medicine* 356, no. 19 (May 10, 2007): 1915–27.

50. George F. Sawaya and Karen Smith-McCune, "HPV Vaccination—More Answers, More Questions," *New England Journal of Medicine* 356, no. 19 (May 10, 2007): 1991.

51. John Carreyrou, "Questions on Efficacy Cloud a Cancer Vaccine," *Wall Street Journal*, April 16, 2007.

52. Gostin and DeAngelis, "Mandatory HPV Vaccination," 1921–23.

53. Rita Rubin, "Study: Cervical Cancer Vaccine Less Effective in Sexually Active," *USA Today*, May 10, 2007, 9D.

54. Runowicz, "Molecular Screening for Cervical Cancer," 1650.

55. Picard, "How Politics Pushed the HPV Vaccine," A1.

56. Diane M. Harper et al., "Efficacy of a Bivalent L1 Virus-like Particle Vaccine in Prevention of Infection with Human Papillomavirus Types 16 and 18 in Young Women: A Randomised Controlled Trial," *Lancet* 364, no. 9447 (November 13, 2004): 1757–65.

57. Gostin and DeAngelis, "Mandatory HPV Vaccination," 1921–23.

58. Eileen F. Dunne et al., "Prevalence of HPV Infection among Females in the United States," *Journal of the American Medical Association* 279, no. 8 (February 28, 2007): 813–19.

59. Ibid.

60. Allan Hildesheim et al., "Effect of Human Papillomavirus 16/18 L1 Viruslike Particle Vaccine among Young Women with Preexisting Infection: A Randomized Trial," *Journal of the American Medical Association* 298, no. 7 (August 15, 2007): 743–53.

61. Lippman et al., "Human Papillomavirus," 485.

62. Charlotte J. Haug, "Human Papillomavirus Vaccination—Reasons for Caution," *New England Journal of Medicine* 359, no. 8 (August 21, 2008): 861.

63. Lopes, "HPV Vaccine Concerns," A01.

64. Diana Zuckerman, interview with author, October 20, 2009.

65. Ibid.

66. Rachel L. Winer et al., "Genital Human Papillomavirus Infection: Incidence and Risk Factors in a Cohort of Female University Students," *American Journal of Epidemiology* 157, no. 3 (2003): 218–26.

67. Rachel L. Winer et al., "Condom Use and the Risk of Genital Human Papillomavirus Infection in Young Women," *New England Journal of Medicine* 354, no. 25 (June 22, 2006): 2645.

68. Lindsey R. Baden et al., "Human Papillomavirus Vaccine—Opportunity and Challenge," *New England Journal of Medicine* 356, no. 19 (May 10, 2007): 1190–91.

69. Haug, "Human Papillomavirus Vaccination," 861.

70. Doctor Gifford-Jones, "Guard against STDs and Cancer Deaths," *Toronto Sun*, April 14, 2007, 30.

71. "Merck's Gardasil Hits a Snag," *Wall Street Journal*, January 12, 2009, B4.

72. "FDA Rejects Wider Patient Age Group for Merck & Co's Gardasil," *Pharma Marketletter*, June 26, 2008.

73. Janelle Miles, "Pap Smears Better Than Vaccines for Older Women, Says Doctor," *Courier-Mail* (Queensland), May 5, 2008, 11.

74. Rita Rubin, "O Babies, Where Are Thou?" *USA Today*, July 3, 2008, 4D.

75. Ginsberg, "Glaxo Asks Cervarix Approval," C01.

76. Matthew M. Davis et al., "Childhood Vaccine Purchase Costs in the Public Sector: Past Trends, Future Expectations," *American Journal of Public Health* 92, no. 12 (December 2002): 1982–87; Andrew Pollack, "In Need of a Booster Shot; Rising Costs Make Doctors Balk at Giving Vaccines," *New York Times*, March 24, 2007, C1.

77. Miriam Hill, "Gardasil for Males? Report Hikes Hopes," *Philadelphia Inquirer*, November 14, 2008, D01.

78. Maria Moscaritolo, "Is It Safe to Inject Our Girls?" *Advertiser* (South Australia), May 24, 2007, 21.

79. Quoted in Melinda Tankard Reist and Renate Klein, "Why Are We Experimenting with Drugs on Australian Girls?" *Age* (Melbourne), May 25, 2007, 13.

80. "Activist Group Reveals Gardasil AE Data," *Pharma Marketletter*, May 31, 2007.

81. Gina S. Ogilvie et al., "Parental Intention to Have Daughters Receive the Human Papillomavirus Vaccine," *Canadian Medical Association Journal* 177, no. 12 (December 4, 2007): 1506.

82. Charlie Fidelman, "Vaccination Push Failing in Ontario," *Gazette* (Montreal), November 22, 2007, A8.

83. André Picard, "Why Politics and Public Health Don't Mix," L6.

84. Rebecca Smith, "Two Girls Die after Cervical Cancer Jab," *Daily Telegraph* (London), January 25, 2008.

85. "Clinical Brief: Gardasil to Continue," *Chemist and Druggist*, February 28, 2009.

86. Anne Karpf, "The State Wants My Daughter to be Vaccinated, but I Want to Know More," *Guardian* (London), March 1, 2008, 5.

87. Ian Munro with Nick Miller, "Link between Cancer Jabs and Deaths in US Rejected," *Age* (Melbourne), July 2, 2008, 11.

88. Julia M. L. Brotherton, et al., "Anaphylaxis Following Quadrivalent Human Papillomavirus Vaccination," *Canadian Medical Association Journal* 179, no. 6 (September 9, 2008): 525–33.

89. Ibid., 529.

90. Neal A. Halsey, "The Human Papillomavirus Vaccine and Risk of Anaphylaxis," *Canadian Medical Association Journal* 179, no. 6 (September 9, 2008): 509.

91. Amy Fagan, "Merck, FDA Expand Gardasil Warnings," *Washington Times*, July 10, 2008, A03.

92. Louise Hall, "Cancer Jab Linked to Pancreas Disease," *Canberra Times*, August 17, 2008, 14.

93. "NVIC [National Vaccine Information Center] Says Government Denies Gardasil Risks," *Drug Week*, November 14, 2008, 2111.

94. "Guillain-Barre Syndrome," Mayo Clinic, May 30, 2009, http://www.mayoclinic.com/health/guillain-barre-syndrome/DS00413.

95. Halsey, "Human Papillomavirus Vaccine," 510.

96. "Sting in Cancer Shot: Girls Report Pain from Gardasil Vaccine," *Herald Sun* (Melbourne, Australia), January 5, 2008.

97. From the Centers for Disease Control and Prevention, Morbidity and Mortality Weekly Report, "Syncope after Vaccination—United States, January 2005–July 2007," *Journal of the American Medical Association* 229, no. 21 (June 4, 2008): 2505.

98. Quoted in Alexandra M. Stewart, letter to the editor, "Mandating HPV Vaccination—Private Rights, Public Good," *New England Journal of Medicine* 356, no. 19 (May 10, 2007): 1998.

99. Lee Hui Chieh, "Safe to Use New Cervical Cancer vaccine," *Straits Times* (Singapore), April 4, 2007.

100. Ogilvie et al., "Parental Intention," 1506.

101. R. Alta Charo, "Politics, Parents, and Prophylaxis—Mandating HPV Vaccination in the United States," *New England Journal of Medicine* 356, no. 19 (May 10, 2007): 1907.

102. Karpf, "The State Wants My Daughter to Be Vaccinated," 5.

103. Ibid.

104. Gostin and DeAngelis, "Mandatory HPV Vaccination," 1921–23.

105. Elizabeth Leyland, "Human Papillomavirus Vaccination: Stabbing in the Dark?" *Lancet* 372, no. 9639 (August 23, 2008): 614.

106. Johnston, "Our Very Modern Dilemma," 26; Fry-Revere, "The Rush to Vaccinate," 17.

107. Gostin and DeAngelis, "Mandatory HPV Vaccination," 1921–23.

108. Quoted in Dawn Rae Downton, "A Cancer Vaccine with Political Will; Marketing Conquers Science, HPV Critics Say," *National Post* (Ontario), August 7, 2007, A1.

109. Carole R. McCann, *Birth Control Politics in the United States* (Ithaca, NY, and London: Cornell University Press, 1994), 44.

110. Quoted in Amy Luft, "Justify Your Existence: Abby Lippman. The Canadian Women's Health Network Has Some Concerns about the Government's Plan to Offer Mass Inoculations against HPV; Has the HPV Vaccine Been Overhyped?" *Gazette* (Montreal), April 26, 2008, B2.

111. Marisa Treviño, "Immigrants Given No Choice on Vaccine," *USA Today*, October 17, 2008, 11A.

112. Quoted in Mary Engel, "Immigrants' Advocates Decry Gardasil Requirement," *Los Angeles Times*, October 22, 2008, A9.

113. Quoted in ibid.

114. Abigail Shefer et al., "Early Experience with Human Papillomavirus Vaccine Introduction in the United States, Canada and Australia," *Vaccine* 26, suppl. 10 (August 19, 2008): K69.

115. Rosenthal, "Drug Makers' Push," A1.

116. Thomas H. Maugh II, "Cervical Cancer Vaccination Rate at 25%, U.S. Says," *Los Angeles Times,* October 10, 2008, A17.

117. Mona Saraiya et al., "Cervical Cancer Incidence in a Prevaccine Era in the United States, 1998–2002," *Obstetrics & Gynecology* 109, no. 2, pt. 1 (February 2007): 360–70.

118. Rosenthal, "Drug Makers' Push," A1.

119. Maggie Fox, "Merck-Sponsored Study Suggests HPV Vaccine Benefits Men Too," *Globe and Mail* (Toronto), November 14, 2008, L4.

120. Quoted in James Cowan, "HPV Vaccine Prevents Genital Lesions in Men, Merck Study Claims; Market Expansion?" *National Post* (Ontario), November 14, 2008, A6.

121. Email to the author, October 21, 2009.

122. Stina Syrjänen, "Human Papillomaviruses in Head and Neck Carcinomas," *New England Journal of Medicine* 356, no. 19 (May 10, 2007): 1994.

123. Zerbisias, "Pap smears Are First Line of Defense," L02.

124. Jan Hoffman, "Vaccinating Boys for Girls' Sake?" *New York Times*, February 24, 2008, Fashion & Style section, 1, http://www.nytimes.com/2008/02/24/fashion/24virus.html.

125. Quoted in ibid.

126. Sue J. Goldie et al., "Cost-Effectiveness of Cervical-Cancer Screening in Five Developing Countries," *New England Journal of Medicine* 353, no. 20 (November 17, 2005): 2158–68.

127. Mark Schiffman and Philip E. Castle, "The Promise of Global Cervical-Cancer Prevention," *New England Journal of Medicine* 353, no. 20 (November 17, 2005): 2101–4.

128. Agosti and Goldie, "Introducing HPV Vaccine in Developing Countries," 1908.

129. Rosenthal, "Drug Makers' Push," A1.

130. Karl Stark, "Cancer Vaccine Donation," *Philadelphia Inquirer*, September 27, 2007, C02.

131. Agosti and Goldie, "Introducing HPV Vaccine in Developing Countries," 1909.

132. Eric J. Suba and Stephen S. Raab, letter to the editor, *New England Journal of Medicine* 357, no. 11 (September 13, 2007): 1155.

133. Anna Koulova et al., "Country Recommendations on the Inclusion of HPV Vaccines in National Immunization Programmes among High-Income Countries, June 2006–January 2008," *Vaccine* 26, no. 51 (December 2, 2008): 6530.

134. Ibid.

Chapter Ten: What About the Boys

1. Barbara Seaman and Gideon Seaman, *Women and the Crisis in Sex Hormones* (New York: Bantam, 1978), 325.

2. Ibid., 301.

3. Interview in *The Pill*, directed by Erna Buffie and Elsie Swerhone (Montreal: National Film Board of Canada, 1999).

4. Elizabeth Siegel Watkins, *On the Pill: A Social History of Oral Contraceptives, 1950–1970* (Baltimore and London: Johns Hopkins University Press, 1998), 20.

5. Gregory Pincus, *The Control of Fertility* (New York: Academic Press, 1965), 194.

6. Nelly Oudshoorn, *The Male Pill* (Durham, NC, and London: Duke University Press, 2003), 23.

7. Lara V. Marks, "Human Guinea Pigs? The History of Early Oral Contraceptive Clinical Trials," *History and Technology* 15, no. 4 (1999): 270–71.

8. Oudshoorn, *Male Pill*, 31.

9. Ibid., 32.

10. Zahra Meghani, "Of Sex, Nationalities and Populations: The Construction of Menstruation as a Patho-Physiology," in *Menstruation: A Cultural History*, ed. Andrew Shail and Gillian Howie (New York: Palgrave Macmillan, 2005), 130–45.

11. *The Pill*, directed by Erna Buffie and Elsie Swerhone (Montreal: National Film Board of Canada, 1999).

12. Y. Wong, Y. Lous, and X. Tang, "Studies on the Antifertility Actions of Cottonseed Meal and Gossypol," *Acta Pharmacologica Sinica* 14 (1979): 662–66.

13. Elsimar Metzker Coutinho, "Gossypol: A Contraceptive for Men," *Contraception* 65, no. 4 (April 2002): 259.

14. G. Z. Liu, C. K. Lyle, and J. Cao, "Trial of Gossypol as a Male Contraceptive," in *Gossypol: A Potential Contraceptive for Men*, ed. S. J. Segal (New York: Plenum Press, 1985), 9–16.

15. Coutinho, "Gossypol," 259.

16. Michelle Goldberg, *The Means of Reproductions: Sex, Power and the Future of the World* (New York: Penguin Press, 2009), 6.

17. Steven W. Sinding, "What Has Happened to Family Planning Since Cairo and What Are the Prospects for the Future?" *Contraception* 78, no. 4 (October 2008): S3–S6.

18. Meika Loe, *The Rise of Viagra: How the Little Blue Pill Changed Sex in America* (New York and London: New York University Press, 2004).

19. Dorothy Bonn, "Male Contraceptive Research Steps Back into Spotlight," *Lancet* 353, no. 9149 (January 23, 1998): 302.

20. Michael J. K. Harper, "Public-Private Partnerships Advance Contraceptive Research and Development," *Contraception* 78, no. 4 (October 2008): S36–S41.

21. C. W. Martin et al., "Potential Impact of Hormonal Male Contraception: Cross-Cultural Implications for Development of Novel Preparations," *Human Reproduction* 15, no. 3 (March 2000): 637–45.

22. A. F. Glasier et al., "Would Women Trust Their Partners to Use a Male Pill?" *Human Reproduction* 15, no. 3 (March 2000): 646–49.

23. *In Their Own Right: Addressing the Sexual and Reproductive Health Needs of Men Worldwide* (New York: Alan Guttmacher Institute, 2003), 29–30.

24. Oudshoorn, *Male Pill*, 122.

25. Klaas Heinemann et al., "Attitudes Toward Male Fertility Control: Results of a Multinational Survey on Four Continents," *Human Reproduction* 20, no. 2 (2005): 549–56.

26. Jacqueline E. Darroch, "Male Fertility Control—Where Are the Men?" *Contraception* 78, no. 4 (October 2008): S12.

27. Ibid., S7–S17.

28. Jacqueline E. Darroch, "Family Planning: A Century of Change," in *Silent Victories: The History and Practice of Public Health in Twentieth Century America*, ed. J. W. Ward and C. Warren (New York: Oxford University Press, 2006), 253–78.

29. Karin Ringheim, "Reversing the Downward Trend in Men's Share of Contraceptive Use," *Reproductive Health Matters* 7, no. 14 (November 1999): 83–96.

30. Darroch, "Male Fertility Control," S7–S17.

31. Barbara Seaman and Laura Eldridge, *The No-Nonsense Guide to Menopause* (New York: Simon and Schuster, 2008), 388.

32. Oudshoorn, *Male Pill*, 108.

33. John K. Amory, "Progress and Prospects in Male Hormonal Contraception," *Current Opinion in Endocrinology, Diabetes and Obesity* 15, no. 3 (June 2008): 255–60.

34. World Health Organization Task Force on Methods for the Regulation of Male Fertility, "Contraceptive Efficacy of Testosterone-Induced Azoospermia in Normal Men," *Lancet* 336, no. 8721 (October 20, 1990): 955–59.

35. World Health Organization Task Force on Methods for the Regulation of Male Fertility, "Contraceptive Efficacy of Testosterone-Induced Azoospermia and Oligozoospermia in Normal Men," *Fertiltiy and Sterility* 65, no. 4 (April 1996): 821–29.

36. D. M. Brady et al., "A Multicentre Study Investigating Subcutaneous Etonogestrel Implants with Injectable Testosterone Decanoate as a Potential Long-Acting Male Contraceptive," *Human Reproduction* 21, no. 1 (January 2006): 285–94.

37. Yi-Qun Gu et al., "A Multicenter Contraceptive Efficacy Study of Injectable Testosterone Undecanoate in Healthy Chinese Men," *Journal of Clinical Endocrinology & Metabolism* 88, no. 2 (February 2003): 562–68.

38. Axel Kamischke et al., "Intramuscular Testosterone Undecanoate and Norethisterone Enanthate in a Clinical Trial for Male Contraception," *Journal of Clinical Endocrinology & Metabolism* 86, no. 1 (January 2001): 303–9.

39. John K. Amory et al., "Acceptability of a Combination Testosterone Gel and Depomedroxyprogesterone Acetate Male Contraceptive Regimen," *Contraception* 75, no. 3 (March 2007): 218–23.

40. David A. Grimes et al., "Steroid Hormones for Contraception in Men: Systematic Review of Randomized Controlled Trials," *Contraception* 71, no. 2 (February 2005): 89–94.

41. Diana Blithe, "Male Contraception: What Is on the Horizon?" *Contraception* 78, no. 4 (October 2008): S23–S27.

42. Stephanie T. Page, John K. Amory, and William J. Bremner, "Advances in Male Contraception," *Endocrine Reviews* 29, no. 4 (2008): 465–93.

43. Regine Sitruk-Ware, "Contraception: An International Perspective," *Contraception* 73, no. 3 (March 2006): 220.

44. Coutinho, "Gossypol," 260.

45. Guang-Hui Cui et al., "A Combined Regimen of Gossypol Plus Methyltestosterone and Ethinylestradiol as a Contraceptive Induces Germ Cell Apoptosis and Expression of its Related Genes in Rats," *Contraception* 70, no. 4 (October 2004): 335–42; Zhan-Jun Yang et al., "Combined Administration of Low-Dose Gossypol Acetic Acid with Desogestrel/Mini-Dose Enthinylestradiol/Testosterone Undecanoate as an Oral Contraceptive for Men," *Contraception* 70, no. 3 (September 2004): 203–11.

46. Bonn, "Male Contraceptive Research," 302.

47. Page, Amory, and Bremner, "Advances in Male Contraception," 481.

48. Dejian Ren et al., "A Sperm Ion Channel Required for Sperm Motility and Male Fertility," *Nature* 413, no. 6856 (October 11, 2001): 603–9.

49. Kathryn Senior, "Non-Hormonal Male Contraceptive on the Horizon?" *Lancet* 358, no. 9289 (October 13, 2001): 1244.

50. Joan Stephenson, "A Hormone-Free Male 'Pill'?" *Journal of the American Medical Association* 289, no. 2 (January 8, 2003): 164.

51. J. K. Amory et al., "Miglustat Has No Apparent Effect on Spermatogenesis in Normal Men," *Human Reproduction* 22, no. 3 (March 2007): 702–7.

52. Eberhard Nieschlag and Alexander Henke, "Hopes for Male Contraception," *Lancet* 365, no. 9459 (February 12, 2005): 554–56.

53. Page, Amory, and Bremner, "Advances in Male Contraception," 482–83.

54. Gregory S. Kopf, "Approaches to the Identification of New Nonhormonal Targets for Male Contraception," *Contraception* 78, no. 4 (October 2008): S18–S22.

55. Quoted in Bridget M. Kuehn, "Male Contraceptives on the Horizon," *Journal of the American Medical Association* 296, no. 21 (December 6, 2006): 2540.

Chapter Eleven: Going Green

 1. Mike Carney, "Pigeons to Get Birth Control Pills," *USA Today*, June 20, 2008.
 2. OvoControl P and similar drugs aren't contraceptives, which prevent fertilization; they are contragestationals, meaning they prevent a fertilized embryo from developing properly.
 3. Quoted in Sewell Chan, "Birth Control for Staten Island's Pigeons?" *New York Times*, October 30, 2007.
 4. David A. Fahrenthold, "Abnormal Fish Found Closer to Washington; Waste Suspected in Egg-Bearing Males," *Washington Post*, December 19, 2004, C01.
 5. Simon Benson, "Gender-Benders Flush Out a Pollution Agenda," *Daily Telegraph* (Surry Hills, Australia), April 2, 2002, 17.
 6. Jon Fogg, "Potomac's Intersex Fish a Puzzle for Scientists," *Washington Times*, July 22, 2005, B01.
 7. Dawn Fallik, "Drinking Water Holds Surprises," *Philadelphia Inquirer*, November 28, 2004, B01.
 8. Dene Moore, "Toxic Drug Traces Detected in River," *Toronto Star*, July 5, 2006, A06.
 9. Quoted in David A. Fahrenthold, "'Human Activity' Blamed for Fish Ills," *Washington Post*, February 8, 2008, B03.
10. Andrew C. Revkin, "Stream Tests Show Traces of Array of Contaminants," *New York Times*, March 13, 2002, A18.
11. Michael Pollan, "Power Steer," *New York Times Magazine*, March 31, 2002, 644.
12. Ibid.
13. David A. Fahrenthold, "Inquiry Turns to Humans on Pollutant, Hormone Tie; Evidence Such as Eggs in Male Fish Spurs Push," *Washington Post*, December 4, 2006, B01.
14. Brian Rademaekers, "Drinking Water Gets a Drug Test," *Philadelphia Inquirer*, February 27, 2006, A01.
15. Quoted in Fallik, "Drinking Water Holds Surprises," B01.
16. Tom Spears, "Flushed Hormones Change Sex of fish: Synthetic Estrogen in Water from Sewage Causes Male Fish to Produce Eggs: Study," *Ottawa Citizen*, January 5, 2002, A1.
17. Seth Borenstein, "Pollution from the Pill Alters Fish; A Study Found that Water Tainted with the Female Hormone Estrogen 'Feminized' Male Fish," *Philadelphia Inquirer*, June 29, 2003, A12.
18. Spears, "Flushed Hormones," A1.
19. Roger Highfield, "'Contraceptive Pill Pollution 'Causes Decline in Fish Numbers,'" *Daily Telegraph* (London), May 22, 2007, 13.
20. Revkin, "Stream Tests," A18
21. Ibid.
22. Ibid.

23. "University of Colorado Opens Lab Focused on Detecting, Treating Pharmaceuticals in Water; Agilent Technologies Provides Core Instrumentation," Agilent Technologies, press release, April 7, 2008, http://www.agilent.com/about/newsroom/presrel/2008/07apr-ca08025.html.

24. Barbara Seaman, *The Greatest Experiment Ever Performed on Women: Exploding the Estrogen Myth* (New York: Hyperion, 2003), 211.

25. Quoted in ibid., 219.

26. Andrew C. Revkin, "F.D.A. Considers New Tests for Environmental Effects," *New York Times*, March 14, 2002, A20.

27. Ibid.

28. Cornelia Dean, "Drugs Are in the Water. Does It Matter?" *New York Times*, April 3, 2007, F1.

29. Ibid.

30. Rademaekers, "Drinking Water Gets a Drug Test," A01.

31. Quoted in "Pill Causes Pollution, Says Report," *Advertiser*, January 25, 2009, 23.

32. Fahrenthold, "Inquiry Turns to Humans," B01.

33. Seaman, *Greatest Experiment*, 214.

34. Devra Davis, interview by Terry Gross, "Chemicals, Cancer and You," *Fresh Air*, National Public Radio, October 4, 2007.

35. Ibid.

36. Fallik, "Drinking Water Holds Surprises," B01.

37. Dean, "Drugs Are in the Water," F1.

38. "Oestrogens Found in Bottled Mineral Water," *ENDS Report*, no. 411, April 1, 2009, 26.

39. Janet Raloff, "Contraceptive-Patch Worry: Disposal Concern Focuses on Wildlife," *Science News* 162, no. 16 (October 19, 2002): 245–46.

40. Quoted in ibid.

41. Janet Raloff, "Contraceptive Ring Could Pose Risks After Its Disposal," *Science News* 163, no. 4 (January 25, 2003): 62.

42. See "Environmentally-Friendly Condom Disposal," Go Ask Alice! December 20, 2002, www.goaskalice.columbia.edu/2311.html.

43. David A. Fahrenthold, "When It Comes to Pollution, Less (Kids) May Be More," *Washington Post*, September 15, 2009.

44. Ibid.

45. Ibid.

Chapter Twelve: Around the World in Twenty-eight Days

1. Quoted in Michelle Goldberg, *The Means of Reproduction: Sex, Power and the Future of the World* (New York: Penguin Press, 2009), 81.

2. Duff Gillespie, "Contraceptive Use and the Poor: A Matter of Choice?" *PLoS Medicine* 4, no. 2 (February 2007): e49.

3. Quoted in Goldberg, *Means of Reproduction*, 81.

4. Arthur Krock, "The Most Dangerous Bomb of All," *New York Times*, October 2, 1959, 28.

5. Goldberg, *Means of Reproduction*, 51.

6. Ibid.

7. Paul Ehrlich, *The Population Bomb* (New York: Ballantine Books, 1968), xi.

8. Goldberg, *Means of Reproduction*, 62.

9. Quoted in ibid., 77.

10. Ibid., 60.

11. Abigail Fee, "Rethinking Fertility: Modern Contraception and the Ewe Women of Ho, Ghana" (undergraduate thesis, Harvard College, 2005).

12. Allan Rosenfield and Karyn Schwartz, "Population and Development—Shifting Paradigms, Setting Goals," *New England Journal of Medicine* 352, no. 7 (February 17, 2005): 647–49.

13. Ibid.

14. Muhammad Yunus, *Banker to the Poor: Micro-Lending and the Battle Against World Poverty* (New York: Public Affairs, 2003), 134.

15. With contraception this happened gradually, and with abortion the process happened relatively rapidly.

16. Rickie Solinger, *Pregnancy and Power: A Short History of Reproductive Politics in America* (New York: New York University Press, 2005), 184.

17. Ibid., 218.

18. Goldberg, *Means of Reproduction*, 98.

19. Rob Stein and Michael Shear, "Funding Restored to Groups That Perform Abortions, Other Care," *Washington Post*, January 24, 2009.

20. Daniel Nasaw, "Obama Reverses 'Global Gag Rule' on Family Planning Organizations," *Guardian* (London), January 29, 2009.

21. Center for Reproductive Justice, "UNFPA Funds Released," news release, March 16, 2009, http://reproductiverights.org/en/press-room/unfpa-funds-released.

22. Adrienne Germain and Jennifer Kidwell, "The Unfinished Agenda for Reproductive Health: Priorities for the Next 10 Years," *International Family Planning Perspectives* 31, no. 2 (June 2005), 90.

23. Joel Achenbach, "At Summit, Dueling Hemispheres; North-South Rift Over Overpopulation," *Washington Post*, June 5, 1992.

24. Quoted in Patrick E. Tyler, "Hillary Clinton, in China, Details Abuse of Women," *New York Times*, September 6, 1995, A1.

25. Shereen El Feki, "The Birth of Reproductive Health: A Difficult Delivery," *PLoS Medicine* 1, no. 1 (October 2004): 13.

26. Ibid.

27. Felicia H. Stewart, Wayne C. Shields, and Ann C. Hwang, "Cairo Goals for Reproductive Health: Where Do We Stand at 10 Years?" *Contraception* 70, no. 1 (July 2004): 1–2.

28. Ibid.

29. "How Bush Treats Women," editorial, *Boston Globe*, March 17, 2004.

30. Steven W. Sinding, "What Has Happened to Family Planning Since Cairo and What Are the Prospects for the Future?" *Contraception* 78, no. 4 (October 2008): S3–S6.

31. Germain and Kidwell, "Unfinished Agenda," 90.

32. Ibid., 91.

33. "World Contraceptive Use, 2007," United Nations, Department of Economic and Social Affairs, Population Division, www.unpopulation.org.

34. John B. Casterline and Steven W. Sinding, "Unmet Need for Family Planning in Developing Countries and Implications for Population Policy," *Population and Development Review* 26, no. 4 (December 2000): 691–723.

35. Emmanuela Gakidou and Effy Vayena, "Use of Modern Contraception by the Poor Is Falling Behind," *PLoS Medicine* 4, no. 2 (February 2007): 381–89.

36. John Bongaarts and Steven W. Sinding, "A Response to Critics of Family Planning Programs," *International Perspectives on Sexual and Reproductive Health* 35, no. 1 (March 2009): 39.

37. Ibid., 40

38. John Bongaarts and Judith Bruce, "The Causes of Unmet Need for Contraception and the Social Content of Services," *Studies in Family Planning* 26, no. 2 (March–April 1995): 57–75.

39. Mohamed Ali and John Cleland, "Contraceptive Discontinuation in Six Developing Countries: A Cause-Specific Analysis," *International Family Planning Perspectives* 21, no. 3 (September 1995): 92–97.

40. Ibid.

41. Regine Sitruk-Ware, "Contraception: An International Perspective," *Contraception* 73, no. 3 (March 2006): 215–22.

42. Ibid.

43. Goldberg, *Means of Reproduction*, 230.

44. Bongaarts and Sinding, "Response to Critics," 40.

45. Ibid.

46. Goldberg, *Means of Reproduction*, 234.

Index

abortion
  African American rates, 318n36
  contraception after, 85
  contraception as, 297–98
  emergency contraception as, 188–90, 192,
    194
  global gag rule on, 193, 299, 302–3, 304
  in health insurance, 193
  history of, 12
  internationally, 306
  IUDs as, 103
  legalization of, 298
  Plan B as, 182, 188–89, 194
  Republican stance on, 298–99
  in United States, 174
abstinence, 6–7, 191
ACOG. *See* American College of Obstetricians
  and Gynecologists
activism, 30–31, 319n50
adrenal gland, 59
Advisory Committee on Immunization Practices, 250
Aetios of Amida, 10
Africa
  contraceptive use in, 304
  female condoms in, 89
  Sub-Saharan, 265, 306
African Americans
  abortion rates of, 318n36
  forced reproduction of, 13
  forced sterilization of, 21, 107, 108, 109
  leadership by, 20
  Pill use by, 46, 320n18
  in slavery, 13, 107
age
  breast cancer risk by, 56
  contraception use by, 5, 84, 124, 125

  HPV rates by, 239, 240
  at menstruation, 152
Agosti, Jan M., 252
A.H. Robins, 95, 96
Alesse, 171–72
Allan, Edgar, 24
Allendale Pharmaceutical, 90
allergies, 85, 91
Allina, Amy, 200, 202
Almost a Woman, 141
7 alpha-methyl-19-nortestosterone (MENT),
  271
aluminum hydroxide, 245
Alvergne, Alexandra, 65
AMA. *See* American Medical Association
amenorrhea, 139
American Association of Pro-Life Obstetricians
  and Gynecologists, 182
American Birth Control League, 18
American Cancer Society, 229, 230, 252
American College of Obstetricians and Gyne-
  cologists (ACOG), 195
American Diabetes Association, 68
American Family Physician, 172
American Indians, 108
American Journal of Obstetrics and Gynecology,
  229
American Medical Association (AMA), 12, 23
American Physiological Society, 67
anaphylaxis, 243–44
Anderson, Richard, 265
androgens, 38, 271
anemia, 70, 160, 167–68, 294
animals, hormonal damage to, 276–80, 281–82,
  287
Annuale, 155
antibiotics, 4

353

About the Author

LAURA ELDRIDGE is a women's health writer and activist living in Brooklyn, New York. Her latest books are *The No-Nonsense Guide to Menopause* and *Body Politic: Dispatches from the Women's Health Revolution*, with Barbara Seaman.

About Seven Stories Press

SEVEN STORIES PRESS is an independent book publisher based in
New York City, with distribution throughout the United States, Canada,
England, and Australia. We publish works of the imagination by such writ-
ers as Nelson Algren, Russell Banks, Octavia E. Butler, Ani DiFranco, Assia
Djebar, Ariel Dorfman, Coco Fusco, Barry Gifford, Hwang Sok-yong, Lee
Stringer, and Kurt Vonnegut, to name a few, together with political titles
by voices of conscience, including the Boston Women's Health Collective,
Noam Chomsky, Angela Y. Davis, Human Rights Watch, Derrick Jensen,
Ralph Nader, Gary Null, Project Censored, Barbara Seaman, Gary Webb,
and Howard Zinn, among many others. Seven Stories Press believes publishers have a special responsibility to defend free speech and human rights,
and to celebrate the gifts of the human imagination, wherever we can. For
additional information, visit www.sevenstories.com.